CONTROLLED RELEASE DOSAGE FORM DESIGN

CONTROLLED RELEASE DOSAGE FORM DESIGN

Cherng-ju Kim, Ph.D.

Associate Professor
School of Pharmacy, Temple University

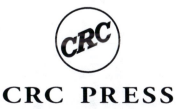

CRC PRESS

Boca Raton   London   New York   Washington, D.C.

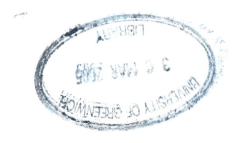

Library of Congress Cataloging-in-Publication Data

Main entry under title:
    Controlled Release Dosage Form Design

This book contains information obtained from authentic and highly regarded sources. Reprinted material is quoted with permission, and sources are indicated. A wide variety of references are listed. Reasonable efforts have been made to publish reliable data and information, but the author and the publisher cannot assume responsibility for the validity of all materials or for the consequences of their use.

Visit the CRC Press Web site at www.crcpress.com

© 2000 by CRC Press LLC

No claim to original U.S. Government works
International Standard Book Number 1-56676-810-1
Library of Congress Catalog Number 99-66000
Printed in the United States of America 1 2 3 4 5 6 7 8 9 0
Printed on acid-free paper

Table of Contents

Chapter I

Introduction

Controlled release dosage forms (CRDF) have been developed for over three decades. They have increasingly gained popularity over other dosage forms in treating disease. Now they are the focus of pharmaceutical dosage form technology. One of the first practically used controlled release oral dosage forms was the Spansule capsule, which was introduced in the 1950s [1]. Spansule capsules were manufactured by coating a drug onto nonpareil particles and further coating with glyceryl stearate and wax. Subsequently, ion exchange resins were proposed for application as sustained release delivery systems of associable drug [2]. Since then numerous products based on various mechanisms and fabrication techniques have been developed for the treatment of diverse diseases and conditions. Transdermal patches delivering scopolamine and nitroglycerin were developed for motion sickness and angina, respectively [3,4]. The oral osmotic pump tablet (OROS®) was introduced and commercialized to deliver phenylpropanol amine HCl for weight control (Accutrim®) [5]. Lately, a variety of nicotine transdermal patches were marketed to help people quit smoking [6]. There is a parenteral (injectable) controlled release system delivering a synthetic analog of luteinizing hormone releasing hormone (LHRH), leuprolide acetate (Lupron Depot®) [7]. This product is administered for prostatic cancer, dometriosis, and central precocious puberty monthly and quarterly.

These products have been developed in order to enhance clinical efficacy and reduce total disease management cost, thereby providing economic merit to the society [8].

I.1. Conventional vs. Controlled Release Dosage Forms (CRDFs)

Controlled release systems provide numerous benefits over conventional dosage forms. Conventional dosage forms, which are still predominant for the pharmaceutical products, are not able to control either the rate of drug delivery or the target area of drug administration and provide an immediate or rapid drug release. This necessitates frequent administration in order to maintain a therapeutic level. As a result, drug concentrations in the blood and tissues fluctuate widely (Fig. I-1). The concentration of drugs may be initially high, that can cause toxic and/or side effects, then quickly fall down below the minimum therapeutic level with time elapse. The duration of therapeutic efficacy is dependent upon the frequency of administration, the half-life of the drug, and the release rate of the dosage form. In contrast, controlled release dosage forms are not only able to maintain therapeutic

1

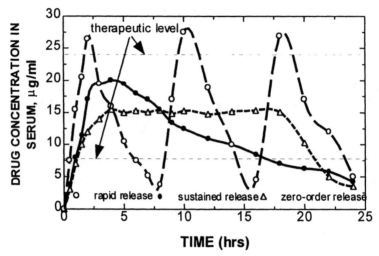

Figure I-1. Hypothetical serum drug concentration of various oral dosage forms.

levels of drug with narrow fluctuations but they also make it possible to reduce the frequency of drug administration. The serum concentration of a drug released from controlled release dosage forms fluctuates within the therapeutic range over a long period of time. The serum concentration profile depends on the preparation technology, which may generate different release kinetics, resulting in different pharmacological and pharmacokinetic responses in the blood or tissues.

Fig. I-2 shows the comparative drug concentration profiles of nifedipine from oral administration of the drug in conventional capsules and the controlled-release OROS push-pull osmotic pump (Procardia® XL). Drug release from OROS push-pull is carefully controlled and is not influenced by gastro-intestinal (GI) conditions (i.e. pH, GI motility, etc.). The mean drug concentration in the plasma is maintained consistently in a range of 30-40 ng/ml for 24 hours following a single dose (60 mg qd) of Procardia® XL. However, after administration of the conventional capsules, a peak drug level above 30-40 ng/ml is reached for a period of 5 hours; after which the drug concentration quickly plummets below the therapeutic level (15 ng/ml). At this time, the patient is advised to take another capsule in order to continue drug therapy. Drug concentration reaches peak level, then quickly falls below 30-40 ng/ml. At peak levels, drugs may cause side effects (e.g. fatigue due to high peaks for β-blocker "metoprolol"), and at low levels they may be below the minimum therapeutic concentration resulting in ineffective therapy.

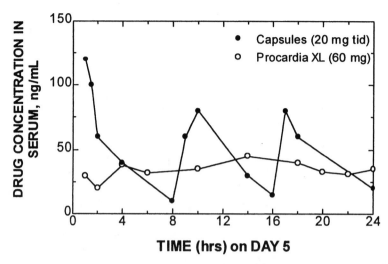

TIME (hrs) on DAY 5

Figure I-2. Comparative mean drug concentration profiles of orally administered nifedipine from conventional capsules and a CRDF (Procardia® XL). (Graph reconstructed from data by Alza Corporation [9].)

I.2. Advantages and Disadvantages of CRDFs

In the literature, different terms have been used to explain the prolonged duration of therapeutic serum levels *in vivo* (e.g. delayed-release, sustained-release, prolonged-release, timed-release, slow-release, extended-release, modified-release forms, etc.). These terms are often ill-defined, misleading, synonymous or used interchangeably when discussing slow release drug formulations and the purely controlled release dosage forms [10]. Here the term "controlled release dosage form" (CRDF) is used to indicate that the drug release kinetics is predictable and reproducible from one unit to another whether or not the release kinetics follow zero order [10].

As mentioned before, there are benefits to using CRDFs. Due to the controlled release of drugs from the dosage forms and less frequent administration, controlled release dosage forms furnish the following advantages over traditional dosage forms [11,12]:

a. Improvement of patient compliance
b. Usage of less total drug
c. Reduction in local or systemic side effects
d. Minimization of drug accumulation (with chronic dosage)
e. Reduction of potentiation or loss of drug activity (with chronic use)
f. Improvement in treatment efficiency
g. Improvement in speed of control of medical conditions
h. Reduction in drug blood level fluctuation

i.   Improvement in bio-availability for some drugs
j.   Improvement in the ability to provide special effects (e.g., morning relief of arthritis through bed-time dosing)
k.   Reduction in cost.

However, CRDFs do not always provide positive effects. Negative effects outweigh benefits in the following circumstances [13,14]:

a.   Dose dumping
b.   Less accurate dose adjustment
c.   Increased potential for first-pass metabolism
d.   Dependence on residence time in GI tract
e.   Delay onset.

The limitations of CRDF technology making some drugs unsuitable for CRDF formulation are as follows [11,13,14]:

a.   There is a risk of drug accumulation in the body if the administered drug has a long half-life, causing the drug to be eliminated at a slower rate than it is absorbed. The half-life of a CRDF drug candidate should be 2-8 hrs to avoid this problem.
b.   Some drugs have a narrow therapeutic index, requiring the serum drug level to be maintained within a narrow range. Such drugs are difficult to prepare as CRDFs.
c.   If the gastro-intestinal tract limits the absorption rate of the drug, the effectiveness of the CRDF is limited.
d.   High dose formulation containing more than 500 mg of active drug are difficult to prepare.
e.   The cost of controlled release formulation technology may be substantially higher than conventional formulation processes.
f.   If a CRDF is required (especially when new polymers are employed for CRDFs), the cost of obtaining government approval is high.
g.   If a drug undergoes extensive first-pass clearance, the drug bio-availability may be reduced.

Although CRDFs offer several advantages over conventional dosage forms, no pharmaceutical manufacturers have declared the clinical efficacy of CRDFs to be superior to conventional dosage forms. In recent years, improvement of safety and efficacy of the new products alone has not been enough to justify introducing new CRDF products. Evaluation of economic benefits, cost, and quality of life impact need to be assessed.

I.3. Pharmacokinetic Consideration of CRDFs

CRDFs are designed to maintain drug plasma concentrations within a therapeutic range. However, pharmacokinetic response from each CRDF varies from product to product. The therapeutic index (TI) is defined as the ratio of the minimum toxic concentration to the minimum effective concentration. Theeuwes and Bayne [15] proposed the dosage form index

(DI) to evaluate the performance of CRDFs. DI is defined as the ratio of the maximum to minimum plasma/serum concentration of the drug at pseudo steady-state (Fig. I-3). The DI is a function of the pharmacokinetics of the drug, the dosing interval, and the delivery rate from the CRDF. The CRDF with the smallest DI is the best design product when compared with others.

The basic concept of CRDFs is that the rate of drug absorption may be controlled through a controlled rate of drug release from the dosage form. However, one has no control over the rate of drug elimination from the body or the rate of metabolism of the drug after it is absorbed. As a result, even though the CRDF is designed to deliver a drug at a constant rate, the therapeutic level of the drug in the blood is not constant. It may not be possible to reach the minimum therapeutic level within a reasonable time frame unless one modifies the original dosage form. In this case, the pharmacokinetic elimination rate of the drug from the body is much slower than the release rate of the drug from the CRDF (e.g. Accutrim®, phenylpropanolamine HCl). The result is that no minimum therapeutic level is reached in a reasonable time frame (24 hrs) [16]. Before one tries to design a CRDF, it is worthwhile to obtain the pharmacokinetic profile of the drug according to the release kinetics of the drug from the CRDF. As shown in Fig. I-4, the simulated plasma concentration (a) of a drug in a one-compartment model reaches the steady-state level in about 24 hrs with an osmotic pump, providing a constant release rate over 24 hrs. However, curve (b) demonstrates that an immediate release (IR) portion of the curve

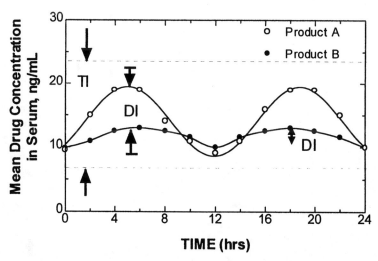

Figure I-3. Drug mean serum concentration-time curve (steady state) of two controlled release formulations. Product A is a higher fluctuation than Product B. The two products are not bio-equivalent.

establishes the early steady-state concentration level within 2 hrs. This can be optimized with a pharmacokinetic model [16].

The drug delivery systems mentioned so far are based on the concept that the human body maintains constant physiology over time. Recently, scientists have found to a good approximation that the human body changes in an orderly and predictable manner over time. Scientific information accumulated or gathered on various disease stages has revealed that some diseases vary with season (seasonal rhinitis) or circadian rhythm (asthma attack at night, high blood pressure after awakening, prevalent myocardial infarction during the early hours of the day) [7]. In the near future, one of the major objectives of CRDF technology should be to match medication delivery in time with the biological rhythm [17]. One such CRDF is Covera-HS® (verapamil HCl) controlled release tablets, which attempt to match the body's circadian rhythm for treatment of blood pressure and heart rate [17]. Covera-HS® is taken at bedtime and the drug release is retarded during the sleep period (4-5 hours) to achieve optimal blood levels between early morning and noon.

I.4. Polymers as Drug Carriers

Generally, natural and synthetic polymers are used as the structural backbone for both controlled release and conventional drug delivery systems.

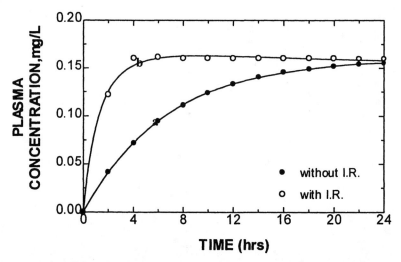

Figure I-4. Effect of adding a bolus dose on theoretical plasma levels to a constant rate delivery profile for a drug: k_e=0.15/hr, k_r=3.0mg/hr, k_a=1.6/hr, distribution volume =125 l, bolus =18.5 mg, total drug=74.0 mg.

These polymers may be swollen, non-swollen, porous, non-porous, semi-permeable, erodible, degradable, bio-adhesive, etc. The main difference between the CRDFs and the conventional systems is disintegration of drugs/systems. Even if the CRDF is eventually dissolved, the dissolution of the polymeric matrix is carefully controlled to maintain its rigidity for a long period of time. Polymers selected in the preparation of the dosage form must comply with the following requirement [18]:

(1) *Biocompatibility*: Harmful/toxic impurities must be removed from polymers before their inclusion in CRDFs. The residual monomers, initiator, and other chemicals used in the polymer synthesis/modification must be removed after the polymerization/modification. The chemicals employed in the polymer fabrication processes (i.e. additives, stabilizers, plasticisers and catalyst residues) are carefully selected to meet regulatory requirements.
(2) *Physical and mechanical properties*: The polymers must possess the necessary mechanical properties required for the dosage form design such as: elasticity, compactability, resistance to tensile, swelling and shear stresses, and resistance to tear and fatigue.
(3) *Pharmacokinetic properties*: Chemical degradation of the polymer matrix should not occur, and if it does, the degradation by-products must be non-toxic, non-immunogenic and non-carcinogenic.

There are many ways to synthesize new polymers and modify existing polymers. Different monomers (for addition polymerization or condensation polymerization) may be used or existing polymers may be modified. However, only a handful of polymers are used in pharmaceutical drug delivery systems due to their commercial availability, established biocompatibility and government registration [18]. Table I-1 lists the polymers used or evaluated for CRDFs. Most polymers used in pharmaceutical dosage forms were not originally designed for this purpose. However, the production of new, life-saving, genetically engineered drugs (peptides and proteins), which have characteristically short half-lives, presents an opportunity for significant research in the area of polymer development in order to prolong their therapeutic effects in the human body [19]. In the future, there will be a variety of polymers, which are commercially available, pharmaceutically acceptable, and specifically designed for CRDFs to control the release of drugs in a variety of applications. Fig. I-5 clearly illustrates the importance of selecting appropriate polymer materials for CRDF design. For a selected polymer, the chemical structure, and molecular properties of polymer materials (M_w, tensile strength etc.) influence the release kinetics of CRDFs.

Table I-1. Natural and Synthetic Polymers Used for Controlled Release Dosage Forms [18].

Polymer	Major functions
Natural polymers	
Gelatin	binder, coacervation
Alginic acid, Na	encapsulation
Xantham gum, arabic gum	matrix, binder
Chitosan	matrix, membrane
Semi-synthetic polymers (cellulose derivatives)	
Methylcellulose	binder, coating
Ethylcellulose	matrix, coating
Hydroxyethylcellulose	binder, coating
Hydroxypropylcellulose	"
Hydroxyethylmethylcellulose	"
Hydroxypropylmethylcellulose	matrix, coating
Carboxymethylcellulose sodium	binder, disintegrant
Cellulose acetate	membrane
Cellulose acetate butyrate	"
Cellulose acetate propionate	"
Cellulose acetatephthalate	enteric
Hydroxypropylmethylcellulose phthalate	"
Synthetic polymers	
ion exchange resins (methacrylic acid, sulfonated polystytrene /divinylbenzene)	matrix
polyacrylic acid (Carbopol)	matrix, bioadhesive
poly(MMA/MAA)	enteric
poly(MMA/DEAMA)	matrix, membrane
poly(MMA/EA)	membrane
poly(vinylacetate phthalate)	enteric
poly(vinyl alcohol)	matrix
poly(vinyl pyrrolidone)	binder
poly(lactic acid)	biodegradable
poly(glycolic acid)	"
poly(lactic/glycolic acid)	"
polyethylene glycol	binder
polyethylene oxide	matrix, binder
poly(dimethyl silicone)	matrix, membrane
poly(hydroxyethyl methacrylate)	matrix, membrane
poly(ethylene/vinyl acetate)	"
poly(ethylene/vinyl alcohol)	matrix, membrane
polybutadiene	adhesive/matrix
poly(anhydride)	bioerodible
poly(orthoester)	biodegradable
poly(glutamic acid)	"

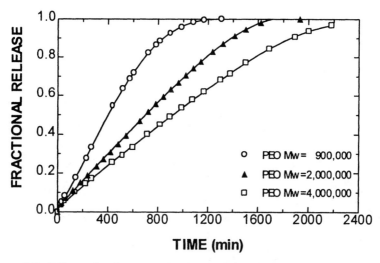

Figure I-5. Effect of polymer molecular weight on the release of salicylic acid from polyethylene oxide tablets.

I.5. Classification of CRDFs

CRDFs may be classified according to their physicochemical, pharmaceutical or clinical aspect [20]. Regardless of the route of drug administration (oral, transdermal, ocular, parenteral, vaginal, etc.), the basic principles involved in fabricating the CRDFs and releasing drugs from them are the same. Controlled release dosage forms can be classified based on their release mechanism and preparation methods as follows [21]:

    A. Physical Systems:
        * Diffusion-controlled systems
            Monolithic systems
                dissolved drug
                disperse drug
                porous system
                hydrogel
                biodegradable/bioerodible system
            Reservoir systems
                constant activity
                non-constant activity
                unsteady-state: time-lag & burst-effect
        * Ion exchange resin systems (cross-linked & uncross-linked)
        * Osmotically controlled systems

                                    OROS systems/microporous osmotic pumps;
                                    push/pull systems
                        * Hydrodynamically balanced systems
                        * Other physical systems (geometry)
        B. Chemical Systems:
                        * Immobilization of drugs
                        * Prodrugs
        C. Biological Systems:
                        * Gene therapy

   In vitro or *in vivo* release characteristics of CRDFs and
pharmacokinetic/pharmacodynamic effects of drugs are highly dependent
upon the principles used to design the CRDF. Fig. I-6 shows the plasma
concentration time profile of diltiazem HCl for Cardizem CD® and Dilacor
XR® [19]. Although both CRDFs are designed to deliver diltiazem HCl, they
are not pharmacokinetically bio-equivalent due to different fabrication
methodologies and physicochemical principles used in their preparation.
   Optimal design of CRDFs requires a detailed knowledge of the
physicochemical principles of release mechanisms, polymer properties,
pharmacokinetics, and physiological constraints.
   The focus of this book will be the exploration of the physicochemical
principles of CRDF design.

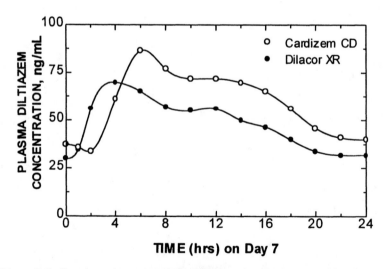

Figure I-6. Steady-state mean plasma diltiazem HCl concentration after 180
mg/day dosing in 23 healthy male volunteers. (Graph reconstructed from data
by Lippert et al [22].)

References

1. R. H. Blythe, U.S. Patent 2,783,303 (1958).
2. L. Saunders, "Sustained Release of Drugs from Ion Exchange Resins," *J. Mond. Pharm.*, 4, 36 (1961).
3. J. Shaw, "Development of Transdermal Therapeutic Systems," *Drug Dev. Ind. Pharm.*, 9, 1957 (1983).
4. W. R. Good, "Transderm-Nitro Controlled Delivery of Nitroglycerin via Transdermal Route," *Drug Dev. Ind. Pharm.*, 9, 647 (1983).
5. F. Theeuwes, "Elementary Osmotic Pump," *J. Pharm. Sci.*, 64, 1987 (1975).
6. C. Repchinsky, "Nicotine Replacement Therapy," *CPJ*, Mar., 87 (1993).
7. Physicians' Desk Reference, 51st Ed., Medical Economics Data, Montvale, New Jersey., 1997, p1534.
8. S. R. Saks and L. B. Gardner, "The Pharmacoecomics Value of Controlled-Release Dosage Forms," *J. Control. Release*, 48, 237 (1997).
9. Alza Corporation, Alza Technology, 1992, p. 6.
10. Y. E. Chien, Novel Drug Delivery Systems, 2nd Ed., Marcel Dekkar, New York, 1992.
11. L. Krowczynski, Extended-Release Dosage Forms, CRC Press, Boca Raton, Fl., 1987, p. 12.
12. Pharmacy Review, L. Shargel et al, Ed., Williams & Wilkins, Baltimore, Md. (1989) p.53.
13. P. G. Welling, "Oral Controlled Drug Administration: Pharmacokinetic Considerations," *Drug Dev. Ind. Pharm.*, 9(7), 1185 (1983).
14. W. A. Ritchel, "Biopharmaceutic and Pharmacokinetic Aspects in the Design of Controlled Release Peroral Drug Delivery Systems," *Drug Dev. Ind. Pharm.* 15 (6&7), 1073 (1989).
15. F. Theeuwes and W. Bayne, "Controlled-Release Dosage Forms," in Controlled Release Pharmaceuticals, J. Urquhart, Ed., APhA, Washington, D.C., (1981) p. 61.
16 W. R. Good and P. I. Lee, "Membrane-Controlled Reservoir Drug Delivery Systems," in Medical Applications of Controlled Release, R. S. Langer and D. L. Wise (Eds.), CRC Press, Boca Raton, FL. (1984) p.1.
17. C. Young, "Chronotherapeutics: The New Way of Delivering Drugs," *Pharm. Times*, May 1996, p19.
18. W. J. Passil, "Synthetic Polymers in Modern Pharmacy," *Prog. Polym. Sci.*, 14, 629 (1989).
19. R. Langer, "Biomaterials in Controlled Drug Delivery: New Perspective from Biotechnological Advances," *Pharm. Tech.*, 13(8), 18 (1989).
20. F. W. H. M. Merkus, "Controlled and Rate-Controlled Drug Delivery: Principal Characteristics, Possibilities, and Limitations," in Rate-Controlled Drug Administration and Action, H. A. J. Stuyker-Boudier (Ed.), CRC Press, Boca Raton, Fl. 1986, p15.

21. D. Rachev, N. Lambov, and E. Minkov, "Some Aspects of Controlled Release Dosage Forms," *Pharmazie*, 44, 186 (1989).

22. C. Lippert, T. Arumugham, D. Dimmit, M. Eller, and S. Weir, "Steady-State Bioavailability of Dilacor XR Capsules versus Cardizem CD Capsules in Normal Volunteers," *Pharm. Res.*, S-324 (1994).

Chapter II

Monolithic Matrix Controlled Systems

In physicochemical systems, drug release is controlled entirely by physicochemical processes such as diffusion, osmosis, dissolution, etc. The drugs may either be contained within a polymeric membrane or immobilized within a polymer matrix. Drug molecules encapsulated within a polymeric membrane or dissolved/dispersed homogeneously throughout a polymer or other carrier material, exhibit a release which is controlled by the diffusion of the drug through the carrier material and/or the dissolution of the carrier. Drug release can be activated by the osmotic pressure generated by the active ingredient (or osmagent) that controls the diffusion of solvent into the dosage form matrix. Dosage forms based on physicochemical processes are discussed in this section.

A monolithic matrix is the simplest and least expensive system used to control drug delivery. The fabrication processes for these systems are similar to those for conventional dosage forms and are highly reproducible. The polymer or other carrier material is homogeneously distributed with the drug by blending the drug with the polymer material and then molding, extruding, or casting them together. The interstices of the polymeric material control the drug release. The degree of diffusion control of the drug within the matrix is determined by the properties of the polymer and the drug. Ideally, drug can exist in one of two states within the polymeric matrix. Either the drug is completely dissolved in the polymer, or is purely dispersed as discrete solid drug particles within the polymer matrix. The latter condition prevails when the drug concentration is much higher than the drug's solubility in the polymer. In the former condition, the drug is dissolved at or below its solubility in the polymer. The release kinetics of the drug from two states is different. Generally, polymers used for this application either do not respond to changes in the surrounding environment or are rubbery state polymers. A polymer in the rubbery state responds to and adjusts to changes in its environment very rapidly, and the diffusion process of any substance within polymer matrix is Fickian. In addition to diffusion of the drug from the polymer matrix, other physicochemical properties (e.g. M_w, tensile strength, modulus) of the polymer may influence the release kinetics. Release characteristics from monolithic matrix systems depend on the nature of the polymer, the additives, the drug, and the geometry of the system. Controlling the release kinetics of a monolithic matrix system is easier than for other systems, i.e. coated systems.

II.1. Dissolved Drug

Polymers fashioned into slabs, cylinders, or spheres permit drug molecules to diffuse into the matrix, dissolve in the polymer, and remain dissolved when the material is dried. The drug is compounded with the polymer so that the drug content is less than the drug's solubility in the polymer. The dissolution rate of a drug is governed by the penetration of the solvent into the polymer matrix. When a dry, drug loaded polymer is placed in a dissolution medium (e.g. water), the imbibed drug in the polymer dissolves immediately in the penetrating solvent due to its high solubility, forms an unsaturated solution, and diffuses out of the polymer matrix. The following section presents mathematical expressions for solute diffusion through a matrix. This model is only applicable for drug in a matrix dissolved by a penetrating solvent. The mathematical model for the counter-current solvent and solute diffusion is discussed in Chapter IV and references [19,20].

II.1.1. *Diffusion of drug from a matrix*

The mathematical expression for the release of dissolved drug from the polymer matrix (spherical geometry) can be described by Fick's second law as:

$$\frac{\partial C}{\partial t} = \frac{D}{r^2}\left(\frac{\partial}{\partial r}\left(r^2\,\frac{\partial C}{\partial r}\right)\right)\tag{2-1}$$

where D is the diffusion coefficient, C is the drug concentration in the polymer, r is the radial distance from the center of the sphere and t is the time,

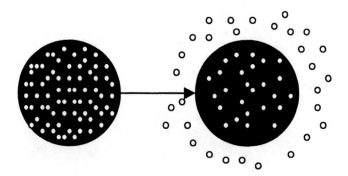

Figure II-1. Release of a drug from a spherical monolithic device.

subject to the following initial and boundary conditions represented by equations (2-2a) and (2-2b),

$$C = C_o \qquad\qquad t = 0 \qquad\qquad 0 \le r \le a \qquad\qquad (2\text{-}2a)$$

$$C = 0 \qquad\qquad t > 0 \qquad\qquad r = a \qquad\qquad (2\text{-}2b)$$

where a is the radius of the sphere and C_o is the initial concentration of drug in the sphere. Several methods [1] may be used to obtain a solution. The Laplace transform technique is most frequently used [1-3]. The Laplace transform of equations (2-1) and (2-2b) is:

$$\frac{1}{r}\frac{d^2 r\overline{C}(r,s)}{dr^2} - \frac{s}{D}\overline{C}(r,s) = -\frac{C_o}{D} \qquad 0 \le r \le a \qquad (2\text{-}3a)$$

$$\overline{C}(r,s) = 0 \qquad\qquad\qquad r = a \qquad (2\text{-}3b)$$

The solution of equations (2-3a) and (2-3b) is:

$$\frac{\overline{C}(r,s)}{C_o} = \frac{1}{s} - \frac{a}{sr}\frac{\sinh(r/\sqrt{s/D})}{\sinh(a/\sqrt{s/D})} \qquad\qquad (2\text{-}4)$$

The inversion theorem gives:

$$\frac{C}{C_o} = 1 - \frac{a}{2\pi i r}\int_{\gamma-i\infty}^{\gamma+i\infty}\frac{e^{\lambda t}\sinh \mu r}{\lambda \sinh \mu a}d\lambda \qquad\qquad (2\text{-}5)$$

The poles of the integrants of equation (2-5) are at $\lambda = 0$ and at those values of λ which make $\sinh \mu a$ zero

$$\mu = n\pi i / a, n = 1,2,3,.....$$

that is $\qquad \lambda = -\dfrac{n^2 \pi^2}{a^2}, \qquad\qquad n = 1,2,3,....... \qquad\qquad (2\text{-}6)$

with residue

$$2(-1)^n \frac{e^{-n^2 \pi^2 / a^2}\sinh(n\pi r / a)}{n\pi} \qquad\qquad (2\text{-}7)$$

Thus, using the contour integration technique, one obtains [2]:

$$\frac{C}{C_o} = -\frac{2a}{\pi r}\sum_{n=1}^{\infty}\frac{(-1)^n}{n}e^{-\frac{n^2\pi^2 D}{a^2}t}\sin(\frac{n\pi r}{a}) \tag{2-8a}$$

Equations (2-8b) and (2-8c) can be obtained for slab and cylindrical geometries, respectively.

$$\frac{C}{C_o} = \frac{4}{\pi}\sum_{n=0}^{\infty}\frac{(-1)^n}{2n+1}e^{-\frac{D(2n+1)^2\pi^2 t}{4l^2}}\cos\left(\frac{(2n+1)n\pi}{2l}\right) \tag{2-8b}$$

$$\frac{C}{C_o} = \frac{2}{a}\sum_{n=1}^{\infty}\frac{e^{-D\alpha_n^2 t}J_o(r\alpha_n)}{\alpha_n J_1(a\alpha_n)} \tag{2-8c}$$

where l is the thickness of the slab, α_n are the root of $J_o(a\alpha_n) = 0$, and J_o and J_1 are a zero-order and first-order Bessel function, respectively.

Fig. II-2 shows the theoretical concentration distributions of drug in a sphere during drug release as a function of τ $(=Dt/a^2)$. Experimental drug concentration profiles of theophylline in a scleroglucan gel slab matrix are shown in Fig. II-2b [4].

Equation (2-8) converges rapidly for large values of Dt/a^2 (or t), but converges very slowly for small values of Dt/r^2 (or t). Therefore, an alternative form of the solution must be determined for small times or small values of Dt/r^2. Instead of inverting equation (2-4) by the inversion formula using the contour integration technique, the *sinh* function is transformed into the exponentials, then inverted [3]. This yields:

$$\frac{\overline{C}(r,s)}{C_o} = \frac{1}{s}+\frac{a}{r}\frac{e^{r\sqrt{s/D}}-e^{-r\sqrt{s/D}}}{s[e^{a\sqrt{s/D}}-e^{-a\sqrt{s/D}}]}$$

$$= \frac{1}{s}-\frac{a}{r}\frac{1}{s}\left[e^{-(a-r)\sqrt{s/D}}-e^{-(a+r)\sqrt{s/D}}\right]\left[1-e^{-2a\sqrt{s/D}}\right] \tag{2-9}$$

$$= \frac{1}{s}-\frac{a}{r}\frac{1}{s}\left[e^{-(a-r)\sqrt{s/D}}-e^{-(a+r)\sqrt{s/D}}\right]\left[\sum_{n=0}^{\infty}e^{-2an\sqrt{s/D}}\right] \tag{2-10}$$

Inverting equation (2-10) by using the Laplace transform table gives:

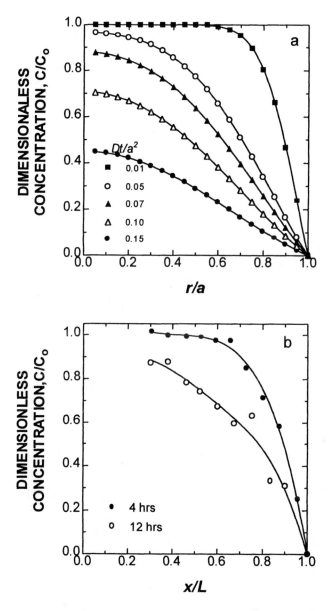

Figure II-2. Dimensionless concentration profile within a sphere (a) and experimental concentration profiles of theophylline in a scleroglucan gel (b). (Graph reconstructed from data by Colombo et al. [4].)

17

$$\frac{C}{C_o} = 1 - \frac{a}{r} \sum_{n=0}^{\infty} \left[erfc \, \frac{(2n+1)a - r}{2\sqrt{Dt}} - erfc \, \frac{(2n+1)a + r}{2\sqrt{Dt}} \right] \qquad (2\text{-}11a)$$

Equations (2-11b) and (2-11c) can be obtained for slab and cylindrical geometries, respectively [1-3].

$$\frac{C}{C_o} = \sum_{n=0}^{\infty} (-1)^n erfc \, \frac{(2n+1)l - x}{2\sqrt{Dt}} + \sum_{n=0}^{\infty} (-1)^n erfc \, \frac{(2n+1)l + x}{2\sqrt{Dt}} \qquad (2\text{-}11b)$$

$$\frac{C}{C_o} = \sqrt{\frac{a}{r}} erfc \, \frac{a - r}{2\sqrt{Dt}} + \frac{(a-r)\sqrt{Dta}}{4ar^{3/2}} \, ierfc \, \frac{a - r}{2\sqrt{Dt}} \, ... \qquad (2\text{-}11c)$$

These solutions converge quite rapidly for small values of Dt/r^2 or t. In equations (2-11a, 2-11b, 2-11c), $erfc$ is the compliment error function as $erfc \, z = 1 - erf \, z$. The error function is defined by:

$$erfz = \frac{2}{\sqrt{\pi}} \int_0^z e^{-t^2} dt = 1 - \frac{2}{\sqrt{\pi}} \int_z^{\infty} e^{-t^2} dt \qquad (2\text{-}11d)$$

and

$$ierfcx = \int_x^{\infty} erfc\xi d\xi = \frac{1}{\sqrt{\pi}} e^{-x^2} - xerfx \qquad (2\text{-}11e)$$

Problem II-1: A semi-infinite medium (a plastic syringe with cut top (length 5 cm, diameter 4.5 mm) filled with a gel) is initially drug-free. The end of the syringe is dipped into a drug solution (C_o) and the following concentration profile (Figure II-3) at two locations x_1 and x_2 is obtained [4]. Calculate the diffusion coefficient of the drug in the gel.
Solution:

$$\frac{\partial C}{\partial t} = D \frac{\partial^2 C}{\partial x^2} \qquad (2\text{-}11f)$$

$$C(x,t) = C_o \qquad\qquad x = 0, \quad t > 0$$

$$C(x,t) = 0 \qquad\qquad x = \infty, \quad t > 0$$

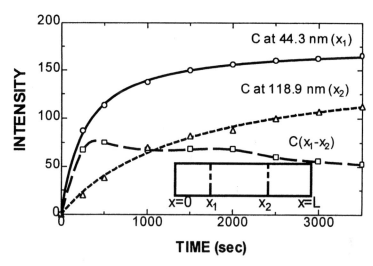

Figure II-3. The concentration time profiles of FTIC-dextran in a 1% agar gel. (Graph reconstructed from data by Henry et al. [5].)

$$C(x,t) = 0 \qquad\qquad t = 0, \quad x > 0$$

By the Laplace transform of equations (2-11f), one obtains the solution [1-3]:

$$\frac{C_i(x,t)}{C_o} = erfc\left(\frac{x}{\sqrt{4Dt}} \right) \tag{2-11g}$$

where $C(x_i,t)$ is the drug concentration in each disk.

$$C(x_1,t) = erfc\left(\frac{x_1}{\sqrt{4Dt}} \right)$$

$$C(x_2,t) = erfc\left(\frac{x_2}{\sqrt{4Dt}} \right)$$

$$C(x_1,x_2;t) = C(x_1,t) - C(x_2,t) = C_o\left\{ erfc\left(\frac{x_1}{\sqrt{4Dt}} \right) - erfc\left(\frac{x_2}{\sqrt{4Dt}} \right) \right\}$$

$$\frac{dC(x_1,x_2;t)}{dt} = 0 \qquad \text{at } t = t_{max}$$

$$x_1 e^{-\frac{x_1^2}{4Dt_{max}}} = x_2 e^{-\frac{x_2^2}{4Dt_{max}}} \tag{2-11h}$$

Rearranging equation (2-11h) yields [4]:

$$\ln\left(\frac{x_2}{x_1}\right) = \frac{x_2^2 - x_1^2}{4Dt_{max}}$$

or

$$D = \frac{x_2^2 - x_1^2}{4\ln\left(\frac{x_2}{x_1}\right)} \frac{1}{t_{max}} = \frac{44.3^2 - 118.9^2}{4\ln\left(\frac{44.3}{118.9}\right)} \frac{1}{495} = 6.23 \times 10^{-8} \ (cm^2/sec)$$

II.1.2. *Amount of drug released in a sink condition*

Although the drug concentration distribution in the matrix provides valuable information for designing a CRDF (see Chapter VI), the total amount of drug diffused out of the CRDF is also important to our discussion. The total amount of drug that is released from the sphere at time t for sink boundary conditions is represented by integrating $-AD\int (\partial c / \partial r)_{r=a} dt$ where A is the surface area [2].

For large values of time [1-3]:

$$\frac{\partial C}{\partial r} = \frac{2}{r} \sum_{n=0}^{\infty} (-1)^n \exp\left(\frac{-Dn^2\pi^2 t}{a^2}\right) \cos\left(\frac{n\pi r}{a}\right) \tag{2-12}$$

$$\frac{M_t}{M_\infty} = 1 - \frac{6}{\pi^2} \sum_{n=0}^{\infty} \frac{1}{n^2} e^{-\frac{n^2\pi^2 Dt}{a^2}} \tag{2-13a}$$

$$\cong 1 - \frac{6}{\pi^2} e^{-\frac{\pi^2 D}{a^2}t} \qquad \text{[Ref. 6]} \tag{2-13b}$$

where M_t is the amount of drug released at time t and $M_\infty = C_o(4\pi a^2 / 3)$. For small values of time [2]:

$$\frac{\partial C}{\partial r} = \frac{1}{4\sqrt{\pi Dt}} \sum_{n=0}^{\infty} (-1)^n \exp\left\{ \frac{-(2n+1)a - r}{2\sqrt{\pi t}} \right\}$$

$$-\left(\frac{1}{2\sqrt{\pi t}}\right) \sum_{n=0}^{\infty} (-1)^n \exp\left\{ \frac{-(2n+1)a + r}{2\sqrt{\pi t}} \right\} \tag{2-14}$$

$$\frac{M_t}{M_\infty} = \frac{6\sqrt{Dt}}{a} [\pi^{-1/2} + 2\sum_{n=1}^{\infty} ierfc \frac{na}{\sqrt{Dt}}] - 3\frac{Dt}{a^2} \tag{2-15a}$$

$$\cong 6(\frac{Dt}{\pi a^2})^{1/2} - 3\frac{Dt}{a^2} \qquad \text{[Ref. 6]} \tag{2-15b}$$

The drug release profile with respect to t (or Dt/a^2) is shown in Fig. II-3. M_t is calculated with the short and long time approximation equations (2-13b) and (2-15b). The simplified equations (2-13b) and (2-15b) are valid within less than 1% error [6]. This method can be applied to other geometries such as the slab and cylinder. The mathematical expressions for the release of drug and their corresponding equations for the release rate can be obtained as shown in Table II-1. For given release data, the diffusion coefficient of a drug can be determined by using equations given in Table II-1. However, except for the slab geometry, it is necessary to use non-linear parameter estimation methods to obtain the diffusivity of the drug for the short time approximation equation because the equation is not linear in time. Therefore,

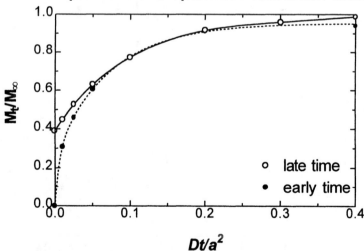

Figure II-4. The fractional release profiles from a sphere calculated with the early-time and late-time approximation.

it is generally recommended to use the long time approximation equations to determine the diffusivity of the drug by rearranging long time equation (2-13b) in Table II-1 into a linear format. For a slab:

$$\ln\left\{\frac{\pi^2}{8}\left(1-\frac{M_t}{M_\infty}\right)\right\} = -\frac{\pi^2 D}{l^2}t \qquad (2\text{-}15c)$$

By plotting the left-hand side term against time t, as shown in Fig. II-5, a straight line can be obtained with a slope of $-\pi^2 D/l^2$ from which the drug diffusivity may be calculated.

   In general, the small time approximation for the three geometries can be simplified for $M_t/M_\infty < 0.2-0.3$ as [7]:

$$\frac{M_t}{M_\infty} = \frac{2}{\sqrt{\pi}}(n+2)\sqrt{\frac{Dt}{l^2(or, a^2)}} \qquad (2\text{-}15d)$$

Table II-1. The Fractional Release and Release Rate of a Slab, Cylinder and Sphere for Dissolved Drug (l= half thickness of a slab, a= radius of a cylinder or sphere [5]).

1.a.   slab

$$\frac{M_t}{M_\infty} = 4\left(\frac{Dt}{\pi l^2}\right)^{1/2} \qquad \frac{dM_t}{dt} = 2M_\infty\left(\frac{D}{\pi l^2 t}\right)^{1/2} \qquad 0 \le M_t/M_\infty \le 0.6$$

$$\frac{M_t}{M_\infty} = 1 - \frac{8}{\pi^2}e^{-\frac{\pi^2 Dt}{l^2}} \qquad \frac{dM_t}{dt} = \frac{8DM_\infty}{l^2}e^{-\left(\frac{\pi^2 Dt}{l^2}\right)} \qquad 0.4 \le M_t/M_\infty \le 1.0$$

1.b.   cylinder

$$\frac{M_t}{M_\infty} = 4\left(\frac{Dt}{\pi a^2}\right)^{1/2} - \frac{Dt}{a^2} \qquad \frac{dM_t}{dt} = 2\left(\frac{D}{\pi a^2 t}\right)^{1/2} - \frac{D}{a^2} \qquad 0 \le M_t/M_\infty \le 0.4$$

$$\frac{M_t}{M_\infty} = 1 - \frac{4}{2.405^2}e^{-\frac{2.405^2 Dt}{a^2}} \qquad \frac{dM_t}{dt} = \frac{4D}{a^2}e^{-\frac{2.405^2 Dt}{a^2}} \qquad 0.6 \le M_t/M_\infty \le 1.0$$

1.c.   sphere

$$\frac{M_t}{M_\infty} = 6\left(\frac{Dt}{\pi a^2}\right)^{1/2} - \frac{3Dt}{a^2} \qquad \frac{dM_t}{dt} = 3\left(\frac{D}{\pi a^2 t}\right)^{1/2} - \frac{3D}{a^2}, 0 \le M_t/M_\infty \le 0.7$$

$$\frac{M_t}{M_\infty} = 1 - \frac{6}{\pi^2}e^{-\frac{\pi^2 Dt}{r^2}} \qquad \frac{dM_t}{dt} = \frac{6}{r^2}e^{-\frac{\pi^2 Dt}{r^2}} \qquad 0.7 \le M_t/M_\infty \le 1.0$$

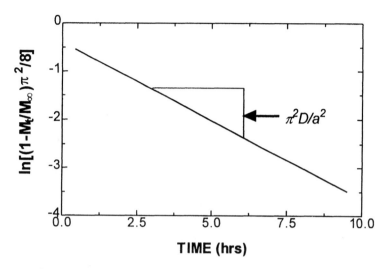

Figure II-5. A linear plot of $\ln\left(\dfrac{\pi^2}{8}(1-\dfrac{M_t}{M_\infty})\right)$ vs. time.

where $n=0$, 1, and 2 for a slab, a cylinder, and a sphere, respectively.

An example of a monolithic dissolved drug matrix system is the nitroglycerin system (NTS, Bolas Pharmaceuticals) which consists of drug dissolved in plasticised poly(vinyl chloride/vinyl acetate) [7]. The polymer matrix is laminated onto an impermeable polymer layer backing. The release of nitroglycerin in perfect sink conditions decreases with time. A linear plot of fractional release vs. the square root of time can be obtained up to 60% of the release and then levels off (Fig. II-6), as would be expected from the equations for early time and late time approximations for slab geometry in Table II-1, respectively.

Problem II-2: Water-soluble drug was released from a spherical bead matrix as shown in Table II-2. However, the duration of the drug release was too short to design the controlled release dosage form based on this matrix. Determine the diffusion coefficient of the drug and the bead size (o.d) needed to deliver 90% of the drug for 12 hrs. [Original bead size = 1.0 mm (diameter)].

Table II-2. Drug Release from a Spherical Bead.

Time (min)	5.5	10.5	15.5	20.5	25.5	30.5	35.5	40.5	50.5
% released	20.3	28.0	32.8	38.7	43.6	47.6	51.4	54.5	60.0
Time (min)	70.5	80.5	90.5	105.5	120.5	135.5	150.5	160.5	170.5
% released	70.8	74.6	77.5	81.8	84.9	87.6	88.9	89.6	90.3

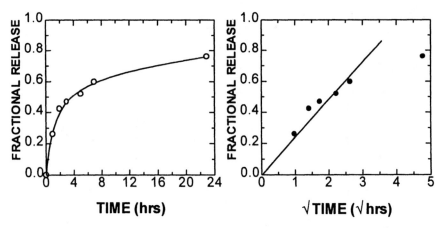

Figure II-6. Release of nitroglycerine from a NTS transdermal patch. (Graphs reconstructed from data by Shah et al. [8].)

Solution: There are two equations (early time and late time approximations) that can be used to determine the diffusion coefficient of the drug. However, the equation for the early time approximation is not linear with respect to time. First the equation for the late time approximation will be used with rearrangement as follows:

$$\ln\left\{\frac{\pi^2}{6}\left(1 - \frac{M_t}{M_\infty}\right)\right\} = -\frac{\pi^2 D}{a^2}t \tag{2-15e}$$

When the left-hand side of equation (2-15e) is plotted against t, the slope can be determined graphically. It is equal to:

$$\text{slope} = -\frac{\pi^2 D}{a^2} \qquad\qquad D = \frac{0.01127a^2}{\pi^2} = 4.76 \times 10^{-6} \text{ mm}^2/\text{sec}$$

In order to increase the duration of drug release, one can vary the size of the bead.

$$a = \sqrt{\frac{-\pi^2 Dt}{\ln\left(\frac{\pi^2}{6}(1 - 0.9)\right)}} = 0.943 \text{ mm} \qquad\qquad \text{diameter} = 1.89 \text{ mm}$$

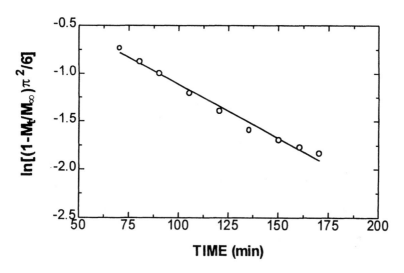

Figure II-7. $\ln\left[\dfrac{\pi^2}{6}\left(1-\dfrac{M_t}{M_\infty}\right)\right]$ vs. time (late time approximation).

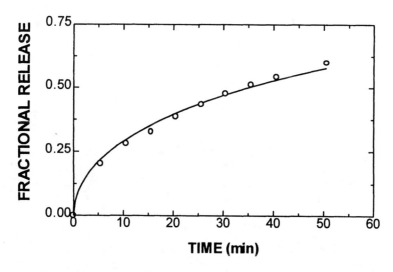

Figure II-8. Experimental release kinetics with the prediction by the early time approximation.

This calculation may be compared with the value obtained using the early time approximation equation with a nonlinear regression analysis, as shown in Fig. II-8. The diffusivity of the drug of 3.64×10^{-6} mm^2/sec is obtained.

It is assumed in the equations derived above that the diffusivity of drug in the matrix is independent of initial drug concentration. As the total amount of drug in the matrix increases, the volume occupied by the drug increases. As the initial drug concentration increases, the state of drug in the polymer matrix may change from the dissolved to the dispersed system (see Chapter II-2). In the dispersed state and dissolved state, interconnecting pores or channels in the matrix, are formed as drug loading increases due to the presence of excess solid drug. Drug release from such a highly loaded system is rapid due to the larger contribution from pore or channel diffusion of the drug. If the drug is highly water soluble, water penetrates into the matrix quickly due to rapid absorption of water by the drug. Hence, the diffusion coefficient of the drug and the release rate increase, as illustrated in Fig. II-9.

II.1.3. *Boundary layer*

The surrounding environment of a CRDF may not be well stirred, and the interfacial boundary layer (mass transfer resistance) may significantly influence drug release from the matrix. For example, dosage forms taken orally travel in the gastro-intestinal tract. The mixing pattern is not well known or the dosage forms are implanted in the confined body cavity where the mixing is minimal with a stagnant layer around the dosage forms. This

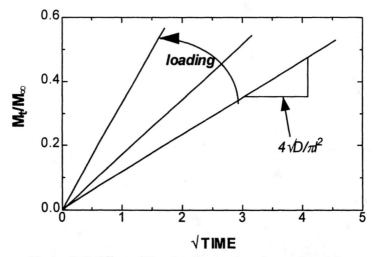

Figure II-9. Effect of drug loading on the release of a solute.

stagnant boundary layer provides additional resistance to drug diffusion into the surrounding environment. Incorporation of external mass transfer resistance in the diffusion equations provides more accurate interpretation of experimental data.

The schematic presentation of this problem for planar geometry is shown in Fig. II-10. The mathematical expression incorporated with the mass transfer boundary in a *semi-infinite medium* is expressed by:

$$\frac{\partial C(x,t)}{\partial t} = D\frac{\partial^2 C(x,t)}{\partial x^2} \qquad 0 < x < \infty, \qquad t > 0 \tag{2-16}$$

$$-D\frac{\partial C}{\partial x} = k(C_\infty - C) \qquad x = 0, \qquad t > 0 \tag{2-17a}$$

$$C = 0 \qquad x \to \infty, \qquad t > 0 \tag{2-17b}$$

$$C = 0 \qquad 0 < x < \infty, \qquad t = 0 \tag{2-17c}$$

where k is the mass transfer coefficient and C_∞ is the concentration of drug in the surrounding environment.

Laplace transform of the above equations is:

$$\frac{d^2\overline{C}(x,s)}{dx^2} - \frac{s}{D}\overline{C}(x,s) = 0 \qquad 0 < x < \infty \tag{2-18a}$$

$$-D\frac{d\overline{C}}{dx} + k\overline{C} = \frac{1}{s}kC_\infty \qquad x = 0 \tag{2-18b}$$

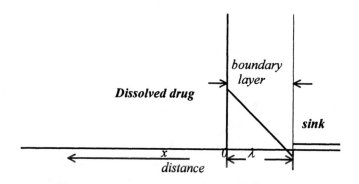

Figure II-10. A schematic diagram of mass transfer resistance in a matrix.

$$\overline{C} = 0 \qquad\qquad\qquad x \to \infty \qquad\qquad (2\text{-}18c)$$

and the solution for equations (2-18a, b, c) is given by [1,3]:

$$\frac{\overline{C}(x,s)}{C_\infty} = H\sqrt{D}\,\frac{e^{-(x\sqrt{D})\sqrt{s}}}{s(H\sqrt{D} + \sqrt{s})} \qquad\qquad (2\text{-}19)$$

where $H=k/D$. The solutions for the concentration distribution and for the total amount of drug released in time t are [1,3]:

$$\frac{C(x,t)}{C_\infty} = erfc\left(\frac{x}{\sqrt{4Dt}}\right) - e^{Hx+H^2Dt}\,erfc\left(H\sqrt{Dt} + \frac{x}{\sqrt{4Dt}}\right) \qquad (2\text{-}20)$$

$$\frac{M_t}{S} = 2C_o\sqrt{\frac{Dt}{\pi}} + \frac{C_oD}{h}e^{k^2t/D}erfc\left(\sqrt{\frac{k^2t}{D}}\right) - \frac{C_oD}{k} \qquad (2\text{-}21)$$

Equation (2-21) may be expanded for short time and long time approximations [9]:

for $t \to 0$

$$\frac{M_t}{S} = C_okt - \frac{4}{3}\frac{k^2t^{2/3}}{(\pi D)^{1/2}} + O(t^2) + \text{.......} \qquad (2\text{-}21a)$$

for $t \to \infty$

$$\frac{M_t}{S} = 2C_o\sqrt{\frac{Dt}{\pi}} - \frac{DC_o}{k} \qquad\qquad (2\text{-}21b)$$

where S is the surface area of the matrix.

Equation (2-21b) has been rearranged as [10]:

$$\frac{M_t}{S} = 2C_o\sqrt{\frac{D}{\pi}}(\sqrt{t} - \sqrt{t_o}) \qquad\qquad (2\text{-}21c)$$

where

$$\sqrt{t_o} = \frac{\sqrt{D\pi}}{2k} \qquad\qquad (2\text{-}21d)$$

The value of the second term of the right-hand side of equation (2-21b) (DC_o/k) increases as the mass transfer coefficient (k) decreases. This results in less of the drug being released. Eventually, the mass transfer resistance is so great that the amount of drug released from the matrix is zero when $2C_o\sqrt{Dt/\pi}$ equals DC_o/k.

Problem II-3: Medley and Andrews [9] studied the uptake rate of Naphthalene Orange G dye by virgin wool. The experimental curve over comparatively large time values is given in Fig. II-11. At $25\,\text{min}^{0.5}$ and on, linearity was established. Calculate the diffusion coefficient of the dye and mass transfer coefficient of the boundary layer.

Solution: From Fig. II-11, the slope and intercept are estimated as $2.38\text{x}10^{-6}$ cm/min$^{0.5}$ and $1.62\text{x}10^{-5}$cm, respectively.   From the asymptote intercept and slope of equation (2-21),

$$\frac{D}{k} = 2.38\text{x}10^{-5}\text{cm} \quad \text{and} \quad 2\sqrt{\frac{D}{\pi}} = 1.62\text{x}10^{-6}\text{cm/min}^{0.5}$$

$$D = 4\times10^{-12}\ \text{cm}^2/\text{min}$$
$$k = 1.7\times10^{-7}\ \text{cm/min}$$

Baker and Lonsdale [6] investigated the effect of the diffusional boundary layer on drug diffusion from a semi-infinite sheet.   Fig. II-12 presents the relative concentration buildup near the surface of a sheet. As time elapses, the external concentration reaches the equilibrium level in an unstirred medium. Eventually, when the external drug concentration reaches the solubility of the drug, the drug release stops. If J_{max} is defined as the flux

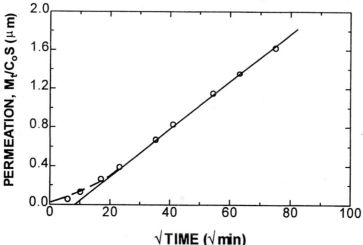

Figure II-11. Penetration of dye into wool plotted against $\sqrt{\text{time}}$.   (Graph reconstructed from data by Medley and Anderson [9].)

of a drug into a well mixed solution in perfect sink condition, then the flux of the drug at time t, J, in an unstirred solution is expressed by [6]:

$$J_t = J_{max}(1 - C_{x=0}/C_s) \tag{2-21e}$$

The flux of drug through the stagnant boundary layer is given by Fick's first law as:

$$J = D\frac{C_{x=0} - C_{x=\lambda}(=0)}{\lambda} \tag{2-21f}$$

Combining equations (2-21e) and (2-21f) yields [6]:

$$\frac{J}{J_{max}} = \frac{1}{1 + J_{max}\lambda/C_s D} \tag{2-21g}$$

In Fig. II-12, the flux in a well-stirred solution at perfect sink conditions is set equal to the solubility of the drug. As the thickness of the boundary layer increases, the flux decreases drastically. For example, when an implant is inserted in a body cavity, limited stirring occurs. This results in the slow transport of the active drug from the implant. The diffusion boundary layer effect is significant for sparsely water-soluble drugs for which the drug concentration in the receiving environment approaches the drug's solubility. This results in a slow drug release or diffusion.

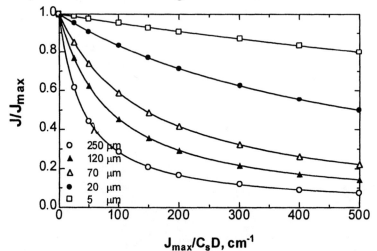

Figure II-12: The concentration buildup near the surface of a sheet in an unstirred medium.

The mathematical expression for the mass transfer resistance in a *finite slab*, $0 \le x \le l$ is given as:

$$\frac{\partial C(x,t)}{\partial t} = D \frac{\partial^2 C(x,t)}{\partial x^2} \quad 0 < x < l, \quad t > 0 \qquad (2\text{-}22a)$$

$$\frac{\partial C}{\partial x} = 0 \qquad x = 0, \quad t > 0 \qquad (2\text{-}22b)$$

$$D \frac{\partial C}{\partial x} + kC = 0 \qquad x = l, \quad t > 0 \qquad (2\text{-}22c)$$

$$C = C_o \qquad t = 0, \quad 0 \le x \le l \qquad (2\text{-}22d)$$

After taking the Laplace transform of these equations, the solution is given for the late time approximation [3]:

$$\frac{\overline{C}(x,s)}{C_o} = \frac{1}{s} - H_2 \frac{\cosh(x\sqrt{s/D})}{s\left(\sqrt{\frac{s}{D}} \sinh\left(L\sqrt{\frac{s}{D}}\right) + H_2 \cosh\left(L\sqrt{\frac{s}{D}}\right)\right)} \qquad (2\text{-}23)$$

$$\frac{C(x,t)}{C_o} = 2\sum e^{-D\beta_m^2 t} \frac{H_2}{L(\beta_m^2 + H_2) + H_2} \frac{\cos \beta_m x}{\cos \beta_m L} \qquad (2\text{-}24a)$$

$$\beta_m \tan \beta_m L = H_2 \qquad (2\text{-}25a)$$

where $H_2 = k/D$.
The fractional release of drug at time t is given as [1-3]:

$$\frac{M_t}{M_\infty} = 1 - \sum_{n=1}^{\infty} \frac{2L^2 \exp(-\beta_m^2 Dt / l^2)}{\beta_m^2 (\beta_m^2 + L^2 + L)} \qquad (2\text{-}26a)$$

For the short times [1-3]:

$$\frac{\overline{C}(x,s)}{C_o} = \frac{1}{s} - \frac{H}{s} \frac{e^{-(l-x)\sqrt{s/D}} + e^{-(l+x)\sqrt{s/D}}}{H + \sqrt{s/D}} \left[\sum_{n=0}^{\infty} (-1)^n \left(\frac{H - \sqrt{s/D}}{H + \sqrt{s/D}}\right)^n e^{-2\ln\sqrt{s/D}}\right] \qquad (2\text{-}27)$$

$$\frac{C(x,t)}{C_o} = 1 - \left(erfc \frac{l-x}{\sqrt{4Dt}} \right) - e^{H(l-x)+H^2Dt} erfc\left(H\sqrt{Dt} + \frac{l-x}{\sqrt{4Dt}} \right)$$

$$- \left(erfc \frac{l+x}{\sqrt{4Dt}} - e^{H(l+x)+H^2} erfc\left(H\sqrt{Dt} + \frac{l+x}{\sqrt{4Dt}} \right) \right) + \dots \qquad (2\text{-}24b)$$

The fractional release expressions for a cylinder are given by the following equations [1-3]:

for short times for the cylinder:

$$\frac{M_t}{M_\infty} = \frac{2DtL}{a^2} - \frac{8L^2}{3\pi^{1/2}} \left(\frac{Dt}{a^2} \right)^{1/2} - L\left(\frac{Dt}{a^2} \right)^2 (\tfrac{1}{2} - L) - \dots \qquad (2\text{-}26b)$$

for long times:

$$\frac{M_t}{M_\infty} = 1 - \sum_{m=1}^{\infty} \frac{4L^2 \exp(-\beta_m^2 Dt / a^2)}{\beta_m^2 (\beta_m^2 + L^2)} \qquad (2\text{-}26c)$$

where $L = ah/D$ and the β_ms are the roots of:

$$\beta_m J_1(\beta_m) - L J_0(\beta_m) = 0 \qquad (2\text{-}25b)$$

in which J_1 and J_0 are the first order and zero order Bessell function, respectively. If longitudinal diffusion is important, the fractional release is given by [11]:

$$\frac{M_t}{M_\infty} = 1 - \sum_{n=1}^{\infty} \frac{2R_1^2}{\beta_m^2(\beta_m^2 + R_1^2 + R_1^2)} \exp\left(-\frac{\beta_m^2}{L^2} Dt \right) \sum_{n=1}^{\infty} \frac{4R_r^2}{\beta_n^2(\beta_n^2 + R_r^2)} \exp\left(-\frac{\beta_n^2}{R_r^2} Dt \right)$$

$$(2\text{-}25c)$$

$$\beta_n \tan \beta_n = R_1, \qquad R_1 = \frac{Lh}{D}, \qquad R_r = \frac{Rh}{D}$$

The corresponding equation for the sphere is [1-3]:

$$\frac{M_t}{M_\infty} = 1 - \sum_{m=1}^{\infty} \frac{6L^2 \exp(-\beta_m^2 Dt / a^2)}{\beta_m^2(\beta_m^2 + L(L-1))} \qquad (2\text{-}26d)$$

where $L = ah/D$ and the β_ms are the root of:

$$\beta_m \cot \beta_m + L - 1 = 0 \qquad (2\text{-}25d)$$

The short time approximation equations were proposed by [12]:

$$\frac{M_t}{M_\infty} = 3L\tau - \frac{4}{\sqrt{\tau}} L^2 \tau^{2/3} - \frac{3L^2}{2}(1-L)\tau^2 \qquad (2\text{-}26e)$$

$$= 3L\tau \qquad \text{for small } L \qquad (2\text{-}26f)$$

The long time approximation can be given by [20]:

$$\frac{M_t}{M_\infty} = 1 - \exp\left(-3L(1 - \frac{L}{5}\tau)\right) \qquad (2\text{-}26g)$$

Problem II-4: Eudragit® RL (a copolymer of dimethylaminoethyl acrylate and methacrylate) and sodium salicylate was blended homogeneously and ethanol was added to the mixture to form a viscous paste [13]. A spherical bead was fabricated in a mold. The evaporation of ethanol was carried out at 20°C, as shown in Fig. II-13. Calculate the mass transfer coefficient. The diffusivity of ethanol from the bead was determined to be 4.0×10^{-8} cm²/sec from the initial rate of evaporation.

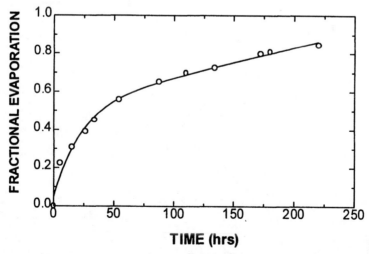

Figure II-13. Fractional evaporation of ethanol from a Eudragit RL bead. (Graph reconstructed from data by Khatir et al. [13].)

Solution: For the long time approximation, terms corresponding to $n \geq 2$ in equation (2-26d) are negligible and the first term becomes predominant, resulting in [13,14]:

$$\frac{M_t}{M_\infty} = 1 - \frac{6L^2}{\beta_1^2(\beta_1^2 + L^2 - L)} e^{-\beta_1^2 Dt/a^2}$$

or

$$\ln\left(1 - \frac{M_t}{M_\infty}\right) = -\frac{\beta_1^2}{a^2} Dt + \ln\left(\frac{6L^2}{\beta_1^2(\beta_1^2 + L^2 - L)}\right)$$

By plotting $\ln(1 - M_t / M_\infty)$ vs. t, a straight line can be obtained with a slope of $\beta_1^2 D/a^2$ (=0.0069) as shown in Fig. II-14. β_1 and k can be determined by the above equation and (2-25c). The mass transfer coefficient is determined to be 2.5×10^{-4} cm/sec [14].

II.1.4. *Diffusion and release in a limited volume*

The equations derived so far apply to a perfect sink, or a constant external solute concentration is assumed. If there is to be some observable concentration change in the liquid phase due to the solute uptake or release, the solute content within the solid and liquid phases should be measured as a function of time. Moreover, the validity of the perfect sink condition assumption fails when the ratio of the liquid phase to sample volume is small.

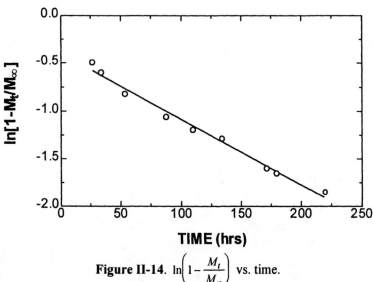

Figure II-14. $\ln\left(1 - \dfrac{M_t}{M_\infty}\right)$ vs. time.

This is the case for the release of a drug from a matrix into a body cavity, having a limited volume. Another case amenable to mathematical analysis is to load the drug into hydrogel beads by placing them in a concentrated drug solution. In order to avoid the waste of solvent and drug, the volume of the drug solution should be kept as small as possible. In this situation, the ratio of drug solution volume to hydrogel bead volume is small.

When a single sphere containing drug is suspended in a limited volume of a well-stirred dissolution medium initially free of the drug or when the drug diffuses into a sphere initially free of the drug, then equation (2-1) is subject to the following initial and boundary conditions:

$$\frac{\partial C_s}{\partial t} = D_e \left(\frac{1}{r^2} \frac{\partial}{\partial r} r^2 \frac{\partial C_s}{\partial r} \right) \tag{2-27a}$$

$$t = 0; \qquad\qquad 0 < r < R; \qquad\qquad C_s = const. \tag{2-27b}$$

$$t = 0; \qquad\qquad r > R; \qquad\qquad C_L = 0 \tag{2-27c}$$

$$t > 0; \qquad\qquad r = 0; \qquad\qquad \frac{\partial C_s}{\partial r} = 0 \tag{2-27d}$$

$$t > 0; \qquad\qquad r = R; \qquad\qquad V_L \frac{\partial C_L}{\partial t} = K_p A_s D_e \left. \frac{\partial C_s}{\partial r} \right)_{r=R} \tag{2-27e}$$

where A_s is the surface of sphere, V_L the volume of a dissolution volume, K_p the distribution factor, and R the radius of a sphere.

The Laplace transform of equation (1) is:

$$\bar{C} = \frac{(1+\alpha)}{R} \frac{\sinh \sqrt{s} R}{(3\alpha - s)\sinh \sqrt{s} - 3\alpha\sqrt{s} \cosh \sqrt{s}} + \frac{1}{s} \tag{2-27f}$$

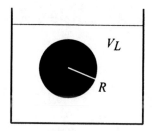

Figure II-15. Drug release from a sphere (radius R) in a finite volume (V_L).

The solution of equation (2-27a) under the above boundary conditions is given by Crank [2] as:

$$\frac{M_t}{M_\infty} = 1 - \sum_{n=1}^{\infty} \frac{6\alpha(1+\alpha)}{9 + 9\alpha + \alpha^2 q_n^2} e^{-\frac{D_e q_n^2 t}{R^2}} \tag{2-28a}$$

or

$$C_p = \frac{C_{po}}{1+\alpha} \left(1 - \sum_{n=1}^{\infty} \frac{6\alpha(1+\alpha)}{9 + 9\alpha + \alpha^2 q_n^2} e^{-\frac{D_e q_n^2 t}{R^2}} \right) \tag{2-28b}$$

where

$$\alpha = \frac{3V_L}{4\pi R^3 K_p} \tag{2-28c}$$

C_p and C_{po} are the transient concentration of drug in the solution and an initial concentration of drug, respectively, and the q_n's are successive, nonzero, positive roots of the function [1-3]:

$$\tan q_n = \frac{3q_n}{3q_n + \alpha q_n^2} \tag{2-28d}$$

Abu-khalaf and Soliman [12] extended the above analysis to short and long time approximations. For short time (large s),

$$\sinh \sqrt{s} \approx \cosh \sqrt{s} \approx e^{\sqrt{s}} / 2$$

A general approximation solution yields:

$$\frac{C}{C_o} = 1 - \frac{6(1+\alpha)}{\sqrt{\pi}} \sqrt{\tau} \left[be^{bh} e^{b^2\tau} erfc\left(b\sqrt{\tau} + \frac{h}{2\sqrt{\tau}} \right) - de^{dh} e^{d^2\tau} erfc\left(d\sqrt{\upsilon} + \frac{h}{2\sqrt{\tau}} \right) \right] \tag{2-29a}$$

where $b = (3\alpha+c)/2$, $c = \sqrt{9\alpha^2 + 12\alpha}$, $d = (3\alpha-c)/2$, and $h = 1-R$. For small α,

$$\frac{M_t}{M_\infty} = \frac{6(1+\alpha)}{\sqrt{\pi}} \sqrt{\tau} - \alpha\left(\frac{89}{4}\alpha + 24 \right)\tau \tag{2-29b}$$

The mathematical solutions for other geometries can be found in Crank [2]. When the release time is large (long time approximation), terms corresponding to $n \geq 2$ in equation (2-28a) are negligible, resulting in the following linear form [13]:

$$\frac{M_t}{M_\infty} = 1 - \frac{6(1+\alpha)}{9\alpha(1+\alpha) + \lambda_1^2} \exp(-\lambda_1^2 \tau) \qquad (2\text{-}28\text{d})$$

$$\ln\left(1 - \frac{C_p(1+\alpha)}{C_{po}}\right) = \ln\left(\frac{6\alpha(1+\alpha)}{9 + 9\alpha + q_1^2\alpha^2}\right) - \left(\frac{D_e q_1^2}{a^2}\right) t \qquad (2\text{-}28\text{e})$$

A plot of the left-hand side of equation (2-28e) vs. time t yields a straight line with a slope of ($D_e q_1^2 / a^2$). Since a is known, the diffusivity of the drug can be determined from the slope of the straight line. Solution (2-28b) is a series form and one has to obtain the root of equation (2-28c). From the intercept of equation (2-28e), q_1^2 may be determined and D_e can then be obtained.

Problem II-5:   Pu and Yang [17] conducted the diffusion experiment of sucrose from calcium alginate beads. The average bead diameter was 3.6 mm. The beads (V=15 ml) containing sucrose (C_{po} = 30 g/l) were added to 37.5 ml distilled water. The transient concentration change of sucrose in the solution is given in Fig. II-16. Calculate the diffusivity of the solute by the linear plot method.

Solution: Applying equation (2-28e) to Fig. II-16, the slope and intercept is determined by the linear regression of the late-time data as shown in Fig. II-17.

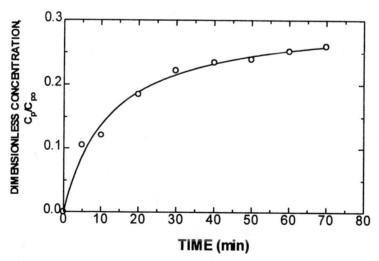

Figure II-16. Diffusion of sucrose from Ca alginate beads.   (Graph reconstructed from data by Pu and Yang [17].)

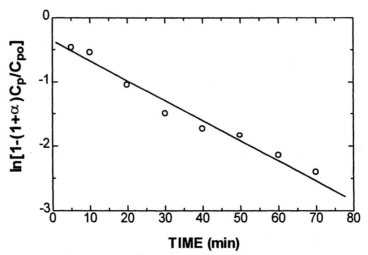

Figure II-17. $\ln\left(1-(1+\alpha)\dfrac{C_p}{C_{po}}\right)$ vs. time. (Graph reconstructed from data by Pu and Yang [17].)

$$\alpha = 2.5 \qquad \ln\left(\frac{6\alpha(1+\alpha)}{9+9\alpha+q_1^2\alpha}\right) = -0.81 \qquad -\frac{D_e q_1^2}{a^2} = -0.02223/\min$$

$$q_1^2 = 34.61 \qquad\qquad D_e = 3.47\times10^{-7}\,\text{cm}^2\,/\sec$$

Lee [16] found accurate approximate solutions for planar, cylindrical, and spherical geometries utilizing the refined heat balance integral approach as follows:

slab: $\qquad\qquad \dfrac{M_t}{M_\infty} = (1+\alpha)(1-\chi)$ $\qquad\qquad$ (2-30a)

where $\alpha = \dfrac{V_L}{K_p \pi A_s l}$ and χ can be obtained from:

$$\frac{Dt}{l^2} = \frac{3\alpha^2}{4}\left(\ln\chi + \frac{1}{2\chi} - \frac{1}{2}\right) \qquad\qquad (2\text{-}30\text{b})$$

cylinder: $\qquad\qquad \dfrac{M_t}{M_\infty} = (1+\alpha)(1-\chi)$ $\qquad\qquad$ (3-31a) where $\alpha = \dfrac{V_L}{K_p \pi R^2 h}$ and χ can be obtained from:

$$\frac{Dt}{a^2} = \frac{3}{40}\alpha^3\left(\frac{1}{\chi}-1\right)^3 + \frac{3(3\alpha+5)}{160}\alpha^2\left(\frac{1}{\chi}-1\right)^2$$

$$+\frac{3\alpha^2(5-3\alpha)}{80}\left[\frac{1}{\chi}-1-\ln\left(\frac{1}{\chi}\right)\right] \quad (2\text{-}31b)$$

sphere: $\qquad \dfrac{M_t}{M_\infty} = (1+\alpha)\left(1 - \dfrac{4\alpha}{4(1+\alpha)-(2-\chi)^2}\right) \quad (2\text{-}32a)$

where $\alpha = \dfrac{3V_L}{4K_p \pi R^3}$ and χ can be obtained from:

$$\frac{Dt}{a^2} = -\frac{\chi}{3} - \left(\frac{\alpha+2}{3}\right)\ln\left(\frac{4\alpha+4-(\chi-2)^2}{4\alpha}\right) + \frac{2}{3}$$

$$\sqrt{1+\alpha}\,\ln\left(\frac{\left(2\sqrt{1+\alpha}+(\chi-2)\right)\left(\sqrt{1+\alpha}+1\right)}{\left(2\sqrt{1+\alpha}-(\chi-2)\right)\left(\sqrt{1+\alpha}-1\right)}\right) \quad (2\text{-}32b)$$

Equations (2-30)-(2-32) start to deviate only at the tail end of the release [16]. For α value larger than 10, the values calculated by equations (2-30)-(2-32) are not significantly different from those calculated for perfect sink conditions. The analytical solution of C_s in the liquid phase is given by:

$$C_s = \frac{\alpha}{1-\alpha}\frac{M_t}{M_\infty}$$

These approximate solutions are easier to use compared to equation (2-28) which is a transcendental equation. To determine the diffusion coefficient of a drug, first calculate χ's from M_t / M_∞ data and then plot the values of the right-hand side of equations (2-30a), (2-31a) and (2-32a) versus time. This provides a straight line with a slope of D/a^2 from which D can be determined.

Problem II-6. A large Ca-alginate bead of diameter ($d_t = 1.239$ cm) was immersed in 2% (w/v) aqueous solution of D-glucose. After 360 min, the equilibrated Ca-alginate bead was removed from the glucose solution and immersed in distilled water to allow the diffusion of the glucose from the bead. The experimental fractional release data plotted against time are shown in Fig. II- 18a [17]. Calculate the diffusion coefficient of the glucose from the Ca-alginate bead in 4 ml of water.

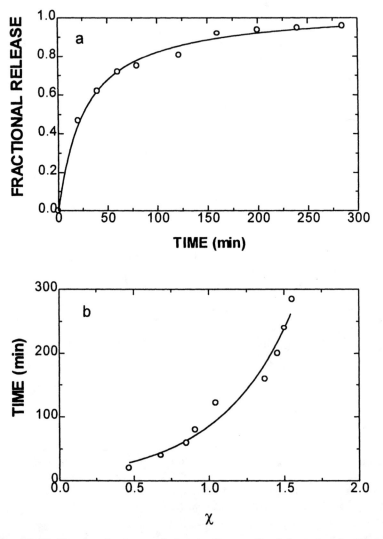

Figure II-18. Fractional release of glucose from a Ca-alginate bead. (Graph reconstructed from data by Merchant et al. [15].)

Solution: Equation (2-32a) for a sphere can be transformed to:

$$\chi = 2\left[1 - \sqrt{(1+\alpha)\left\{\frac{1 - M_t/M_\infty}{1 + \alpha - M_t/M_\infty}\right\}}\right]$$

$$\alpha = \frac{3 \times 4}{4\pi 0.6298^2} = 3.82, \qquad \text{assuming } K_p = 1$$

From Fig. II-18a and the above equation, χ's are determined at different times and plotted against time, as shown in Fig. II-18b. Non-linear regression analysis of equation (2-32b) was used to determine D to be 5.42×10^{-6} cm^2/sec.

The mathematical expressions given in equations (2-30)-(2-32) do not take into account the *boundary layer resistance* at the liquid-solid interface in a *finite volume*. Ruggeri et al. [18] included the external diffusional resistance in their solution of equation (2-1) for the sphere. Another boundary condition regarding the external resistance is added to those given in equations (2-2c)-(2-2f):

$$K_L(C_L - k_p C_s(R)) = D_e\left(\frac{\partial C_s}{\partial r}\right)_{r=R} \qquad (2\text{-}33)$$

where C_L, C_s and K_L are the drug concentration in liquid, solid phases, and the mass transfer coefficient, respectively. By applying Laplace transforms, the expression for the concentration of drug in the liquid phase is found to be [16]:

$$\frac{C_L}{C_{so}} = \frac{1}{k_p}\left[\frac{1}{1+\alpha} - \frac{6}{\alpha}\sum_{n=1}^{\infty} G(q_n)e^{-D_e q_n^2 t/R^2}\right] \qquad (2\text{-}34)$$

where

$$G(q_n) = \left\{\left(\frac{3}{\alpha} - \frac{q_n^2}{Bi}\right)^2 + 3\left(\frac{3}{\alpha} - \frac{q_n^2}{Bi}\right) + \left(1 + \frac{2}{Bi}\right)q_n^2\right\}^{-1} \qquad (2\text{-}35)$$

and q_n are the nth non-zero roots of the following equation:

$$\tan q_n + \left(\tan q_n - q_n\right)\left(\frac{3}{\alpha}q_n^2 + \frac{1}{Bi}\right) = 0 \qquad (2\text{-}36)$$

The Biot number ($Bi = K_L R / D_e$) takes account of the external mass transfer resistance. Equation (2-34) is identical to Crank's equation (2-8a) when $\alpha \to \infty$ or $\alpha \neq \infty$ provided that $Bi \to \infty$. Fig. II-19 shows the release of glucose from alginate beads (diameter = 3.18 mm and V=6.0x10^{-6} m^3) in water (V_L=20.56x10^{-6} m^3). The initial drug concentration in the beads was 62.0 mg/L.

II.1.5. *Release of dissolved drug via matrix-drug conjugate cleavage*

When covalently conjugated drugs in matrices are cleaved enzymatically or hydrolytically, the cleaved free drugs are released from the matrices by diffusion [21,22]. The release of a drug freed by first order cleavage of matrix-drug conjugate in slab geometry is given by Pitt and Schindler [21]:

$$\frac{\partial C}{\partial t} = D \frac{\partial^2 C}{\partial x^2} + kC_o e^{-kt} \qquad (2\text{-}37)$$

where C_o and k are the initial matrix-drug conjugate and the first order rate constant of cleavage of the matrix-drug conjugate. Taking Laplace transformation of equation (2-37) yields:

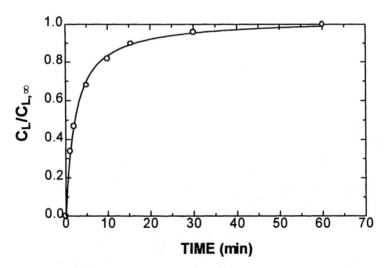

Figure II-19. Diffusion of glucose from Ca alginate beads. (Graph reconstructed from data by Ruggerri et al. [18].)

$$\overline{C} = \frac{kC_o}{s(s+k)}\left(1 - \frac{\cosh(q(L-2x)/2)}{\cosh(qL/2)}\right) \tag{2-38}$$

where $q = \sqrt{\frac{s}{D}}$ and L is the thickness of slab. The freed-drug concentration distribution in the matrix is obtained by taking the inverse transformation:

$$C = \frac{4kC_o}{\pi}\sum_{n=1}^{\infty}\frac{(e^{-\alpha_n t} - e^{-kt})\sin[(2n-1)\pi x/L]}{(2n-1)(k-\alpha_n)} \tag{2-39}$$

where
$$\alpha_n = \frac{(2n-1)^2\pi^2 D}{L^2} \tag{2-40}$$

The fractional release of the freed drug may be determined from:

$$\frac{M_t}{M_\infty} = \frac{8kD}{L^2}\sum_{n=1}^{\infty}\frac{(1/\alpha_n)(1-e^{-\alpha_n t}) - (1/k)(1-e^{-kt})}{(k-\alpha_n)} \tag{2-41}$$

The fractional amount of the freed drug remaining in the matrix (Q_t) at time t is then given by:

$$\frac{Q_t}{M_\infty} = \frac{8k}{\pi}\sum_{n=1}^{\infty}\frac{1}{(2n-1)^2}\frac{e^{-\alpha_n t} - e^{-kt}}{k-\alpha_n} \tag{2-42}$$

The relative contribution of drug diffusion in the matrix and cleavage kinetics can be evaluated by investigating the ratio of the drug release rate of the freed drug to the first order cleavage rate:

$$\frac{J}{d(LC)/dt} = 8\phi\sum_{n=1}^{\infty}\frac{2^{(1-\alpha_n/k)(t/\tau)} - 1}{1-\alpha_n/k} \tag{2-43}$$

where $\phi = (D/L^2)/k$ and τ is the half-life of cleavage.

For high or low values of ϕ, drug release from a polymer-conjugate film matrix is non-linear as shown in Fig. II-20. At high ϕ ($=1.0$) the drug bound to the polymer is not completely dissociated (hydrolyzed) or the freed drug concentration in the film is low. On the other hand, at low ϕ ($=0.01$) the bound drug is hydrolyzed completely in a short time period, resulting in high drug concentration in the film matrix. For high or low values of ϕ, hydrolysis or drug diffusion determines the drug release mechanism, respectively.

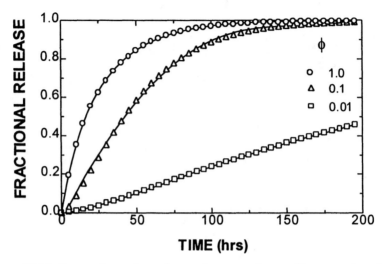

Figure II-20. Drug release from drug-polymer conjugate films as a function of ϕ.

However, for intermediate range of ϕ (=0.1), the relative contributions of hydrolysis and drug diffusion are balanced, leading to a linear release with a slight sigmoidal profile [22].

II.1.6. *Tablet geometry*

Common oral dosage forms for pharmaceutical applications are tablets. Mathematically, tablets may be treated as slabs or cylinders. However, depending upon the ratio of thickness to diameter, the tablet geometry is intermediate between a slab and a cylinder. Also, drug diffusion occurs from all surfaces rather than from a single surface. In a cylindrical geometry the drug release occurs through circular surfaces whereas in the slab geometry, the release occurs through the top and bottom surfaces. Fu et al. [23] took into consideration the drug release from all surfaces (Fig. II-21) and derived the following mathematical equation after rigorous manipulation as follows:

$$\frac{\partial C}{\partial t} = D\left(\frac{\partial^2 C}{\partial r^2} + \frac{1}{r}\frac{\partial C}{\partial r} + \frac{\partial^2 C}{\partial z^2}\right) \tag{2-44}$$

$$C = C_o \qquad \text{at} \qquad t = 0$$

$$C = 0 \qquad \text{at} \qquad z = l, r = a, t > 0$$

In these conditions, the concentration distribution in the tablet matrix has been described by Jaegar and Caslaw [3]:

$$C = C_o \varphi(z,l) \chi(r,a) \tag{2-45}$$

where

$$\varphi(z,l) = \frac{4}{\pi} \sum_{n=0}^{\infty} \frac{(-1)^n}{(2n+1)} \exp\left(-D(2n+1)^2 \pi^2 t / 4l^2\right) \cos\left(\frac{(2n+1)\pi z}{2l}\right) \tag{2-46}$$

$$\chi(r,a) = \frac{2}{a} \sum \exp(-\alpha_m^2 / t) \frac{J_o(r\alpha_m)}{J_1(a\alpha_m)} \tag{2-47}$$

The expressions for the release rate and the total mass release across all the surfaces (circular and lateral) have been found by Fu et al [23] after a vigorous manipulation of mass conservation equations to be:

$$\frac{dM_t}{dt} = \frac{16\pi c_o D}{l} \left[\sum \exp(-D\alpha_m^2 t) \sum \exp(-D\beta_n^2 t) / \beta_n^2 \right]$$

$$+ \sum \exp(-D\alpha_m^2 t) / \alpha_m^2 \sum \exp(-D\beta_n^2 t) \tag{2-48}$$

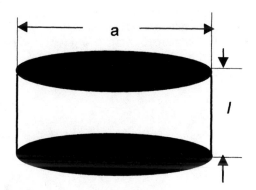

Figure II-21. A schematic diagram of a tablet.

$$\frac{M_t}{M_\infty} = 1 - \frac{8}{l^2 a^2} \sum_{m=1}^{10} \frac{e^{-D\alpha_m^2 t}}{\alpha_m^2} \sum_{n=0}^{10} \frac{e^{-D\beta_n^2 t}}{\beta_n^2} \tag{2-49}$$

where l is the thickness of the tablet, a is the radius of the tablet, α_n are the root of $J_0(a\alpha_n) = 0$; a α_n may be found in standard tables [ref.(3)], J_0 is a zero-order Bessel function, and

$$\beta_n = \frac{(2n+1)\pi}{2l} \tag{2-50}$$

        This equation presents a comprehensive method for the prediction of a CRDF release tablet, when the drug is distributed homogeneously throughout the polymer matrix. The long time approximation equation is given by [23]:

$$\frac{M_t}{M_\infty} = 1 - \frac{32}{(2.048)^2 \pi^2} \exp\left(-D(\alpha_1^2 + \beta_0^2)t\right) \tag{2-51a}$$

where $\alpha_1 = 2.4048/a$, and $\beta_0 = \pi/2l$.

        The short time approximation is obtained by the sum of the short time approximation solutions for the slab and cylinder with the addition of coupling term as [24]:

$$\frac{M_t}{M_\infty} = 8\sqrt{\frac{Dt}{\pi a^2}} - 4\frac{Dt}{\pi a^2} - \frac{8\pi}{3}\left(\frac{Dt}{\pi a^2}\right)^{3/2} + 4\sqrt{\frac{Dt}{\pi l^2}} - \frac{a}{l}\left[32\frac{Dt}{\pi a^2} - 16\pi\left(\frac{Dt}{\pi a^2}\right)^{3/2} - \frac{32\pi}{3}\left(\frac{Dt}{\pi a^2}\right)^2\right] \tag{2-51b}$$

Problem II-8: The diffusion coefficient of a drug was determined to be 7.0×10^{-7} cm²/sec by a membrane permeation study, which is intrinsic to polymer/drug systems. Compare the fractional releases calculated at 10 hrs from equation (2-51) with those based on slab and cylindrical geometries (equations for slab and cylinder in Table II-1). a=10 mm and l=4.5 mm.

Solution:

For slab $\dfrac{M_t}{M_\infty} = 1 - \dfrac{8}{\pi^2} e^{-\frac{\pi^2 D}{l^2}t} = 0.994$

For cylinder $\dfrac{M_t}{M_\infty} = 1 - \dfrac{4}{2.405^2} e^{-\frac{2.405^2 D}{a^2}t} = 0.614$

For tablet
$$\frac{M_t}{M_\infty} = 1 - \frac{32}{2.405^2 \, \pi^2} \, e^{-D(\alpha_1^2 + \beta_o^2)t} = 0.91$$

References

1. M. N. Oziak, Heat Conduction, Wiley Intersciences, New York, 1980.
2. J. Crank, The Mathematics of Diffusion, 2nd Ed., Clarendon Press, Oxford, 1975.
3. H.S. Carlow and J. C. Jaegar, Conduction of Heat in Solids, Clarendon Press, Oxford, 1959.
4. I. Colombo, M. Grassi, R. Lapasin, and S. Pricl, "Determination of the Drug Diffusion Coefficient in Swollen Hydrogel Polymeric Matrices by Means of the Inverse Sectioning Method," *J. Control. Rel.*, 47, 305 (1997).
5. B. T. Henry, J. Adler, S. Hibberd, M. S. Cheema, S. S. Davis, T. G. Rogers, "Epi-fluorescence Microscopy and Image Analysis Used to Measure Diffusion Coefficient in Gel Systems," *J. Pharm. Pharmacol.*, 44, 543 (1992).
6. R. W. Baker and H. K. Lonsdale, "Controlled Release: Mechanism and Rate," in Controlled Release of Biologically Active Agents, A. C. Tranquany and R. E. Lacey (Eds.), Plenum Press, New York, 1974, p15.
7. I. Singh and M. E. Weber, "Kinetics of One Dimensional Gel Swelling and Collapse for Large Volume Change," *Chem. Eng. Sci.*, 51, 4499 (1996).
8. V. P. Shah, N. W. Tynes, and J. P. Skelley, "Comparative In-Vitro Release Profiles of Marketed Nitroglycerin Patches by Different Dissolution Methods," *J. Control. Rel.*, 7, 79 (1988).
9. J. A. Medley and M. W. Anderson, "The Effect of a Surface Barrier on Uptake Rate of Dye in Wool Fibers," *Textile Res. J.*, 29, 398 (1959).
10. D. R. Paul and S. K. McSpadden, "Diffusional Release of a Solute from a Polymer Matrix," *J. Membr. Sci.*, 1, 33 (1976).
11. B. Nia, E. M Vunemchi, and J. M Vergnaud, "Calculation of the Blood Level of a Drug Taken Orally with a Diffusion Controlled Dosage Form," *Int. J. Pharm.*, 119, 165 (1995).
12. A. M. Abu-khalaf and M. A. Soliman, "Drug Release from Spherical Particles under Nonsink Conditions. I. Theoretical Evaluation," *Drug. Dev. Ind. Pharm.*, 22, 465 (1996).
13. Y. Khatir, J. Bouzon, and J. M. Vergnayd, "Liquid Sorption by Rubber Sheets and Evaporation. Models and Experiments," *Polym. Test.*, 6, 253 (1986).
14. J.-M. Vergnaud, Controlled Drug Release of Oral Dosage Forms, Ellis Horwood, New York, 1993, p93.
15. F. J. A. Merchant, A. Marganitis, J. B. Wallace, and A. Vardanis, "A Novel Technique for Measuring Solute Diffusivities in Entrappent Matrices Used in Immobilization," *Biotech. Bioeng.* 30, 936 (1987).
16. P.I. Lee, "Determination of Diffusion Coefficient by Sorption from a Constant Finite Volume," in Controlled Release of Bioactive Materials, R. W. Baker (Ed.), Academic Press, New York, 1980, p135.

17. H. T. Pu and R. Y. K. Yang, "Diffusion of Sucrose and Yohimbine in Calcium Alginate Gel Beads with or without Entrapped Plant Cell," *Biotech. Bioeng.*, 32, 891 (1988).

18. B. Ruggeri, A. Gianetto, S. Sicardi, and V. Specchia, "Diffusion Phenomena in the Spherical Matrices Used for Cell Immobilization," *Chem. Eng. J.*, 46, B21 (1991).

19. N. A. Peppas, R. Gurny, E. Doelker, and P. Buri, "Modelling of Drug Diffusion through Swellable Polymeric Systems," *J. Membr. Sci.*, 7, 241 (1980).

20. H. L. Frisch, "Simultaneous Nonlinear Diffusion of a Solvent and Organic Penetrant in a Polymer," *J. Polym. Sci. Polym. Phys. Ed.*, 16, 1651 (1978).

21. C. G. Pitt and A. Schindler, "The Kinetics of Drug Cleavage and Release from Matrices Containing Covalent Polymer-Drug Conjugates," *J. Control. Rel.*, 33, 393 (1995).

22. C. G. Pitt and S. S. Shah, "Manipulation of the Rate of Hydrolysis of Polymer-Drug Conjugates: the Degree of Hydration", *J. Control. Rel.*, 33, 397 (1995).

23. J. C. Fu, C. Hagemeir, D. L. Mayer, and E. W. Ng, "A Unified Mathematical Model for Diffusion from Drug-Polymer Composite Tablets," *J. Biomed. Mater. Res.*, 10, 743 (1976).

24. P. L. Ritger and N. A. Peppas, "A Simple Equation for Description of Solute Release I. Fickian and non-Fickian Release from non-Swellable Devices in the Form of Slabs, Spheres, Cylinders or Discs," *J. Control. Rel.*, 5, 23 (1987).

II.2. Dispersed Drug

II.2.1. *Higuchi's approach (pseudo steady-state approximation)*

If the solubility of a drug in a polymer is very low, most of the drug is homogeneously dispersed within the polymer matrix and the rest is dissolved in the polymer. Release kinetics of this type of system has been schematically diagrammed for slab geometry by T. Higuchi [1], as shown in Fig. II-22. In Higuchi's model, the concentration gradient between the drug receding section and the drug dissolution section are assumed to be linear (pseudo-steady state approximation). The dissolution front moves inward after the drug molecules at that front are exhausted. The mathematical derivation of the release of dispersed drugs from polymer matrix follows:

From Fick's first law of diffusion:

$$J = D\frac{\partial c}{\partial \delta} = D\frac{\Delta c}{\Delta x} = \frac{DC_{s,m}}{\xi} \tag{2-52}$$

$$\frac{dM_t}{dt} = SJ = \frac{SDC_{s,m}}{\xi} \tag{2-53a}$$

where $C_{s,m}$ is the drug concentration in the polymer matrix and S is the surface area (one side). The total amount of drug released at time t through either side of the matrix and up to the drug dissolution front position is $2\xi/l$, which is the sum of the amount of drug in the receding section, M_t, and the remaining drug in the depleted region $(0-\xi)$, $S(\xi C_{s,m}/2)$. Therefore, the

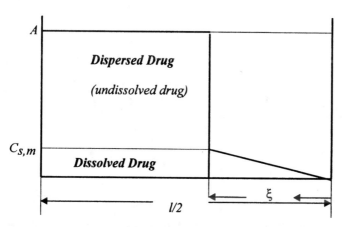

Figure II-22. A schematic diagram of dispersed drug in a matrix.

mass balance of the amount of drug released yields:

$$\frac{2\xi}{l} = \frac{M_t + S\xi C_{s,m}/2}{M_\infty} \tag{2-53b}$$

$$\xi\left(\frac{2}{l} - \frac{SC_{s,m}/2}{M_\infty}\right) = \frac{M_t}{M_\infty} \tag{2-54}$$

$$\xi = \frac{M_t}{M_\infty} \Big/ \left(\frac{2}{l} - \frac{SC_{s,m}/2}{M_\infty}\right) \tag{2-55}$$

Substituting equation (2-55) into equation (2-53) yields:

$$\frac{dM_t}{dt} = \frac{SDC_{s,m}M_\infty}{M_t}\left(\frac{2}{l} - \frac{SC_{s,m}}{2M_\infty}\right) \tag{2-56}$$

Integrating equation (2-56) gives:

$$M_t^2 = 2SDC_{s,m}\left(\frac{2}{l} - \frac{SC_{s,m}}{2M_\infty}\right)M_\infty t \tag{2-57}$$

However, the total amount of drug loaded in the matrix is $M_\infty = SAl/2$ where A is the initial drug concentration in the matrix. Therefore equation (2-57) can be written as:

$$M_t = S[DtC_{s,m}(2A - C_{s,m})]^{1/2} \cong S(2DtC_{s,m}A)^{1/2}, \quad A \gg C_s \tag{2-58}$$

The corresponding release rate and depleted region at time t are then:

$$\frac{dM_t}{dt} = \frac{S}{2}\left[\frac{DC_{s,m}}{l}(2A - C_{s,m})\right]^{1/2} \cong \frac{S}{2}\left(\frac{DC_{s,m}}{l}2A\right)^{1/2} \tag{2-59}$$

$$\xi = \frac{S\sqrt{2DtC_{s,m}A}}{M_\infty} \Big/ \left(\frac{2}{l} - \frac{SC_{s,m}/2}{M_\infty}\right) \tag{2-60}$$

respectively. Contrary to the case of dissolved state of drug, one may calculate the time taken for dispersed drug to be exhausted as:

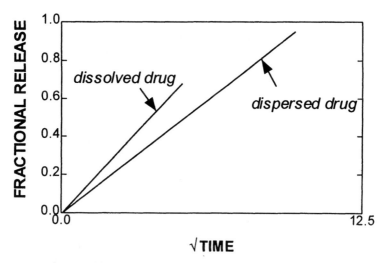

Figure II-23. Drug release kinetic profiles of dissolved drug and dispersed drug in matrices.

$$M_\infty = \frac{SAl}{2} = S(2Dt_\infty C_{s,m} A)^{1/2} \tag{2-61}$$

$$t_\infty = \frac{l^2 A}{8DC_{s,m}} \tag{2-62}$$

$C_{s,m}$ can be calculated by KC_s in which K and C_s are the partition coefficient and the drug solubility in water, respectively.

Equation (2-61) is similar to equation (2-15d) for the short time approximation for the release of a dissolved drug in terms of the square root of time. However, the difference between the dissolved and the dispersed state of drug in a slab geometry is that for the dispersed state of drug, M_t vs. square root of t is linear all the way to t_∞ but for the dissolved state of drug linearity is lost around 60%, as shown in Fig. II-23. Under the assumption that the amount of drug remaining in the drug depleted layer is negligible, mathematical expressions for the release rate in other geometries (cylinder and sphere), the amount of drug released at time t, and the exhaustion time (t_∞) are shown in Table II-3. The derivation of these expressions can be found elsewhere [2]. The moving front of the drug depleted region for a cylinder (radius r_0 and length h) and a sphere (radius r_0) may be expressed by [3]:

$$\frac{Dt}{r_o^2} = \frac{1}{4}\left(\frac{A}{C_s}\right)\left(1-\left(\frac{r}{r_o}\right)^2\right)+\frac{1}{2}\left(\frac{A}{C_s}\right)\ln\frac{r}{r_o} \tag{2-63}$$

$$\frac{Dt}{r_o^2} = -\frac{1}{6}\left(\frac{r}{r_o}\right)+\frac{1}{2}\left(\frac{A}{C_s}-\frac{2}{3}\right)\left(\frac{r}{r_o}\right)^2 -\frac{1}{3}\left(\frac{A}{C_s}-1\right)\left(\frac{r}{r_o}\right)^3 -\frac{1}{6}\ln\left(1-\frac{r}{r_o}\right) \tag{2-64}$$

respectively. The amount of drug released at time t for a cylinder and a sphere is given by equations (2-65) and (2-66a), respectively:

$$M_t = \pi h A(r_o^2 - r^2)+\frac{\pi h C_s}{\ln\frac{r_o}{r}} - \pi L C_s r^2 \tag{2-65}$$

Table II-3. Fractional Drug Release and Release Rates from Dispersed Matrices [2].

cylinder:

$$\frac{d(M_t/M_\infty)}{dt} = \frac{-4DC_{s,m}}{r_o^2 A \ln(1-M_t/M_\infty)} \tag{2-67a}$$

$$\ln\left(1-\frac{M_t}{M_\infty}\right)d\left(M_t/M_\infty\right) = -\frac{4DC_{s,m}}{r_o^2}dt \tag{2-67b}$$

$$\left(1-\frac{M_t}{M_\infty}\right)\ln\left(1-\frac{M_t}{M_\infty}\right)+\frac{M_t}{M_\infty} = \frac{4DC_{s,m}t}{Ar_o^2} \tag{2-67c}$$

$$t_\infty = \frac{Ar_o^2}{4DC_{s,m}} \tag{2-67d}$$

sphere:

$$\frac{d(M_t/M_\infty)}{dt} = \frac{3DC_{s,m}}{r_o^2 A}\left[\frac{\left(1-M_t/M_\infty\right)^{1/3}}{1-\left(1-M_t/M_\infty\right)^{1/3}}\right] \tag{2-68a}$$

$$\left[1-\left(1-\frac{M_t}{M_\infty}\right)^{2/3}\right]-\frac{2}{3}\frac{M_t}{M_\infty} = \frac{2DC_{s,m}}{r_o^2 A}t \tag{2-68b}$$

$$t_\infty = \frac{r_o^2 A}{6DC_{s,m}} \tag{2-68c}$$

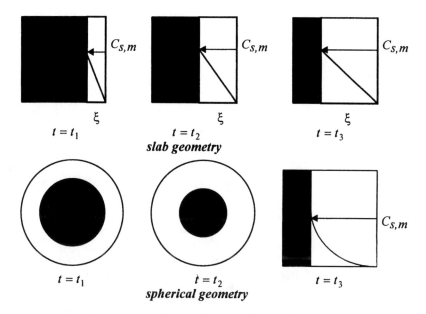

Figure II-24. A schematic diagram of drug concentration profiles and drug depleted layer in slab and cylindrical dispersed matrices.   (Graph reconstructed from figure by Cardinal [5].)

$$M_t = \frac{4\pi r_o^3}{3} A \left[3\left(\frac{A}{C_s} - \frac{1}{2}\right)\frac{r}{r_o} - 3\left(\frac{A}{C_s} - \frac{5}{6}\right)\left(\frac{r}{r_o}\right)^2 + \left(\frac{A}{C_s} - 1\right)\left(\frac{r}{r_o}\right)^3 \right]\left/\left(\frac{A}{C_s}\right)\right. \quad (2\text{-}66a)$$

Equation (2-66a) is further approximated as [3]:

$$M_t \cong 4\pi r_o^2 \left[\sqrt{2(A - C_s)C_s Dt} + \frac{4C_s}{9r_o}\left(\frac{C_s}{2A - C_s} - 3\right)Dt \right] \qquad (2\text{-}66b)$$

Simple forms of these equations for drug release kinetics are shown in Table II-3.

A schematic representation of the variation of the moving boundary of the depleted zone as a function of time in slab and spherical geometries is presented in Fig. II-24.   Under pseudo-steady-state conditions, the concentration gradient in slab geometry is linear; however, it is not linear in cylindrical or spherical geometry due to the decrease in releasing area with time. The photograph taken by Roseman and Higuchi [4] clearly illustrates

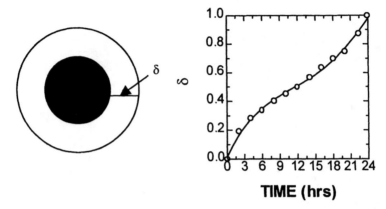

TIME (hrs)

Figure II-25. A schematic presentation of the drug dissolution front movement in a bead and normalized drug-depleted layer thickness with time.

the moving boundary front in a cylinder. Initially, the transparent silicone rubbery material is rendered opaque by the presence of the drug, medroxyprogesterone acetate. As the drug diffuses out of the matrix, the clear depleted drug zones appear. A longer release time shows a thicker depleted zone [4]. Fig. II-25 shows the slow moving boundary of the drug-depleted layer of a hydrogel bead loaded with a drug.

From equation (2-58), the amount of drug released at time t is proportional to the square root of the initial drug concentration, A, in the polymer matrix. However, the amount of drug released at time t is much larger than that predicted by equation (2-58) as the initial concentration increases. As the drug loading increases, the area occupied by the drug molecules increases and there are more chances for adjacent drug molecules to come in contact with each other. Beyond a critical loading level, the drug molecules are so close to each other that they form channels. Therefore, the drug molecules that dissolved upon contact with the solvent (water) diffuse out through the pores or channels created by the occupied drug molecules. The release rate of drug is much faster than that only through the polymer matrix. According to equation (2-58), the plot of $M_t / \sqrt{A}$ vs $\sqrt{t}$ should be superimposable regardless of the drug loading level. As shown in Fig. II-26, the plots are not superimposeable as the drug loading increases due to the increase of the diffusion coefficient via open pore and/or channels.

The interconnecting pore (or channel) network is a very important release pathway for macromolecules from the hydrophobic matrix system. A majority of the macromolecules are dispersed within and surrounded by the polymer, which is impermeable to macromolecules but not to smaller molecules. At low drug loading, the macromolecule is never released. Only drugs at or near the surface of the matrix (burst period) are released.

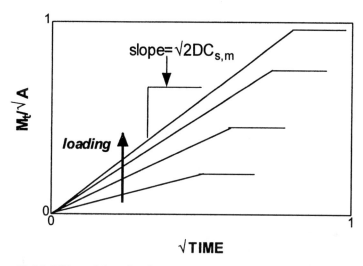

Figure II-26. Effect of drug loading on release kinetics in a dispersed matrix.

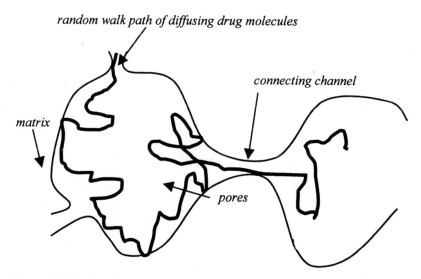

Figure II-27. A schematic presentation of the pore structure in a polymer matrix with a high drug loading. Macromolecules do not diffuse out of the matrix through the narrow channels easily. (Graph reconstructed from figure by Siegal and Langer [6].)

However, at sufficiently high drug loading, the spaces occupied by the drugs create pores or channels that are interconnected, so that the macromolecule is released by aqueous diffusion through the channel [6]. The release of proteins is controlled by the interconnected protein particles. The total fraction of the releasable protein in a matrix increases as the volumetric loading level of the protein increases. As shown in Fig. II-27, the macromolecules, unlike small molecules, diffuse by a random walk [6]. If the channel diameter is smaller than the pore diameter, it will be difficult for the macromolecules to find a channel to diffuse out through. At high drug loading, the channel diameter is large enough to release 100% of drug. However, at intermediate loading, only the portion of the drug which is connected to the surface is released. The rest of the drug is trapped by the polymer and never released. There is a threshold volumetric loading level above which the releasable fraction significantly increases to near complete release [6]. As a consequence, the release rate of the protein increases. On the other hand, only a small amount of the potent protein is required for therapeutic efficacy (i.e. low loading); therefore only a small portion of the protein drug is released. To increase the total fraction of lightly loaded protein drug releasable without increasing the release rate, water-soluble pore forming excipients have been incorporated [7]. Classical percolation theory has been applied to account for many of the qualitative features of the release of macromolecules [8,9].

Cardinal [5] developed a kinetic expression, using Higuchi's pseudo-steady-state approximation, for the release of drug from tablets (radius r_o and thickness l_o) for which the drug release occurs from all surfaces. From the mass balance of a dispersed drug tablet, one can show that:

$$\frac{M_t}{M_\infty} = \frac{\pi r_o^2 l_o A - \pi r l A}{\pi r_o^2 l_o A} = 1 - \frac{r^2}{r_o^2} \frac{l}{l_o} \tag{2-69}$$

where r and l are the radius and the thickness of the tablet at the moving boundary at the time t, respectively. l can be calculated as:

$$l = l_o - 2\sqrt{\frac{2DC_{s,m}t}{A}} \tag{2-70}$$

Substitution of equations (2-70) into (2-69) and rearranging gives:

$$\left(\frac{r}{r_o}\right)^2 = \frac{1 - M_t/M_\infty}{1 - b\sqrt{2Kt}} \tag{2-71}$$

where K and b are defined as $4C_s D / A l_o^2$ and r_o / l_o, respectively. Substitution of equations (2-71) into (2-63) and rearranging yields:

$$1 + \frac{1 - \dfrac{M_t}{M_\infty}}{1 - b\sqrt{2Kt}} \ln\left[\frac{1 - \dfrac{M_t}{M_\infty}}{1 - b\sqrt{2Kt}} \right] - \frac{1 - \dfrac{M_t}{M_\infty}}{1 - b\sqrt{2Kt}} = Kt \qquad (2\text{-}72)$$

Equation (2-72) was evaluated with the experimental data of Fu et al. [10] for the release of hydrocortisone from an 18% loaded polycaprolactone tablet matrix of $a = 1.5$ cm and $l = 0.17$ cm and $b = 4.41$. Fig. II-28 compares the results of Song et al.'s equation (2-72) with Higuchi's equation (2-58). The open triangles were obtained using Higuchi's equation (2-58) in conjunction with the determined value of D by (2-72). It showed that Higuchi's equation falls short of the experimental results. However if one uses Higuchi's equation to estimate the product of $DC_{s,m}$ for hydrocortisone from polycaprolactone, there is excellent agreement between experimental and predicted results. The value of D obtained from Higuchi's equation was much higher (by about 30%) than that estimated by equation (2-72).

Problem II-9: A methoxyprogesterone acetate cylinder, 4 cm long and 0.5 cm in radius was prepared by levigating the required amount of drug with

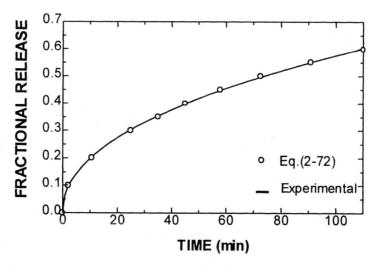

Figure II-28. Release of hydrocortisone from an 18% loaded polycaprolactone tablet. (Graph reconstructed from data by Cardinal [5].)

Table II-4. Release of Methoxyprogesterone from a Silicone Rubber Cylinder

Time (wks)	1	2	3	4	6
Amount released (mg)	16.6	22.1	26	31.2	40.0

elastomer (silicone) and polymerizing with a catalyst [4]. The mixture was then forced into tubing and allowed to cure. The solubility of methoxyprogesterone acetate in water at 37°C is 3.25×10^{-3} mg/ml. The value of the partition coefficient K was determined to be 0.033. Experimental data are given in Table II-4. (1) Calculate the diffusion coefficient of methoxyprogesterone acetate and the cumulative amount of drug released in 8 wks. (2) Determine the required time for the entire drug to be completely exhausted. The initial drug concentration in the polymer matrix was 30 mg/cm^3 (24% loading) [4]. (3) Calculate the time required for 50% of a drug to be released from a spherical bead matrix. (4) Calculate the cumulative amount of drug released in 5 wks.

Solution:

(1)   volume of the cylinder $= \pi \times (0.5\text{cm})^2 \times 4\text{cm} = 3.14 \text{ cm}^3$

$$C_{s,m} = KC_s = 0.033 \times 3.25 \times 10^{-3} \text{ mg/ml} = 1.07 \times 10^{-4} \text{ mg/ml}$$

$$M_\infty = 30 \text{ mg/ml} \times 3.14 \text{ cm}^3 = 94.2 \text{ mg}$$

Drug release equation for a cylindrical geometry

$$\left(1 - \frac{M_t}{M_\infty}\right)\ln\left(1 - \frac{M_t}{M_\infty}\right) + \frac{M_t}{M_\infty} = \frac{4DC_{s,m}}{Ar_o^2} t$$

t	M_t	M_t / M_∞	above equation
0	0	0.0	0.0
1	16.6	0.176	-0.0165
2	22.1	0.235	-0.0300
3	26	0.276	-0.0422
4	31.2	0.331	-0.0621
6	40	0.425	-0.1070

$$\frac{4DC_{s,m}}{Ar_o^2} = 0.0166 / \text{wk} \quad D = \frac{0.0166 \times Axr_o^2}{4C_{s,m}} = 290.9 \text{ cm}^2 / \text{wk}$$

(2) $t = 8 \text{ wks}$

$$\left(1 - \frac{M_t}{M_\infty}\right)\ln\left(1 - \frac{M_t}{M_\infty}\right) + \frac{M_t}{M_\infty} = \frac{4DC_{s,m}}{Ar_o^2} 8(\text{wk})$$

By trial and error, $\dfrac{M_t}{M_\infty} = 0.47$,　　$M_t = 0.47 \times 94.2 \text{ mg} = 46.4 \text{ mg}$

(3)　　Drug release equation for a sphere

$$\frac{3}{2}\left[1-\left(1-\frac{M_t}{M_\infty}\right)^{2/3}\right]-\frac{M_t}{M_\infty}=\frac{3DC_{s,m}}{Ar_o^2}t\,,$$

$$M_\infty = \frac{4}{3}\pi r_o^3 \times A = 15.7 \text{ mg}$$

$$\frac{M_t}{M_\infty}=0.5\,,\qquad t=\frac{0.055\,Ar_o^2}{3DC_{s,m}}=4.5 \text{ wks}$$

(4)　　$t = 5$ wks

$$\frac{3}{2}\left[1-\left(1-\frac{M_t}{M_\infty}\right)^{2/3}\right]-\frac{M_t}{M_\infty}=\frac{3DC_{s,m}}{Ar_o^2}5(\text{wk})$$

By trial and error, $\dfrac{M_t}{M_\infty} \cong 0.52$, $M_t = 0.52 \times 15.7 \text{ mg} = 8.2 \text{ mg}$

Syncro-Mate-B: Polymer rods are prepared by the free-radical polymerization of 2-hydroxyethyl methacrylate with ethylene glycol dimethacrylate. They are loaded with various amounts of norgestromet by equilibration in aqueous drug solutions [11]. The amount of drug

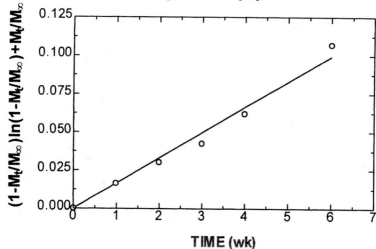

Figure II-29. $\left(1-\dfrac{M_t}{M_\infty}\right)\ln\left(1-\dfrac{M_t}{M_\infty}\right)+\dfrac{M_t}{M_\infty}$ vs. time.

incorporated in the polymer rod is much greater than the drug's solubility in the polymer (0.266 mg/ml). The majority of the drug in the polymer rod matrix is in the dispersed state. Non-linear release kinetics are observed as shown in Fig. II-30. However the experimental data becomes linear if the amount of drug released is plotted versus the square root of time. This polymer rod can be easily implanted subcutaneously in an animal's ear by a special implanter.

Nitro-Dur: This transdermal system is manufactured by mixing the lactose triturate of nitroglycerin with a polyvinyl alcohol and polyvinyl pyrollidone solution [12]. Upon cooling, the nitroglycerin disperses in the diffusion-controlled matrix medium to form a drug reservoir. The drug is partitioned between the binding sites on the lactose and the two polymers. Fig. II-31 presents the in-vitro release kinetics of nitroglycerin from Nitro-Dur systems. A linear relationship is observed in the plot of the amount of drug release versus the square root of time.

II.2.2. *Boundary layer*

A schematic representation of the diffusional boundary layer of a monolithic matrix consisting of dispersed drugs is illustrated in Fig. II-32. The solute dissolved at the dissolution front diffuses through a drug-depleted zone ($0 \leq x \leq l$) and then through the boundary layer (mass transfer

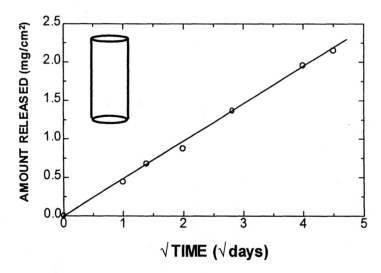

Figure II-30. Drug release from Syncro-Mate-B. (Graph reconstructed from data by Chien and Lau [11]).

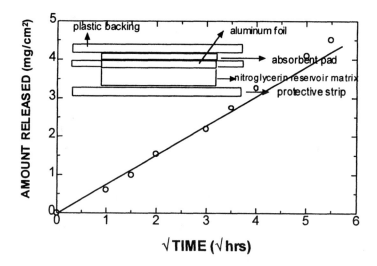

Figure II-31. Cross-sectional view of matrix controlled transdermal delivery systems. (Graph reconstructed from data by Chien [12].)

coefficient k) in series. It is assumed that the outside boundary layer is maintained under perfect sink conditions. Under the pseudo-steady state approximation, Higuchi's approach can include a mass transfer resistance of an outer stagnant boundary layer. The drug concentration profile within the drug-depleted layer is given by Fick's first law:

$$\frac{1}{S}\frac{dM_t}{dt} = D\frac{C_s - C_o}{\xi} \tag{2-73}$$

For the boundary layer, the assumption that the drug concentration outside the boundary layer is zero (sink condition) yields:

$$\frac{1}{S}\frac{dM_t}{dt} = \frac{k}{K}C_o \tag{2-74}$$

The mass balance equation is given by:

$$\frac{1}{S}\frac{dM_t}{dt} = (A - C_s/2)\frac{d\xi}{dt} \tag{2-75}$$

Combining equations (2-73), (2-74) and (2-75) and integrating the resulting equation yields:

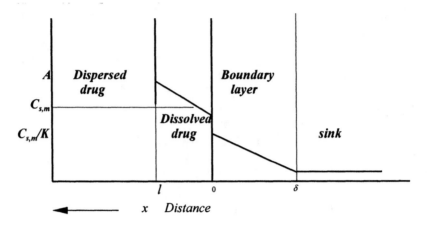

Figure II-32. Schematic diagram for the diffusional boundary layer of a monolithic matrix containing a dispersed drug.

$$\xi = \left[\left(\frac{DK}{k} \right)^2 + \frac{2C_s Dt}{A - C_s/2} \right]^{1/2} - \frac{DK}{k} \tag{2-76}$$

By taking $d\xi/dt$ from equation (2-76) and substituting the result into equation (2-75), the amount of drug released, M_t, can be calculated by [12]:

$$\frac{M_t}{S} = (A - C_s/2) \left[\sqrt{\left(\frac{DK}{k} \right)^2 + \frac{2DC_s t}{A - C_s/2}} - \frac{DK}{k} \right]$$

$$+ \frac{C_s}{2} \left[\frac{(DK/k)^2}{\sqrt{\left(\frac{DK}{k} \right)^2 + \frac{2DC_s t}{A - C_s/2}}} - \frac{DK}{k} \right] \tag{2-77}$$

For the long time approximation, equation (2-77) may be given as:

$$\frac{M_t}{S} = \sqrt{2DC_s(A - C_s/2)t} - \frac{ADK}{k} \tag{2-78a}$$

or

$$\frac{M_t}{S} = \sqrt{2DC_s(A - C_s/2)}(\sqrt{t} - \sqrt{t_o})$$ (2-78b)

where

$$\sqrt{t_o} = \frac{KA}{kC_s}\sqrt{\frac{D}{2(A - C_s/2)}}$$ (2-78c)

Cylindrical geometry [13]:

$$\frac{r^2}{2}\ln\left(\frac{r}{r_o}\right) + \frac{1}{4}\left(r_o^2 - r^2\right) + \frac{DK}{2kr}\left(r_o^2 - r^2\right) = \frac{C_sD_st}{A}$$ (2-79a)

$$\frac{M_t}{S} = \pi h_c A(r_o^2 - r^2)$$ (2-79b)

Spherical geometry [13]:

$$r_o^3 - 3r_or^2 + 2r^3 - \frac{2DK}{kr_o}(r^3 - r_o^3) = \frac{6r_o DC_st}{A}$$ (2-80a)

$$\frac{M_t}{S} = \frac{4}{3}\pi A(r_o^3 - r^3)$$ (2-80b)

Tojo [14] presented an exact solution to evaluate the intrinsic release rate from a matrix-type drug delivery system while considering the effect of the hydrodynamic diffusional layer on the rate of drug release. When $A \gg C_s$, the cumulative amount of drug released per unit area (Q_t) may be calculated by:

$$Q_t = \left[\left(\frac{bD}{a}\right)^2\left(A - \frac{C_s}{2}\right)^2 + 2D\left(A - \frac{C_s}{2}\right)C_st\right]^{1/2} - \frac{Db}{a}\left(A - \frac{C_s}{2}\right)$$ (2-81)

where

$$a = k/K, \qquad\qquad b = (A - C_s)/(A - C_s/2)$$

when the drug loading (A) is much higher than the drug's solubility. If the following condition is satisfied:

$$\frac{k^2 t}{K^2} \gg \frac{D}{2}\left(\frac{A}{C_s} - \frac{1}{2}\right)$$

equation (2-81) is reduced to equation (2-82) which was originally derived by Roseman and Higuchi [4].

$$Q_t = \sqrt{(2A - C_s)D\ C_s t} - (A - C_s/2)KD\ /k \qquad (2\text{-}82)$$

Evaluating equation (2-82) against the intrinsic equation $(Q_i = \sqrt{(2A - C_s)DC_s t}\,)$ yields:

$$\gamma = \frac{Q_t}{Q_i} = \sqrt{1 + \left(\frac{Q_i}{2C_s k_m t}\right)^2} - \frac{Q_i}{2C_s k_m t} \qquad (2\text{-}83)$$

Differentiation of the intrinsic release (Higuchi's equation) from the actual release including the mass transfer resistance can then be obtained. The ratio of the intrinsic and apparent release rate, η, is given by:

$$\eta = \frac{dQ/d\sqrt{t}}{(dQ/d\sqrt{t})_i} = \left[1 + \frac{Q_i^2}{(2C_s \ln t)^2}\right]^{-\frac{1}{2}} = \frac{2\gamma}{\gamma^2 + 1} \qquad (2\text{-}84)$$

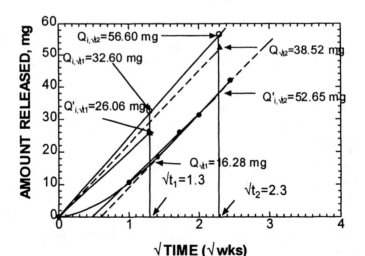

Figure II-33. Graphic evaluation of intrinsic release profile.

where $(dQ/d\sqrt{t})_i$ is the intrinsic release rate.
Equation (2-82) can be rearranged:

$$\frac{Q_i}{Q_i'} = \frac{Q_i' + \Delta Q}{Q_i'} = \frac{\left[Q/(Q_i' + \Delta Q)\right]^2 + 1}{2Q/(Q_i' + \Delta Q)} \tag{2-85}$$

or

$$\frac{\Delta Q}{Q} = \sqrt{\xi/(2-\xi)} - \xi \tag{2-86}$$

where $Q_i = Q_i' + \Delta Q$ and $\xi = Q'_i/Q$.

From the experimental plot of Q versus $\sqrt{t}$, Q_i' can be obtained easily by drawing a parallel line to the slope at the point along the release curve as shown in Fig. II-33. It is better to fit the plots of cumulative release versus time to a polynomial equation of the actual release curve and take its derivative at $\sqrt{t}$. The intrinsic release amount Q_i is then calculated simply by $Q_i = Q_i' + \Delta Q$ since ξ is already determined. The entire intrinsic release profile can be constructed by determining Q_i at all data points and connecting them.

II.2.3. *Exact analysis (unsteady state)*

To avoid Higuchi's approximation of the "pseudo-steady-state", for which the limit of $A > C_s$ does not precisely predict the release kinetics for $A < C_s$ or $A = C_s$, Paul and McSpadden [15] remove the "pseudo-steady-state" approximation with Fick's second law giving a result that merges correctly with the unsaturated core in the limit $A \to C_s$ as follows:

$$\frac{\partial C}{\partial t} = D\frac{\partial^2 C}{\partial x^2} \tag{2-87}$$

in the region $0 < x < \xi$ using the boundary conditions:

$$x = 0, \qquad\qquad C = 0 \tag{2-88a}$$

$$x = \xi, \qquad\qquad C = C_s \tag{2-88b}$$

However, at the interface there is an additional boundary condition:

$$(A - C_s)\frac{\partial \xi}{\partial t} = D\frac{\partial C}{\partial x} \tag{2-89}$$

We can assume a solution in the form of:

$$C = C_o + Berf\left[x/2(Dt)^{\frac{1}{2}}\right]$$

(2-90)

where B is an arbitrary constant and the differential equation (2-87) and boundary conditions (2-88) are satisfied since $erf(0) = 0$. In order to use this solution and satisfy the boundary conditions (2-88) at the interface, we must incorporate the expression:

$$C_s = C_o + Berf(\lambda)$$

(2-91)

where

$$\lambda = \frac{\xi}{2\sqrt{Dt}}, \qquad \text{or} \qquad \xi = 2\lambda(Dt)^{1/2}$$

(2-92)

Combining equations (2-91) and (2-92) yields:

$$C = C_s \frac{erf(\eta)}{erf(\lambda)}$$

(2-93)

where

$$\eta = \frac{x}{\sqrt{Dt}}$$

(2-94)

The following transcendental equation must be satisfied in order to solve equation (2-93):

$$\sqrt{\pi}\lambda e^{\lambda^2} erf(\lambda) = \frac{C_s}{A - C_s}$$

(2-95)

and λ is the root of this equation. Knowing λ, x can be determined from equation (2-94) and C from equation (2-93).

The amount of drug released at time t can be obtained using:

$$M_t = -D\int\left(\frac{\partial c}{\partial x}\right)_{x=l} dt = \frac{2C_s}{erf(\lambda)}\sqrt{\frac{Dt}{\pi}}$$

(2-96)

In this equation M_t is linear with respect to the square root of time as it is in equation (2-58), but the dependence on drug loading A is different. The finite mass transfer resistance can be incorporated into this approach by applying a similar form of equation (2-21b) to equation (2-96) which produces:

$$M_t = \frac{2C_s}{erf(\lambda)} \sqrt{\frac{Dt}{\pi}} - A\frac{D}{h} \tag{2-97}$$

From equation (2-95), a λ value can be calculated numerically by Newton-Ralph's method and then M_t can be evaluated from equation (2-96). When $A = C_s$, equation (2-96) and equation (2-58) are identical since λ becomes infinity.

However, it is not convenient to use both equations (2-95) and (2-96) to evaluate the drug release kinetics. Koizumi et al. [16] derived an approximate solution of equations (2-95) and (2-96). Expansion of equations (2-95) and (2-96) in λ produces equations (2-98a) and (2-98b), respectively.

$$\left[\frac{Q}{\sqrt{Dt}\,2(A - C_s)}\right]^2 = \lambda^2 + 2\lambda^4 + 2\lambda^6 + \ldots\ldots\ldots \tag{2-98a}$$

$$\frac{C_s}{A - C_s} = 2\lambda^2 + \frac{4}{3}\lambda^4 + \frac{8}{15}\lambda^6 + \ldots\ldots\ldots \tag{2-98b}$$

Elimination of λ, term by term, gives [3]:

$$Q = \sqrt{DtC_s\left(2A - \frac{2}{3}C_s - \frac{1}{45}\frac{C_s^2}{A - C_s} + \frac{2}{189}\frac{C_s^2}{(A - C_s)} - \ldots\ldots\right)} \tag{2-99}$$

Equation (2-99) was simplified further as [3]:

$$Q = \sqrt{DtC_s\left(2A - \frac{2}{3}C_s\left(\frac{A - 0.0066C_s}{A - 0.89C_s}\right)\right)} \tag{2-100a}$$

or

$$Q = \sqrt{\left(2A - \frac{2}{3}C_s\right)C_s Dt} \tag{2-100b}$$

Table II-5 clearly shows that the values of $Q/C_s\sqrt{Dt}$ calculated by the approximate equation [equation (2-100a)] and by the explicit equation [equation (2-96)] coincide within <0.05% error. For $A/C_s > 1.5$, differences between equations (2-100b) and (2-96) are less than 0.5%.

Table II-5. Comparison of the Explicit Solution and the Approximation Solutions [3].

C_0/C_s	Eq.(2-96)	Eq. (2-100a)	Eq. (2-100b)	Eq. (2-58)
1.00	1.1284	1.1282	1.1547	1.0000
1.10	1.2205	1.2254	1.2383	1.0954
1.50	1.5198	1.5239	1.5275	1.4142
2.00	1.8216	1.8241	1.8257	1.7321
2.50	2.0789	2.0807	2.0817	2.0000
3.00	2.3074	2.3087	2.3094	2.2361
3.50	2.5151	2.5161	2.5166	2.4495
4.00	2.7068	2.7076	2.7080	2.6458
6.00	3.3659	3.3663	3.3665	3.3166
8.00	3.9154	3.9157	3.9158	3.8730
10.00	4.3967	4.3969	4.3970	4.3589
20.00	6.2715	6.2716	6.2716	6.2450

Lee [17] derived another analytical solution for equations (2-87), (2-88a), and (2-88b) using the heat balance integral method. For slab geometry:

$$M_t = C_s \left[\frac{1+H}{\sqrt{3H}} \right] \sqrt{Dt} \tag{2-101}$$

where

$$H = 5\left(\frac{A}{C_s} \right) + \left[\left(\frac{A}{C_s} \right)^2 - 1 \right]^{1/2} - 4 \tag{2-102}$$

For spherical geometry:

$$\frac{M_t}{M_\infty} = [1 - (1-\delta)^3](1 - \frac{C_s}{A}) + 3\delta(\frac{C_s}{A})[(a_1 + \frac{a_2}{2} + \frac{a_3}{3}) - (\frac{a_1}{2} + \frac{a_2}{3} + \frac{a_3}{4})\delta] \tag{2-103}$$

$$\frac{Dt}{a^2} = \frac{1}{12}\left[6\frac{A}{C_s} - 4 - a_3 \right]\delta^2 - \frac{1}{3}(\frac{A}{C_s} - 1)\delta^3 \tag{2-104}$$

where $a_1 = 1$, $a_2 = -a_3 - 1$, and,

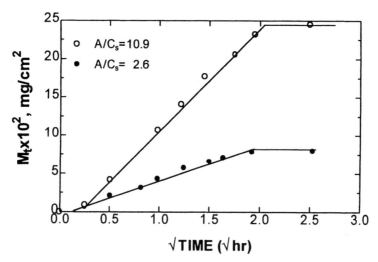

Figure II-34. Effect of drug loading on release kinetics. (Graph reconstructed from data by Paul and McSpadden [15].)

$$a_3 = 1 - (1 - \frac{A}{C_s})(1-\delta) - \left\{ \left[1 - (1 - \frac{A}{C_s})(1-\delta) \right]^2 - 1 \right\}^{1/2} \qquad (2\text{-}105)$$

where δ is the dimensionless thickness of the drug depleted zone.

As observed in equations (2-96), (2-100a), and (2-101), the cumulative amount of drug released at time t is directly proportional to the square root of time for each method. The solutions based on Fick's second law have some advantages over the Higuchi model (pseudo-steady-state approximation) for the drug release kinetics when the loading level is close to the level of drug solubility in the polymer matrix. However, when the drug loading is much higher than the drug solubility, the three methods become virtually identical as shown in Table II-4. These solutions are applicable to the drug release kinetics of dispersed drug, provided the dissolution of un-dissolved drug is not the rate-determining step (rapid dissolution). The dissolution-diffusion controlled (slow dissolution) kinetics of drug release is discussed in Chapter II-3.

Problem II-11: Paul and McSpadden [15] studied the release of Sudan A dye dissolved in acetone from a loaded membrane (diameter = 8 cm, thickness ≐ 0.15 cm). The cumulative release, M_t, was plotted against the square root of time at different loading levels (Fig. II-34). Calculate the diffusion coefficient of the dye assuming the solubility of Sudan A is 0.274 g/l. The diffusivity of the drug was determined independently to be 2.68×10^{-6} cm^2/sec.

Solution: A finite external mass transfer boundary layer can be incorporated into equation (2-95) in analogy to equation (2-21c) as [15]:

$$M_t = \frac{2C_s}{erf(\eta)}\sqrt{\frac{Dt}{\pi}} - A\frac{D}{h} = \frac{2C_s}{erf(\eta^*)}\sqrt{\frac{D}{\pi}}(\sqrt{t} - \sqrt{t_o})$$

$$A \gg C_s, \quad \sqrt{t_o} \cong \frac{1}{\alpha}\frac{A}{C_s}\sqrt{\frac{D}{2(\frac{A}{C_s} - 1)}} \cong \frac{1}{\alpha}\sqrt{\frac{DA}{2C_s}}$$

For $A/C_s = 10.9$, $\qquad \sqrt{t_o} = 0.171 = \frac{K}{k}\sqrt{\frac{DA}{2C_s}}$

$$k = 4.7 \times 10^{-5} \text{ cm/sec}$$
For $A/C_s = 2.6$, $\qquad k = 3.7 \times 10^{-5} \text{ cm/sec}$

II.2.4. *Release of dispersed drug in a finite volume*

Exact solution: When dispersed drug in a slab matrix diffuses out in a finite volume, the concentration of the drug in the depleted layer can be expressed by:

$$\frac{\partial C}{\partial t} = D\frac{\partial^2 C}{\partial x^2} \tag{2-1}$$

subject to the following initial and boundary conditions:

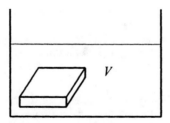

Figure II-35.   Release of a drug in a finite volume.

$$C = C_o \qquad\qquad t=0 \qquad\qquad\qquad (2\text{-}106a)$$

$$C = kC_b \qquad\qquad x = 0\,,\, t > 0 \qquad\qquad (2\text{-}106b)$$

$$C = C_s \qquad\qquad x = R(t)\,,\, t > 0 \qquad (2\text{-}106c)$$

$$D\frac{\partial C}{\partial r} = (A - C_s)\frac{dR}{dt} \qquad x = R(t)\,,\, t > 0 \qquad (2\text{-}106d)$$

$$R = S \qquad\qquad t = 0 \qquad\qquad\qquad (2\text{-}106e)$$

where k is the distribution coefficient between the external solution and the matrix and C_b is the drug concentration in the bulk with time t.

Equation (2-106d) can be combined with a total mass balance at time t as:

$$A\left(1 - \frac{R}{S}\right) = C\lambda + \frac{\alpha+1}{S}\int_R^S C\left(\frac{x}{S}\right)^\alpha dx \qquad (2\text{-}106e)$$

$$\lambda = \frac{V}{2k\sigma S} \qquad\qquad (2\text{-}106f)$$

where σ is the surface area of a slab and V is the volume of external solution.

Abdekhodie and Cheng [18] solved the above equations for the drug concentration distribution (θ) and the dissolution front position (Γ) at time t as:

$$\theta = 1 - \frac{[K(1-\Gamma) - \lambda]\sqrt{\pi}\left(erf(\frac{1-\varsigma}{2\sqrt{\tau}}) - erf(\frac{1-\Gamma}{2\sqrt{\tau}})\right)}{\sqrt{\pi}\lambda erf(\frac{1-\Gamma}{2\sqrt{\tau}}) + 2\sqrt{\tau}\left(1 - \exp(-\frac{(1-\Gamma)^2}{2\sqrt{\tau}})\right)} \qquad (2\text{-}107)$$

$$K\frac{d\Gamma}{d\tau} = \frac{[K(1-\Gamma) - \lambda]\exp\left(-\frac{(1-\Gamma)^2}{4\tau}\right)}{\sqrt{\pi}\lambda\sqrt{\tau}erf(\frac{1-\Gamma}{2\sqrt{\tau}}) + 2\tau\left(1 - \exp(-\frac{(1-\Gamma)^2}{4\tau})\right)} \qquad (2\text{-}108)$$

where $\tau = \dfrac{Dt}{S^2}$, $\varsigma = \dfrac{x}{S}$, $\Gamma = \dfrac{R}{S}$, $K = \dfrac{A}{C_s} - 1$, and $\theta = \dfrac{C}{C_s}$.

The cumulative amount of drug released (M_t) can be expressed by [17]:

$$\frac{M_t}{M_\infty} = \frac{\lambda}{A/C_s} \frac{[K(1-\Gamma)-\lambda]\sqrt{\pi}\exp\left(-\dfrac{1-\Gamma}{2\sqrt{\tau}}\right)}{\sqrt{\pi}\lambda erf(\dfrac{1-\Gamma}{2\sqrt{\tau}})+2\sqrt{\tau}\left(1-\exp(-\dfrac{(1-\Gamma)^2}{4\tau})\right)} \qquad (2\text{-}109)$$

where $M_\infty = 2\sigma SA$.

Abdekhodie and Cheng [18] derived also the analytical solutions for spherical geometry similar to equations (2-107) to (2-109) as follows:

$$\theta = \Gamma + B_1\sqrt{\pi}\left(erf\left(\frac{1-\varsigma}{2\sqrt{\tau}}\right) - erf\left(\frac{1-\Gamma}{2\sqrt{\tau}}\right)\right) \qquad (2\text{-}110)$$

$$B_1 = \frac{(1-\Gamma^3)\dfrac{A}{C_s} - \lambda\Gamma - \dfrac{3}{2}\Gamma(1-\Gamma^2)}{\sqrt{\pi}(3\tau-\lambda)erf\left(\dfrac{1-\Gamma}{2\sqrt{\tau}}\right) - 6\sqrt{\tau} + 3\sqrt{\tau}(1+\Gamma)\exp\left(-\dfrac{(1-\Gamma)^2}{4\tau}\right)} \qquad (2\text{-}111)$$

$$K\frac{d\Gamma}{d\tau} = -\frac{B_1\exp\left(-\dfrac{(1-\Gamma)^2}{4\tau}\right)}{\Gamma\sqrt{\tau}} - \frac{1}{\Gamma} \qquad (2\text{-}112)$$

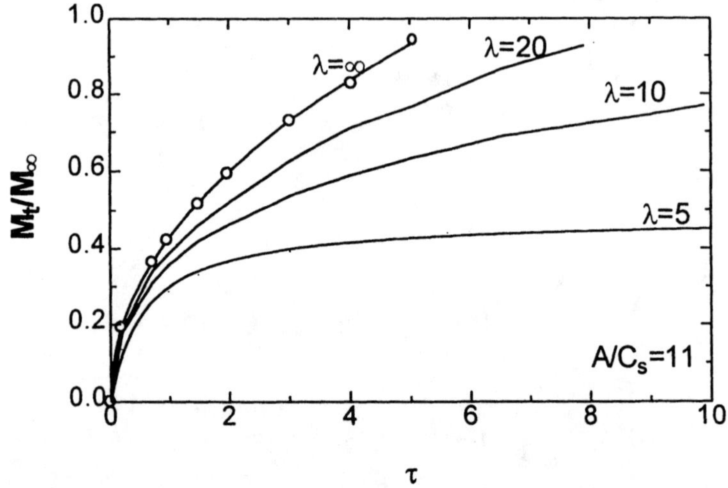

Figure II-36. Effect of finite volume on drug release of dispersed matrix. (Graph reconstructed from data by Abdekhodie and Cheng [18].)

The fractional release from a sphere is given by:

$$\frac{M_t}{M_\infty} = \frac{\lambda}{A/C_s}\left(\Gamma - B_1\sqrt{\pi}\,erf\left(\frac{1-\Gamma}{2\sqrt{\tau}}\right)\right) \tag{2-113}$$

Equations (2-108) and (2-112) provide the dimensionless moving front position with time. However, the initial condition [equation (2-106e)] prohibits calculating $d\Gamma/d\tau$ at $\tau = 0$. Therefore other values of Γ at $\tau = 0$ are needed as an initial condition for the calculation of the moving front position as a function of time. Abdekhodie and Cheng [18] proposed to use equation (2-95) derived under a perfect sink condition for a planar and spherical matrix to calculate Γ for a small value of τ. It has been shown that $\Gamma(\tau)$ is insensitive to the initial conditions selected over a wide range of τ [18].

References

1. T. Higuchi, "Rate of Release of Medicaments from Ointment Bases Containing Drugs in Suspension," *J. Pharm. Sci.*, 50, 874 (1961).
2. R. W. Baker and H. K. Lonsdale, "Controlled Release: Mechanism and Rate" in Controlled Release of Biologically Active Agents, A. C. Tranquany and R. E. Lacey (Eds.), Plenum Press, New York, 1974, p15.
3. T. Koizumi and S. P. Panomsuk, "Release of Medicaments from Spherical Matrices Containing Drug in Suspension: Theoretical Aspects," *Int. J. Pharm.*, 116, 45 (1995).
4. T. J. Roseman and W. I. Higuchi, "Release of Medroxyprogesterone Acetate from a Silicone Matrix," *J. Pharm. Sci.*, 59, 353 (1970).
5. J. R. Cardinal, "Drug Release from Matrix Devices," In Recent Advances in Drug Delivery Systems, J. M. Anderson and S. W. Kim (Eds.), Plenum Press, New York, 1984, p229.
6. R. A. Siegal and R. Langer, "Controlled Release of Polypeptides and Other Macromolecules," *Pharm. Res.*, 1, 2 (1984).
7. R. A. Siegal, J. Kost, and R. Langer, "Mechanistic Studies of Macromolecular Drug Release from Macroporous Polymer. I. Experiments and Preliminary Theory Concerning Completeness of Drug Release," *J. Control. Rel.*, 8, 223 (1989).
8. R. A. Siegal and R. Langer, "Mechanistic Studies of Macromolecular Drug Release from Macroporous Polymer. II. Models for the Slow Kinetics of Drug Release," *J. Control. Rel.*, 14, 153 (1990).
9. B. G. Amsden and Y.-L. Cheng, "Enhanced Fraction Releasable above Percolation Threshold from Monoliths Containing Osmotic Excipients," *J. Control. Rel.*, 31, 21 (1994).

10. J. C. Fu, C. Hagemeir, D. L. Mayer, and E. W. Ng., "A Unified Mathematical Model for Diffusion from Drug-Polymer Composite Tablets," *J. Biomed. Mater. Res.*, 10, 743 (1976).

11. Y. W. Chien and E.-P. K. Lau, "Controlled Release from Polymeric Delivery Devices (IV): In Vitro-In-Vivo Correlation on the Subcutaneous Release of Norgestromet from Hydrophilic Implants," J. Pharm. Sci., 68, 689 (1979).

12. Y. W. Chien, Novel Drug Delivery Systems, 2nd Edition, Marcel Dekker, Inc., New York, 1992, p346.

13. T. J. Roseman and N. F. Cardarelli, "Monolithic Polymer Devices," In Controlled Release Technologies: Methods, Theory and Applications. Vol. I., A. Kydonieus, Ed., CRC Press, Boca Raton, Fl., 1980, p21.

14. K. Tojo, "Intrinsic Release Rate from Matrix-Type Drug Delivery Systems," *J. Pharm. Sci.*, 74, 685 (1985).

15. D. R. Paul and S. K. McSpadden, "Diffusional Release of a Solute from a Polymer Matrix," *J. Membr. Sci.*, 1, 33 (1976).

16. T. Koizumi, M. Ueda, M. Kakemi, and H. Kameda, "Rate of Release of Medicaments from Ointment Bases Containing Drugs in Suspension," *Chem. Pharm. Bull.*, 23, 3288 (1975).

17. P. I. Lee, "Diffusional Release of a Solute from a Polymeric Matrix - Approximate Analytical Solutions," *J. Membr. Sci.*, 7, 255 (1980).

18. M. J. Abdekhodie and Y.-L. Cheng, "Diffusional Release of a Dispersed Solute from Planar and Spherical Matrices into Finite External Volume," *J. Control. Rel.*, 43, 175 (1997).

II.3. Drug Dissolution/Diffusion Controlled Systems

Higuchi's model and exact analytical methods cannot adequately describe the drug release kinetics from a dispersed drug matrix in some situations. It is reasonable to anticipate that the solubility of a drug and its dissolution rate can significantly influence the drug release kinetics. For a dispersed drug it is assumed that the dissolution rate of the drug is minimal compared to the diffusion rate of drug. When the dissolution rate is slower than the diffusion rate of the drug, the former rate markedly influences the drug release. In this case the results based on Higuchi's model are not consistent with the experimental data.

Drug release from a matrix containing a drug with slow dissolution follows a two-step process. The drug first dissolves in water (solvent) in the matrix and then diffuses out of the matrix. The relative magnitude of the two processes (dissolution and diffusion) controls the release kinetics. A combined dissolution- and diffusion-controlled release system is shown in Fig. II-37.

The equation describing drug dissolution and diffusion for semi-infinite slab geometry can be transformed to a first order expression as follows [1,2]:

$$\frac{\partial C}{\partial t} = D \frac{\partial^2 C}{\partial x^2} - k_d (C_s - C)\delta(C_d - C_s) \tag{2-114}$$

with

$$\delta(C_d - C_s) = \begin{cases} 0 \\ 1 \end{cases}, \qquad \begin{matrix} C_d \le C_s \\ C_d > C_s \end{matrix} \tag{2-115}$$

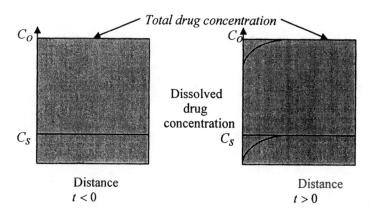

Figure II-37. Dissolved drug concentration in a matrix containing a crystalline drug [1].

where k_d is the dissolution rate constant.

The appropriate boundary conditions for a dissolved drug are:

$$C = 0 \qquad\qquad x = 0 \qquad\qquad t > 0 \qquad\qquad (2\text{-}116a)$$

$$C = C_s \qquad\qquad t = 0 \qquad\qquad 0 \le x \le l \qquad\qquad (2\text{-}116b)$$

If C is defined as:

$$\overline{C} = C_s - C \qquad\qquad (2\text{-}117)$$

Equation (2-114) can be transformed to:

$$\frac{\partial \overline{C}}{\partial t} = D \frac{\partial^2 \overline{C}}{\partial x^2} - k_d \overline{C} \qquad\qquad (2\text{-}118)$$

with boundary conditions:

$$\overline{C} = C_s \qquad\qquad x = 0 \qquad\qquad t > 0 \qquad\qquad (2\text{-}119a)$$

$$\overline{C} = 0 \qquad\qquad t = 0 \qquad\qquad 0 < x < l \qquad\qquad (2\text{-}119b)$$

The analytical solution of equation (2-118) can be found in equation (2-120)

$$\frac{\overline{C}}{C_s} = \frac{1}{2} e^{-x\sqrt{k_d/D}} \, erfc\left(\frac{x}{2\sqrt{Dt}} - \sqrt{k_d t} \right) + \frac{1}{2} e^{x\sqrt{k_d/D}} \, erfc\left(\frac{x}{2\sqrt{Dt}} + \sqrt{k_d t} \right)$$

$$(2\text{-}120)$$

and

$$M_t = C_s \sqrt{\frac{D}{k_d}} \left[(k_d t + \frac{1}{2}) erf\sqrt{k_d t} + \sqrt{\frac{k_d t}{\pi}} e^{-k_d t} \right] \qquad\qquad (2\text{-}121)$$

The fractional release at any time t is then:

$$\frac{M_t}{M_\infty} = 2 \frac{C_s}{C_o} \sqrt{\frac{D}{k_d l^2}} \left[(k_d t + \frac{1}{2}) erf\sqrt{k_d t} + \sqrt{\frac{k_d t}{\pi}} e^{-k_d t} \right], \text{ for } C_s k_d t \le C_o$$

$$(2\text{-}122)$$

where $M_\infty = C_o l / 2$ (2-123)

Simplifications of equation (2-122) may be made for large values of $k_d t$ (or small times) and dissolution controlled systems [1-3]:

$$\frac{M_t}{M_\infty} = 2\frac{C_s}{C_o}\sqrt{\frac{Dk_d}{l^2}}\left(\frac{1}{2k_d} + t\right)$$ (2-124)

$$\frac{dM_t}{dt} = C_s\sqrt{Dk_d}\left[\frac{k_d t}{\pi} + (1+\frac{k_d t}{2})\frac{1}{\sqrt{\pi_d kt}}\right]$$ (2-125)

and for $k_d t > 4$,

$$\frac{M_t}{M_\infty} = 4C_s\sqrt{Dk_d}\,(t + \frac{1}{2k_d})$$ (2-126)

$$\frac{dM_t}{dt} = C_s\sqrt{Dk_d}$$ (2-127)

Equation (3-13) is good within 2% error [3].

Kurnik and Potts [4] showed other forms of equation (2-120) for dissolution controlled systems in a *finite length slab* (thickness L). The concentration of a slowly dissolving drug in a finite matrix is given by:

$$\frac{C}{C_s} = 2\sum_{n=0}^{\infty}\left\{\frac{(-1)^n \cos(\eta\varsigma)}{\eta}\left[\left(1+\frac{\varsigma}{\vartheta}\right)\exp(\vartheta\varsigma) - \frac{\varsigma}{\vartheta}\right]\right\}$$ (2-128)

and for the amount of drug released at time t:

$$M_t = 2LC_o\sum_{n=0}^{\infty}\frac{1}{\vartheta^2}\left\{\eta^2(1-\exp(\vartheta\tau)) - \varsigma\vartheta\tau\right\}$$ (2-129)

where $\tau = \frac{Dt}{L^2}$, $\varsigma = \frac{x}{L}$, $\zeta = \frac{k_d L^2}{D}$, $\eta = \frac{(2n+1)\pi}{2}$, and $\vartheta = -\eta^2 - \varsigma$.

Kumik and Potts [4] applied the equation (2-129) to evaluate the effect of crystal particle size on the release of estradiol from polymer matrices in water. They determined the diffusion coefficient of soluble estradiol using equation (2-33). The drug dissolution rate constant was obtained from the diffusion coefficient by using equation (2-121). They observed that crystal size significantly influenced the rate of drug release as shown in Fig. II-38.

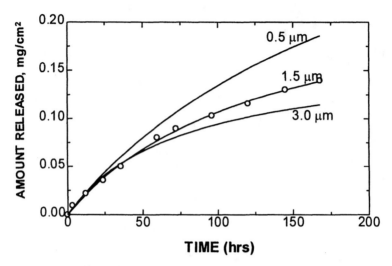

Figure II-38. Effect of crystal particle size on the release of estradiol into water. (Graph reconstructed from data by Kumi and Potts [4].)

The dissolution rate constant was evaluated with:

$$k_d = ANk'$$

where k' is the dissolution rate per unit surface area, A is the surface area of an individual crystal, and N is the number of crystals. The amount of drug released is increased by about 40% simply by decreasing the crystal size from 3 μm to 0.5 μm.

Harland et al. [5] applied a mathematical model based on a spherical geometry (radius r_o) from Crank [2] to the drug release. The solution for the drug diffusion is the same as equation (2-114). However, the following boundary conditions were used:

$t = 0$	$0 < r < r_o$	$C = C_s$	(2-130a)
$t > 0$	$r = 0$	$\dfrac{\partial C}{\partial r} = 0$	(2-130b)
$t > 0$	$r = r_o$	$C = 0$	(2-131c)

The solution to equations (2-130a), (2-130b), and (2-130c) can be found in Crank [2] and Harland et al. [5]. The amount of drug released at time t is given by:

$$M_t = 8\pi r_o DC_o \sum_{n=1}^{\infty} \frac{k_d r_o^2 + Dn^2\pi^2}{k_d r_o^2 + Dn^2\pi^2} \exp\{-t(k_d + Dn^2\pi^2/2)\} \qquad (2\text{-}132a)$$

For long times:

$$M_t = \frac{2\pi r_o^3 C_s}{\sqrt{k_d}} \left[\frac{\sqrt{D}}{r_o} \coth\left(r_o\sqrt{\frac{k_d}{D}}\right) - \sqrt{k_d}\, \csc^2 h\left(r_o\sqrt{\frac{k_d}{D}}\right) \right] +$$

$$8\pi r_o DC_s \left(\frac{k_d r_o}{2D}\sqrt{\frac{D}{k_d}} \coth\left(r_o\sqrt{\frac{k_d}{D}}\right) - \frac{1}{2} \right) t \qquad (2\text{-}132b)$$

The rate of drug released may be expressed as [5]:

$$\frac{dM_t}{dt} = 8\pi r_o DC_o \sum_{n=1}^{\infty} \frac{k_d r_o^2 + Dn^2\pi^2 \exp\left(-(k_d + Dn^2\pi^2/r_o^2)t\right)}{k_d r_o^2 + Dn^2\pi^2} \qquad (2\text{-}133)$$

Chang and Himmelstein [6] also performed a numerical simulation of simultaneous dissolution- and diffusion-controlled systems. As Fig. II-39 shows, zero-order drug release is not obtained for systems which have a high dissolution rate constant ($k_d > 10^{-3}$ /sec) and a diffusion coefficient of 10^{-9} cm^2/sec; whereas, it is achieved for systems having a low dissolution rate constants $k_d \ll 10^{-4}$ /sec even for a spherical geometry. It is interesting to note that in principle, zero-order release can not be attained for systems of spherical geometry which have a decreasing releasing surface area. However, geometry is not an important factor for a drug dissolution controlled system. As will be discussed later in Chapter VII, generally an initial drug distribution following a sigmoidal pattern (where the drug is distributed more toward the core of the sphere) allows for zero-order release kinetics. When the delivery system is controlled by the dissolution of drug, the sigmoidal and other initial drug distributions do not yield a zero-order release rate [6]. Van Bommel et al. [7] also included position-dependent diffusion coefficient on their model:

$$\frac{\partial c}{\partial t} = \frac{\partial}{\partial x} D(x,t)\frac{\partial c}{\partial x} - k_d(C_s - C)\delta(C_d - C_s) \qquad (2\text{-}134)$$

$$D(x,t) = D_o(1 + MC_{sd}^o(x)) \qquad (2\text{-}135)$$

where D_o is the initial diffusion coefficient of a drug in the matrix, C_{sd}^o is the initial drug concentration in a solid phase, and M is a proportionality constant. The effective diffusivity of the dissolved drug in the matrix

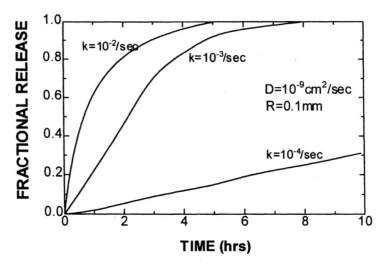

Figure II-39. Drug release profiles from matrices containing a crystalline drug. (Graphs reconstructed from data by Chang and Himmelstein [6].)

increases by the generation of void volume in the matrix by drug dissolution. However, the increasing drug diffusivity does not influence the release kinetics controlled by drug dissolution ($k_d \leq 10^{-4}$ / sec). The dissolution controlled kinetic equations may be applied to obtain zero-order release kinetics for a drug with very low solubility in a hydrophilic polymer matrix. This position and time-dependent diffusivity method has been applied to the release of acetophenophen from triple layer tablets (one side opening) [7].

Problem II-11: Gurny et al. [3] studied the release of KCl (Fig. II-40) from an ethyl cellulose tablet matrix having a total weight of 0.8 g, diameter of 1.5 cm and uniform thickness of 0.4 cm. the tablet's cross-sectional area is 1.77 cm^2; the total amount of drug in the tablet is 0.4 g and $C_s = 0.395$ g/cm^3. The dissolution rate constant was determined to be 1.7×10^{-3}/sec. Determine the diffusion coefficient of KCl from the ethyl cellulose tablet.

Solution:

$$C_o = \frac{0.48}{0.4 x 1.77} = 0.565 g / cm^3$$

If one includes the porosity (ε=0.296) and tortuosity (τ=3) of the tablet, equation (2-124) can be expressed by [3]:

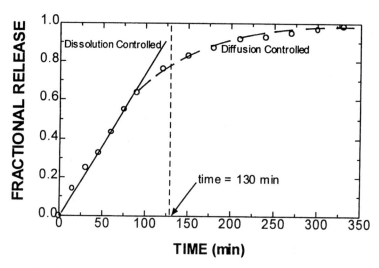

Figure II-40. Release of KCl from an ethyl cellulose tablet. (Graph reconstructed from data by Gurney et al. [3].)

$$\frac{M_t}{M_\infty} = 2\frac{\varepsilon C_s}{C_o}\sqrt{\frac{D\varepsilon k_d}{\tau l^2}}\left(\frac{1}{2k_d} + t\right)$$

From the slope of Fig. II-40, the diffusivity of the drug can be obtained:

$$\text{slope} = 0.006513\text{fraction} / \min = 2\frac{\varepsilon C_s}{C_o}\sqrt{\frac{D\varepsilon k_d}{\tau l^2}}$$

$D = 4.1 \times 10^{-4}$ cm²/sec

References

1. S. K. Chandrasekren and D. R. Paul, "Dissolution-Controlled Transport from Dispersed Matrices," *J. Pharm. Sci.*, 71, 1399 (1982).
2. J. Crank, <u>The Mathematics of Diffusion</u>, 2nd Edition, Oxford Press, 1975.
3. R. Gurney, E. Doelkar and N. A. Peppas, "Modelling of Sustained Release of Water Soluble Drugs from Porous Hydrophilic Polymers," *Biomaterials*, 3, 27 (1982).

4. R. T. Kurmik and R. O. Potts, "Modeling of Diffusion and Crystal Dissolution in Controlled Release Systems," *J. Control. Rel.,* 45, 257 (1997).
5. R. S. Harland, C. Dubernet, J.-P. Benoit, and N. A. Peppas, "A Model of Dissolution-Controlled, Diffusional Drug Release from Non-swellable Polymer Microsphere," *J. Control. Rel.,* 7, 207 (1988).
6. N. J. Chang and K. J. Himmelstein, "Dissolution-Diffusion Controlled Constant-Rate Release from Heterogeneously Loaded Drug-Containing Materials," *J. Control. Rel.,* 12, 201 (1990).
7. E. M. G. van Bommel, N. J. Chang, and K. Himmelstein, "In Vitro Release Kinetics of Heterogeneously Loaded Gradient Matrix System," *Proceed. Inter. Symp. Control. Rel. Bioact. Mater.,* 17, 148 (1990).

Chapter III

Membrane Controlled Systems

III.1. Constant Activity Reservoir

Drug molecules or chemicals are encapsulated and separated by a membrane into upstream and downstream sections. This membrane controls the movement of drug or solvent between the two sides. The membrane permeability of the solvent and the drug as well as the geometry of the device determines the diffusion rate of molecules through the membrane. A system (slab or plane) having a constant activity reservoir maintains a constant concentration gradient across the membrane under steady-state conditions as illustrated in Fig. III-1.

Fick's first law of diffusion controls the amount of drug molecules that travel through the membrane:

$$J = -D\frac{\partial C}{\partial x} \qquad (3\text{-}1)$$

where J is the flux of drug molecules, C is the concentration of the drug in the membrane, x is the travel distance within the membrane, and D is the membrane diffusion coefficient of the drug. The negative sign in the equation indicates that the movement of drug occurs from a higher concentration to a lower concentration. Integrating equation (3-1) over the thickness of the membrane under steady-state condition yields:

$$J = \frac{(C_1^m - C_2^m)D}{l} \qquad (3\text{-}2)$$

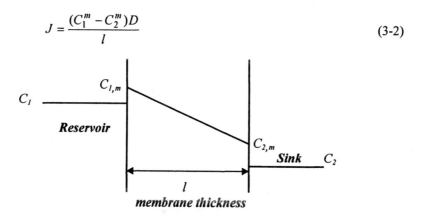

Figure III-1. Schematic model for a membrane-reservoir system.

83

where l is the thickness of the membrane; however the concentration of the upstream and downstream sides inside the membrane are not known. Equation (3-2) can be written in terms of known values for drug concentrations in the upstream and downstream sides as:

$$J = \frac{k(C_1 - C_2)}{l} D \qquad (3-3)$$

where k is the partition coefficient, assumed to be independent of concentration and position. Noting $J = (dM_t / dt) / S$ equation (3-3) can be rewritten as:

$$\frac{dM_t}{dt} = \frac{k(C_1 - C_2)SD}{l} \qquad (3-4)$$

where M_t is the amount of drug diffused through the membrane at time t, dM_t / dt is the release rate of the drug, and S is the surface area of the membrane. Integrating equation (3-4) gives:

$$M_t = \frac{k(C_1 - C_2)SDt}{l} \qquad (3-5)$$

However, if the membrane thickness is unknown or if there are other parameters (D or K) to be obtained, the permeability coefficient, P, can be substituted, giving:

$$M_t = P(C_1 - C_2)St \qquad (3-6)$$

If the perfect sink conditions can be assumed (i.e. $C_2 = 0$):

$$M_t = PC_1St, \quad \text{or} \quad M_t = \frac{kC_1SDt}{l} \qquad (3-7a)$$

For other geometries (cylinder and sphere) a similar method can be applied to obtain the release rate and the cumulative amount of drug released at time t as shown in Table III-1.

Problem III-1: Calculate the drug release rate for perfect sink conditions (under steady state) from a device having the following properties: membrane area = 2.5 cm², diffusion coefficient of drug through the membrane = 10^{-6} cm²/sec, constant reservoir concentration (saturated) = 35 mg/cm³, partition coefficient of drug in the membrane = 5, and the membrane thickness = 75 mm. How many mg of drug have been released after 2 hrs?

Table III-1. Cumulative Drug Release and Release Rates through a Membrane from a Constant Activity Reservoir.

slab	$M_t = \dfrac{SDkC_s}{l} t,$	$\dfrac{dM_t}{dt} = \dfrac{SDkC_s}{l}$	(a)
cylinder	$M_t = \dfrac{2\pi hDkC_s}{\ln(r_o/r_i)} t,$	$\dfrac{dM_t}{dt} = \dfrac{2\pi hDkC_s}{\ln(r_o/r_i)}$	(b)
sphere	$M_t = \dfrac{4\pi DkC_s r_o r_i}{r_o - r_i} t,$	$\dfrac{dM_t}{dt} = \dfrac{4\pi DkC_s r_o r_i}{r_o - r_i}$	(c)

Solution:

$$dM_t / dt = (2.5 \text{ cm}^2)\,(10^{-6} \text{ cm}^2/\text{sec})\, 5\, (35 \text{ mg/cm}^3)/(75\times10^{-4} \text{ cm})$$
$$M_t = (0.35 \text{ mg/min}) \times 2 \text{ hrs } (60 \text{ min/hr}) = 42 \text{ mg}.$$

To evaluate the effect of membrane thickness on the permeation of drug through the membrane under the steady-state condition, the normalized flux ($flux_{norm}$) can be used as [1]:

$$flux_{norm} = \frac{M_t l}{tS} = DKC_s \qquad (3\text{-}7b)$$

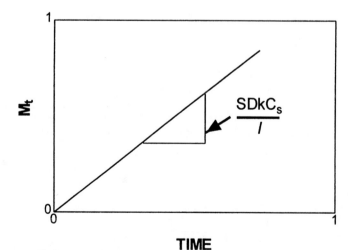

TIME

Figure III-2. Drug release under steady state condition through a membrane from a constant activity reservoir.

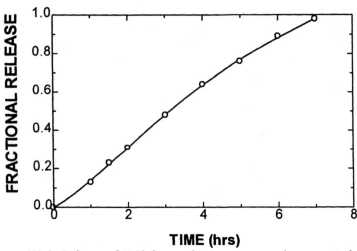

TIME (hrs)

Figure III-3. Release of KCl from micro-porous membrane coated tablets. (Graph reconstructed from data by Kallstrand and Ekmano [2].)

Both KC_s and D are intensive properties of a drug/polymer system.

Micro-porous Membrane Coated Tablets: Potassium chloride (KCl) granulated with a 50% solution of poly(vinyl pyrrolidone) was compressed to produce 12 mm diameter circular bi-convex tablets containing 1000 mg of KCl. Polyvinyl chloride solutions containing different amounts of micronized sugar were sprayed onto the KCl tablets using a pan coater. *In vitro* release profiles of KCl from the membrane-coated tablets are shown in Fig. III-3. The water-soluble substance (sugar) creates the micro-porous structure of tablets. The water in the dissolution medium penetrates the tablets through their micro-porous membrane and dissolves the drug, allowing the dissolved drug to diffuse out of the tablet through the pores. Approximately 70-80% of KCl is released at a constant rate until the drug concentration reaches a level below its saturation concentration (i.e. no solid drug is left within the tablet). Afterwards, the rate of release declines with decreasing concentration within the tablet (see next section).

Micro-encapsulated Mating Control: Microcapsules that release a pheromone were produced for controlling insect population. Fig. III-4 represents the release of disparlure from the microcapsules. As the equation in Table III-1 may predict, the release rate should be constant as long as the pheromone concentration in the microcapsules is constant. The release is reasonably constant even if there are variations of membrane wall thickness and microcapsule size.

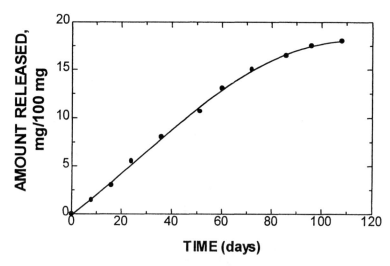

Figure III-4. Release of disparlure from microcapsules. (Graph reconstructed from data by Smith et al. [3].)

III.2. Non-Constant Activity Reservoir

The drug activity inside the reservoir is not constant level the entire period because more water diffuses in with time, resulting in the dilution of drug concentration or the continuous diffusion of drug. For limited periods of time, a saturated level (suspension) in the reservoir may be maintained. As soon as the solid drug disappears, the drug concentration in the reservoir falls below the saturation concentration. As a result, the drug concentration in the reservoir falls below the saturated level. The rate of change of drug concentration in the membrane for a non-constant activity system (sphere) can be written under the steady state assumption as:

$$\frac{D}{r^2}\frac{d}{dr}\left(r^2\frac{dC}{dr}\right) = 0 \tag{3-8}$$

The boundary conditions are:

$$t > 0, \qquad r = a, \qquad C = C_{1,m} \tag{3-9a}$$

$$r = b \qquad C = C_{2,m} \tag{3-9b}$$

where a and b are the radius of the core reservoir and the radius of the entire sphere, respectively and $C_{1.m}$ and $C_{2.m}$ are the drug concentration at the interface between the reservoir and the film, and the film and bulk medium, respectively. Equation (3-8) can be solved to yield:

$$C = \frac{aC_{1,m} - bC_{2,m}}{a-b} - \frac{1}{r}\frac{ab}{a-b}\left(C_{1,m} - C_{2,m}\right) \tag{3-10}$$

From Fick's first law of diffusion (equation (3-1)), the drug release rate is as:

$$\frac{dM_t}{dt} = 4\pi D \frac{abK}{b-a}\left(C_1 - C_2\right) \tag{3-11}$$

The drug concentration in the reservoir and in the bulk medium is:

$$C_1 = (M_1 - M_t)/V_1, \qquad C_2 = (M_2 + M_t)/V_2 \tag{3-12}$$

where V_1 and V_2 are the volume of the sphere and the bulk medium, respectively.

By substituting equations (3-12) into (3-11) and assuming $V_2 >> V_1$, the following equation (3-13) results:

$$\frac{M_t}{M_\infty} = 1 - \exp\left(\frac{-3bDK}{a^2(b-a)}t\right) \tag{3-13}$$

where M_∞ is the initial amount of drug in the reservoir which is equivalent to $C_1^o V_1$. For other geometries, a similar approach can be applied to obtain the release rate and fractional release of a drug as presented in Table III-2. Fig. III-5 shows the fractional release profiles both from a non-constant activity reservoir.

Table III-2. Fractional Release and Release Rate through a Membrane from a Non-constant Activity Reservoir.

slab	$\dfrac{M_t}{M_\infty} = 1 - e^{-SDkt/V_1 l}$, $\qquad \dfrac{dM_t}{dt} = \dfrac{SDkC_1}{l}e^{-SDkt/V_1 l}$
cylinder	$\dfrac{M_t}{M_\infty} = 1 - e^{-2Dkt/a^2 \ln(b/a)}$, $\dfrac{dM_t}{dt} = \dfrac{2\pi h DkC_1^o}{\ln(b/a)}e^{-2Dkt/a^2 \ln(b/a)}$
sphere	$\dfrac{M_t}{M_\infty} = 1 - e^{-3bDkt/a^2(b-a)}$, $\dfrac{dM_t}{dt} = \left[\dfrac{4\pi ab DkC_1^o}{(b-a)}\right]e^{-3bDkt/a^2(b-a)}$

Problem III-2: Watano et al. [4] studied the controlled release of a water soluble dye (pigment blue No. 1) from spherical particles coated with an aqueous acrylate methacrylate copolymer as shown in Fig. III-5. The average size of core particles is 600 μm and the coated film thickness is 4.5 μm. Calculate the permeability coefficient ($K_p = KD /(a - b)$). Design film thickness of coated-particles from which 95% of the drug is released in 22 hrs.

Solution:

$$slope = \frac{3bDk}{a^2(b-a)} = 0.1493 / hr \qquad P = \frac{0.1493 \times 0.03^2}{3x0.0305} = 1.47x10^{-3} \, cm/hr$$

$$DK = 7.34 \times 10^{-7} \, cm^2/hr \qquad 0.95 = 1 - \exp\left(-\frac{3b \times 7.34 \times 10^{-7}}{0.03^2(b - 0.03)}\right)$$

$$b = 0.030025 \, cm \qquad b-a = 25 \, μm$$

III.3.   Release of a Drug from a Membrane-Reservoir in a Finite Volume (Steady State Condition)

When drug is released from a coated particle in a finite volume, the drug concentration in the bulk medium at the steady state can be obtained by rearranging equation (3-10) [5]:

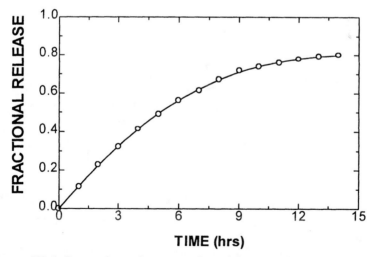

Figure III-5. Drug release from coated particles (Graph reconstructed from data by Watano et al. [4].)

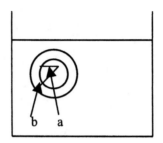

Figure III-6. Release of a drug from a membrane reservoir in a finite volume V_e.

$$\frac{dC_2}{dt} = \frac{4\pi D}{V_2} \frac{abK}{a-b}(C_1 - C_2) \tag{3-14}$$

When solid drug maintains in the reservoir until t_s at which time the solid drug is disappeared, equation (3-14) can be integrated to give:

$$\frac{C_2}{C_s} = 1 - \exp\left(-\frac{4\pi D}{KV_2}\frac{ab}{a-b}t\right) \tag{3-15}$$

The cumulative release of drug is given by:

$$M_t = V_2 C_2 = V_2 C_s\left(1 - \exp\left(-\frac{4\pi D}{KV_2}\frac{ab}{a-b}t\right)\right) \tag{3-16}$$

The time t_s then can be obtained by:

$$t_s = -\frac{KV_2}{4\pi D}\frac{a-b}{ab}\ln\left(1 - \frac{V_1}{V_2}\left(\frac{M_o}{V_1 C_s} - 1\right)\right) \tag{3-17}$$

where M_o is the initial amount of drug in the reservoir.

When the release time is larger than t_s, the change of drug concentration in the reservoir can be expressed by:

$$-\frac{dC_1}{dt} = \frac{4\pi D}{V_1}\frac{ab}{a-b}(C_{1,m} - C_{2,m}) \tag{3-18}$$

Integrating equation (3-18) yields:

$$C_{1,m} - C_{2,m} = \left(\frac{C_s}{K} - C_{a,s}\right)\exp\left(-\frac{V_1 + V_2}{V_1 V_2}\frac{\pi D}{K}\frac{ab}{a-b}(t-t_s)\right) \quad (3\text{-}19)$$

Substituting equation (3-19) into equation (3-14) and integrating from t_s to t yields:

$$\frac{C_2}{C_s} = \frac{V_1}{V_2}\left(\frac{M_o}{V_1 C_s} - 1\right) + \frac{V_1}{V_1 + V_2}\left(1 - \frac{V_1}{V_2}\left(\frac{M_o}{V_1 C_s} - 1\right)\right)$$
$$\times\left\{1 - \exp\left(-\frac{(V_1 + V_2)4\pi Dab}{V_1 V_2 K(a-b)}\right)(t-t_s)\right\} \quad (3\text{-}20)$$

The cumulative drug release at time t is [5]:

$$M_t = V_1 C_s\left[\left(\frac{M_o}{V_1 C_s} - 1\right) + \frac{1 - (V_1/V_2)\left(\frac{M_o}{V_1 C_s} - 1\right)}{1 + V_1/V_2}\right.$$
$$\left.\times\left\{1 - \exp\left(-\frac{(V_1 + V_2)4\pi Dab}{V_1 V_2 K(a-b)}(t-t_s)\right)\right\}\right] \quad (3\text{-}21)$$

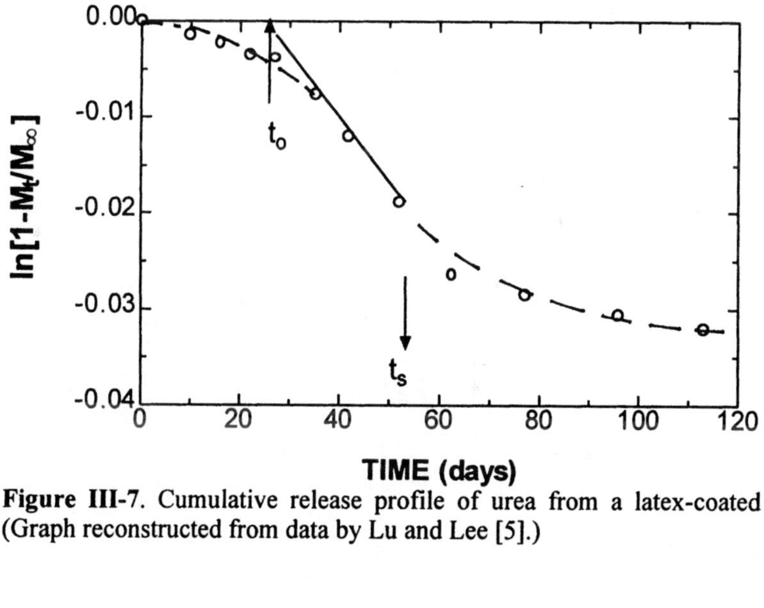

Figure III-7. Cumulative release profile of urea from a latex-coated ball. (Graph reconstructed from data by Lu and Lee [5].)

This approach can also be applied to other geometries to obtain the cumulative drug release, M_t.

Fig. III-7 shows the release of urea from latex film coated balls having diameters of 14.02 mm into a finite volume. The coating thickness was 0.434 mm. A time lag of 21 days was observed followed by a constant release up to t_s and then exponential release. The model and experimental data were in good agreement.

III.4. Unsteady-State Release from a Membrane-Reservoir System (Time Lag and Burst Effect)

The mathematical expressions presented so far are based on the pseudo-steady state approximation, which means that the concentration gradient across the membrane is expressed by Fick's first law, indicating a linear concentration gradient across the membrane. However, it takes some time for a freshly prepared membrane-reservoir system (where the membrane has no drug) to establish a linear gradient. Here we examine the release of a drug prior to reaching steady-state conditions. The concentration gradient across the membrane is shown in Fig. III-8 for a freshly made, or non-drug loaded, membrane. As time proceeds, the concentration gradient changes from the steepest gradient to an ultimately linear gradient. Therefore, Fick's second law of diffusion can be used to express the amount of drug diffused from the upstream to downstream sections of the slab membrane:

$$\frac{\partial C}{\partial t} = D \frac{\partial^2 C}{\partial x^2} \tag{3-22}$$

with initial and boundary conditions given by:

$$x = 0 \qquad\qquad\qquad C = C_1 \tag{3-23a}$$

$$x = l \qquad\qquad\qquad C = C_2 \tag{3-23b}$$

Equation (3-22) has been solved by Crank [6] and Lee [7]:

$$\frac{C}{C_s} = k\left(1 - \frac{x}{l}\right) - \frac{2kC_s}{\pi} \sum_{n=1}^{\infty} \frac{1}{n} \sin\left(\frac{n\pi x}{l}\right) e^{-n^2\pi^2 Dt/l^2} \tag{3-24a}$$

The total amount of drug that has diffused through the membrane into the sink in time t is obtained by integrating $-D\partial c/\partial x \big|_{x=l}$:

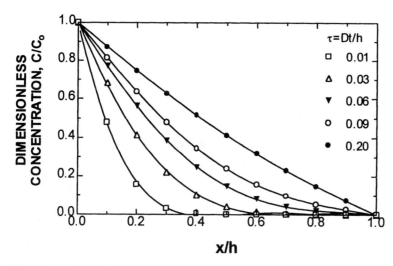

Figure III-8.   Drug concentration profiles vs. time in a membrane.

$$M_t = \frac{SDkC_1}{l}\left[t - \frac{l^2}{6D}\right] - \frac{2lSDkC_1}{\pi^2}\sum_{n=1}^{\infty}\frac{(-1)^n}{n^2}e^{-n^2\pi^2Dt/l^2} \qquad (3\text{-}24\text{b})$$

During storage time, the drug molecules migrate into the membrane. Drug that migrates into the membrane diffuses out first even before drug diffuses from the upstream to downstream sections. In this case, the drug release is faster than initially expected prior to reaching steady state conditions (burst effect). This situation can be described by [7]:

$$M_t = \frac{SDkC_1}{l}\left[t + \frac{l^2}{3D}\right] - \frac{2lSkC_1}{\pi^2}\sum_{n=1}^{\infty}\frac{(-1)^n}{n^2}e^{-n^2\pi^2Dt/l^2} \qquad (3\text{-}25)$$

As time goes to infinity (steady state), the amount of drug released at time t is given by:

$$M_t = \frac{SDkC_1}{l}\left[t - \frac{l^2}{6D}\right] \qquad (3\text{-}26\text{a})$$

for the freshly prepared membrane (time lag). Likewise for the stored membrane under steady state (burst effect) conditions drug release may expressed by:

$$M_t = \frac{SDkC_1}{l}\left[t + \frac{l^2}{3D}\right] \qquad\qquad (3\text{-}26b)$$

Fig. III-9 illustrates the plot of the amount of drug released versus time t for two cases: time lag and burst effect. For the time lag case, the time intercept is given by $l^2/6D$; whereas for the burst effect case the time intercept is given by $l^2/3D$. From the time intercept, one can determine the diffusion coefficient of a drug through the membrane from the reservoir. The analytical solutions for the other geometries (cylinder and sphere) are presented in Table III-3.

Equations (3-24) to (3-26b) may be normalized in order to evaluate permeation properties of different membranes with respect to the membrane thickness [8]:

$$\frac{M_t}{l} = SkC_1\left[\frac{Dt}{l^2} - \frac{1}{6}\right] - \frac{2SDkC_1}{\pi^2}\sum_{n=1}^{\infty}\frac{(-1)^n}{n^2}e^{-n^2\pi^2 Dt/l^2} \qquad (3\text{-}27a)$$

$$\frac{M_t}{l} = SkC_1\left[\frac{Dt}{l^2} + \frac{1}{3}\right] - \frac{2SkC_1}{\pi^2}\sum_{n=1}^{\infty}\frac{(-1)^n}{n^2}e^{-n^2\pi^2 Dt/l^2} \qquad (3\text{-}27b)$$

Under steady-state condition, equations (3-24c) and (3-25c) may be rewritten as:

Table III-3. Cumulative Release from Membrane-Reservoir Systems of Various Geometry.

	Time-lag	Burst-effect

Slab:
$$M_t = \frac{SDkC_1}{l}\left[t - \frac{l^2}{6D}\right] \qquad\qquad M_t = \frac{SDkC_1}{l}\left[t + \frac{l^2}{3D}\right]$$

Cylinder:
$$M_t = \frac{2\pi DkC_1}{\ln(b/a)}\left[t - \frac{a^2 - b^2 + (a^2 + b^2)\ln(b/a)}{4\ln(b/a)}\right]$$

$$M_t = \frac{2\pi DkC_1}{\ln(b/a)}\left[t + \frac{a^2 - b^2 + (a^2 + b^2)\ln(b/a)}{2\ln(b/a)}\right]$$

Sphere:
$$M_t = \frac{4\pi abDkC_1}{(b-a)}\left[t - \frac{(b-a)^2}{6D}\right] \qquad M_t = \frac{4\pi abDkC_1}{(b-a)}\left[t + \frac{b(b-a)^2}{3aD}\right]$$

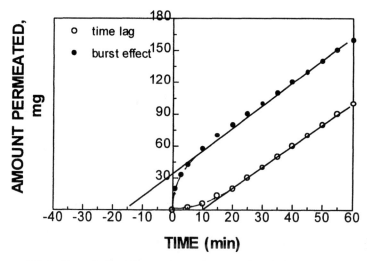

Figure III-9. Cumulative drug release from a membrane-reservoir system (time lag and burst effect).

$$\frac{M_t}{l} = SkC_1\left[\frac{Dt}{l^2} - \frac{1}{6}\right]$$

(3-27c)

$$\frac{M_t}{l} = SkC_1\left[\frac{Dt}{l^2} + \frac{1}{3}\right]$$

(3-27d)

respectively. As shown in Fig. III-10(a), the amount of drug permeated through a membrane is dependent on the thickness of the membrane. When normalized with respect to membrane thickness (M_t/l vs. t/l^2), the three data sets are superimposable, as illustrated in Fig. III-10(b).

In vitro permeation of scopolamine free base through various human skins was tested and the result is shown in Fig. III-11. The postauricular skin site is the most permeable, while the skin of the thigh is the least permeable. As illustrated in Fig. III-11, drug diffusion through skins yields a time lag, which is different from one skin to another. It takes about 10 hrs to reach the steady-state flux for most skins.

The actual release profile from membrane-controlled reservoir systems into a perfect sink is illustrated in Fig. III-12. The release profile exhibits three regions, in which each region accounts for a distinctive release mechanism for the diffusion of drug through the membrane. The first region is the representative release of the burst-effect or time lag. This is followed by the steady-state diffusion of the drug through the constant concentration gradient membrane in the second region. In the third region, a decrease in the

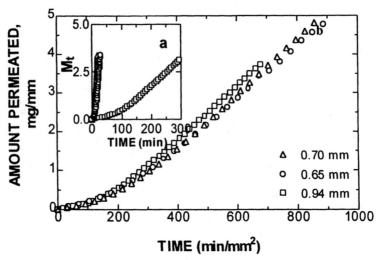

Figure III-10. Permeation of theophylline through poly(2-hydroxyethyl methacrylate) membranes: (a) M_t vs. t; (b) M_t/l vs. t/l^2.

release rate of the drug is observed. Equation (3-26) or (3-27), equation (3-7), and equation (3-13) express the release kinetics for the first, the second, and the third regions, respectively.

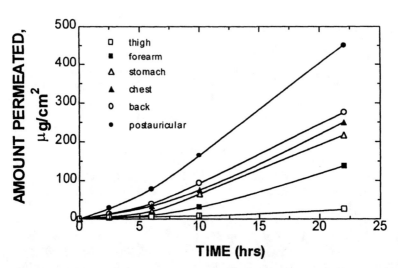

Figure III-11. In vitro permeation of scopolamine through human skins at 30°C. (Graph reconstructed from data by Shaw [9].)

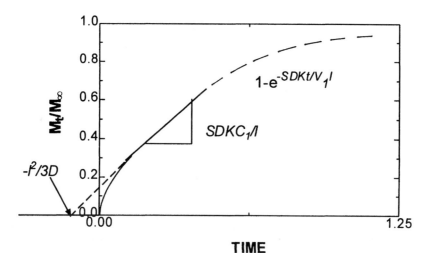

TIME

Figure III-12. Complete release profile from a membrane-reservoir system.

        Equation (3-24b) rapidly converges at long times to a straight line (steady-state establishment). However, if the diffusivity of a drug is very small and the membrane thickness is very large, it takes a long time to reach the steady- state conditions, often beyond the experimental time frame. Under these circumstances, Rogers et al. [10] and Short et al. [11] used another expression of unsteady-state permeation, which converges for short times. For small time values:

$$\ln\left(\frac{Q}{t^{1.5}}\right) = \ln\left(\frac{8C_oC_s}{\sqrt{\pi}L^2 S}\right) + \frac{3}{2}\ln D - \frac{L^2}{4Dt} \qquad (3\text{-}28)$$

where Q is the amount of drug that permeates through the membrane, S is the solubility of the drug in the solvent, C_s is the solubility of drug in the membrane, C_o is the drug concentration in the solvent, and l is the thickness of the membrane. By plotting $\ln(Q/t^{1.5})$ versus $1/t$, a straight line is obtained, as shown in Fig. III-13, and given by:

$$\text{slope} = -\frac{l}{4D} \qquad\qquad y\text{-intercept} = \frac{8C_oKD^{3/2}}{\sqrt{\pi}l^2} \qquad (3\text{-}29)$$

from which the diffusivity of the drug may be calculated. Both short-time and long-time approximations, equations (3-26) and (3-28), render a 15% error at 2.7 t_{lag} [11] corresponding to the onset point of equation (3-26).

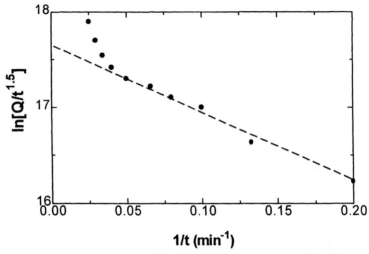

Figure III-13. Plot of $\ln(Q/t^{1.5})$ vs. $1/t$. (Graph reconstructed from data by Short et al. [11].)

If a membrane is placed in contact with a well-stirred solution in a diffusion cell, which has two equal volume compartments, equation (3-30) may be used to determine the diffusion coefficient of the drug [12]:

$$C_1(t) = \frac{C_\sigma}{2}\left(1 - \frac{\lambda}{2} + \frac{\lambda^2}{4} + \left(1 - \frac{\lambda}{6} + \frac{\lambda^2}{60}\right)\exp\left(\frac{-2\lambda Dt(1 - \frac{\lambda}{6} + \frac{\lambda^2}{65})}{l^2}\right)\right)$$

$$+ \sum_{n=1}^{\infty} \frac{4\lambda}{n^2\pi^2}\left(1 - \frac{6\lambda}{n^2\pi^2}\right)\exp\left(\frac{-Dt(n^2\pi^2 + 4\lambda)}{l^2}\right) \tag{3-30}$$

where C_σ is the initial concentration of drug in the upstream source, $C_1(t)$ is the concentration of the drug in the downstream source at time t, and l is the gel thickness.

Ocusert®: The device which is used as a classical example of a constant reservoir membrane system is the Ocusert® delivery system designed by Alza Corporation as shown in Fig. III-14. It consists of a pilocarpine-alginate reservoir core and two rate-controlling PE/VAc (top and bottom) membranes. Upon contact with water, water diffuses through the non-porous, low water permeable membrane and dissolves the drug in the reservoir core. The dissolved pilocarpine is delivered through the membrane at a nearly constant rate. The release rate remains reasonably constant over a week after an initial burst resulting from substantial migration of pilocarpine into the membrane during the storage period.

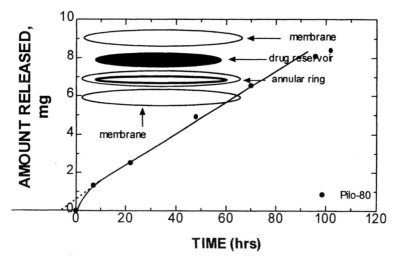

Figure III-14. Schematic diagram of Ocusert® (a) and a release profile of pilocarpine from the Ocusert® systems (b). (Graph reconstructed from data by Amaly and Rao [13].)

IUD: Like the Ocusert® system, the intrauterine therapeutic system (IUD) (contraceptive) was developed using a polymeric membrane that controls the release of drug (progesterone) to the uterus as shown in Fig. III-15. This device is prepared by cutting the downward arm of the T bar and inserting a cylindrical estradiol capsule. The capsule, filled with 6mg estradiol in cocoa butter, is made in polyurethane tubing (2.6 mm o.d. x 380 mm thickness). As shown in Fig. III-15, the drug release rate is constant over 300 days after an initial burst.

Transderm-NITRO®: Nitroglycerine impregnated in silicone ointment is sandwiched between an impermeable backing and a rate-controlling membrane, as illustrated in Fig. III-16. An adhesive is sprayed onto the membrane, allowing intimate contact with human skin. The release of nitroglycerine as represented in Fig. III-16 follows a dynamic release profile of a membrane reservoir system characterized by a burst effect. However, after approximately 15 hrs of release time, the release rate decreases because the drug's concentration within the reservoir falls below saturation.

Problem III-2: Hannoun and Stephanopoulos [16] studied the permeation of glucose in water through a calcium alginate membrane as shown in Fig. III-17. Calculate the diffusion coefficient and partition coefficient of glucose. The thickness of membrane is 0.4 cm. The surface area of the membrane is 0.37 cm². The solubility of glucose is 590 mg/cm³.

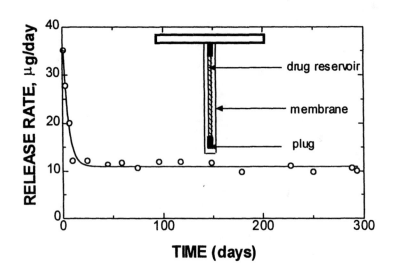

Figure III-15. Schematic diagram of an estradiol releasing IUD and a release rate profile of estradiol from the IUD. (Graph reconstructed from data by Chien [14].)

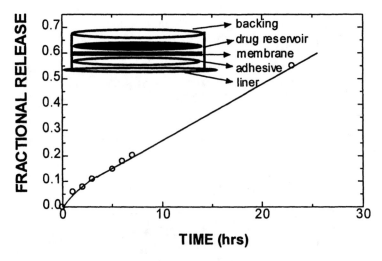

Figure III-16. Cross-sectional view of Transderm-Nitro and *in vitro* release profile from Transderm-Nitro. (Graph reconstructed from data by Shah et al. [15].)

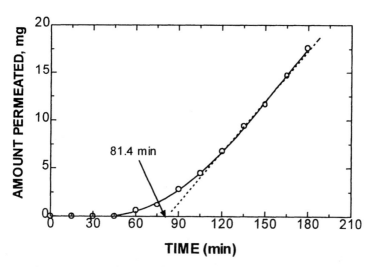

Figure III-17. Dynamic permeation of glucose through a calcium alginate membrane in water. (Graph reconstructed from data by Hannoun and Stephanopoulos [16].)

Solution: From the time-lag plot (Fig III-17),

$\qquad$ time-lag = 81.4 min, $D=(0.4)2/6/81.4/60=5.5 \times 10^{-6} cm^2/sec$

$\qquad$ slope = $SDKC_1/l$ = 0.176 mg/min

$\qquad$ $K = (0.176)(0.4)/0.37/590/(5.5 \times 10^{-6})/60 = 0.98$

Problem III-3: One of the transdermal patch manufacturers carried out in-vitro experiments of a transdermal nitroglycerin patch (Fig. III-18). Determine (a) the diffusion coefficient, (b) the partition coefficient, and (c) the solubility of nitroglycerin C_s. (Physical data given: surface area = 30 cm², thickness of membrane = 0.01 cm, volume of patch = 10 cm³).

Solution: 1). Burst effect
$$M_t = \frac{SDkC_s}{l}\left(t + \frac{l^2}{3D}\right)$$

$$t = -\frac{l^2}{3D} = -2.204 \ hr$$

$$D = 1.51 \times 10^{-5} \ cm^2/hr$$

2). $\qquad\qquad\qquad$ slope = 0.0555 mg/cm²hr

$\qquad\qquad\qquad\qquad$ KC_S = 36.8 mg/cm³

At 15 hrs, M_t = 0.95 mg/cm² x 10 cm² = 9.5 mg

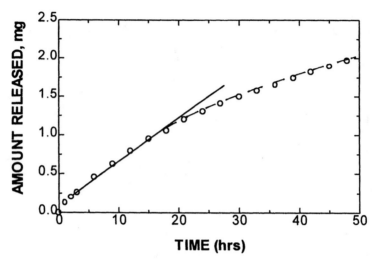

Figure III-18. *In vitro* cumulative release of nitroglycerin under sink conditions. (Graph reconstructed from data by Good [17].)

The total mass of drug loaded in the patch is 25 mg. After 15 hrs, the maximum amount of drug in the system is 25 mg − 9.5 mg = 15.5 mg, which is the new M_∞ in the reservoir. The transdermal patch follows non-constant reservoir release after 15 hrs,

$$\frac{M_t}{M_\infty} = 1 - e^{-\frac{SDkt}{V_1 l}}$$

Transformation of the above equation yields:

$$\ln\left(1 - \frac{M_t}{M_\infty}\right) = \frac{-SDk}{V_1 l} t$$

From the table below and graph, the slope $= -\dfrac{SDk}{V_1 l} = -0.0309$

$$k = \frac{0.0309 V_1 l}{SD} = 2.05$$
$$C_S = 36.8/k = 18.0 \text{ mg/cm}^3$$

t	M_t	new t	new M_t	$\ln(1-{}^{M_t}\!/\!_{M_\infty})$
15	9.5	0.0	0.0	0.0000
18	10.6	3	1.1	-0.0736
21	12.1	6	2.6	-0.1836
24	13.0	9	3.5	-0.2559
27	14.1	12	4.6	-0.3521
30	15.0	15	5.5	-0.4383
33	15.8	18	6.3	-0.5216
36	16.6	21	7.1	-0.6126
39	17.5	24	8.0	-0.7259
42	18.3	27	8.8	-0.8387
45	19.0	30	9.5	-0.9491
48	19.7	33	10.2	-1.0731

III.5. Drug Release from Multi-Layer Membrane Devices

Drug diffusion is applicable to certain situations through a multi-layer membrane. One may consider that a skin layer consists of two layers in which the thin stratum corneum is in contact with the thick viable epidermis. If drug release occurs through skin from a membrane-reservoir device, drug diffusion through the three membranes from a constant activity reservoir, as shown in Fig. III-20, can be expressed by equations (3-31a) to (3-32d):

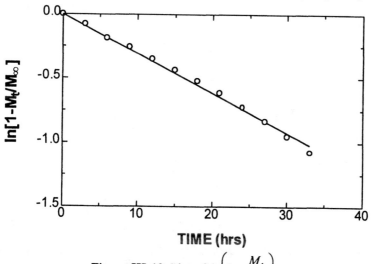

Figure III-19. Plot of $\ln\left(1-\dfrac{M_t}{M_\infty}\right)$ vs. t.

$$\frac{\partial C_1}{\partial t} = \frac{\partial^2 C_1}{\partial x^2}, \qquad -l_1 < x < 0 \qquad\qquad (3\text{-}31a)$$

$$\frac{\partial C_2}{\partial t} = \frac{\partial^2 C_2}{\partial x^2}, \qquad 0 < x < l_2 \qquad\qquad (3\text{-}31b)$$

$$\frac{\partial C_3}{\partial t} = \frac{\partial^2 C_3}{\partial x^2}, \qquad l_2 < x < l_3 \qquad\qquad (3\text{-}31c)$$

$$C_1 = C_2 = C_3 = 0, \qquad t = 0 \qquad\qquad (3\text{-}32a)$$

$$C_1 = C_o, C_3 = 0 \qquad t > 0 \qquad\qquad (3\text{-}32b)$$

$$D_1 \frac{\partial C_1}{\partial x} = D_2 \frac{\partial C_2}{\partial x}, D_2 \frac{\partial C_2}{\partial x} = D_3 \frac{\partial C_3}{\partial x}, \qquad x = 0 \qquad (3\text{-}32c)$$

$$K_2 C_1 = K_1 C_2, x = 0; \qquad , K_3 C_2 = K_2 C_3 \quad x = l_2 \qquad (3\text{-}32d)$$

Barrie et al. [18] solved the above equations by Laplace transforms to yield the time lag given by:

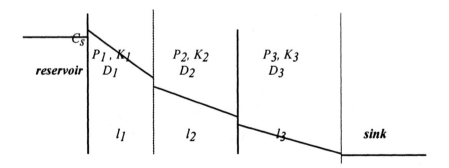

Figure III-20. Schematic diagram of a three-layer membrane reservoir system.

$$t_{lag,3} = \left(\frac{l_1}{D_1 K_1} + \frac{l_2}{D_2 K_2} + \frac{l_3}{D_3 K_3} \right)^{-1} \times \left[\frac{K_2 l_1 l_2 l_3}{D_1 D_3 K_1 K_3} + \frac{l_1^2}{D_1} \left(\frac{l_1}{6 D_1 K_1} + \frac{l_2}{2 D_2 K_2} + \frac{l_3}{2 D_3 K_3} \right) \right.$$

$$\left. + \frac{l_2^2}{D_2} \left(\frac{l_1}{2 D_1 K_1} + \frac{l_2}{6 D_2 K_2} + \frac{l_3}{2 D_3 K_3} \right) + \frac{l_3^2}{D_3} \left(\frac{l_1}{2 D_1 K_1} + \frac{l_2}{2 D_2 K_2} + \frac{l_3}{6 D_3 K_3} \right) - \right]$$

$$(3\text{-}33)$$

The time lag across the two-layer membrane is given by:

$$t_{lag,2} = \frac{\dfrac{l_1^2}{D_1} \left(\dfrac{l_1}{6 D_1 K_1} + \dfrac{l_2}{2 D_2 K_2} \right) + \dfrac{l_2^2}{D_2} \left(\dfrac{l_1}{2 D_1 K_1} + \dfrac{l_2}{6 D_2 K_2} \right)}{\dfrac{l_1}{D_1 K_1} + \dfrac{l_2}{D_2 K_2}} \qquad (3\text{-}34)$$

Permeability (P), lag time (τ) and mean residence time ($\bar{t}$) for a solute in membrane in series can be generalized as [19]:

$$\frac{1}{P} = \sum_{i=1}^{n} \frac{1}{P_i} \qquad (3\text{-}35a)$$

$$\tau = \sum_{i=1}^{n} \frac{\dfrac{1}{P_i} \left(\tau_i + \sum_{i=1}^{n-1} \bar{t}_{i+1} \right)}{\dfrac{1}{P_i}} \qquad (3\text{-}35b)$$

$$\bar{t} = \sum_{i=1}^{n} \bar{t}_i + \sum_{i=2}^{n} \frac{P_{i-1}}{P_i} 2 \bar{t}_{i-1} \qquad (3\text{-}35c)$$

where

$$P_i = \frac{K_i D_i}{l_i}, \qquad \tau_i = \frac{l_i^2}{6 D_i}, \qquad \bar{t}_i = \frac{l_i^2}{2 D_i} \qquad (3\text{-}35d)$$

Tojo et al. [20] used equation (3-34) to determine the drug diffusivity in intact skin and stripped skin. The steady-state rate of diffusion across the two-layer membrane was reported as:

$$\left(\frac{dM_t}{dt}\right)_2 = \frac{C_s}{\dfrac{l_1}{D_1 K_1} + \dfrac{l_2}{D_2 K_2}} = \frac{C_s}{\dfrac{l_2}{D_2 K_2}\left(\dfrac{1}{1-\eta}\right)} \tag{3-36}$$

where $\eta = (dM_t/dt)_2 /(dM_t/dt)_1$. The drug diffusivity in the second layer, D_2, is calculated by:

$$D_2 = \frac{1}{1-\eta}\left(\frac{l_2}{K_2 C_s}\right)\left(\frac{dM_t}{dt}\right)_2 = \frac{1}{1-\eta}\frac{l_2}{C_2}\left(\frac{dM_t}{dt}\right)_2 \tag{3-37a}$$

Combining equations (3-36) and (3-37a) and substituting the result into equation (3-34) yields:

$$t_{lag,2} = t_{lag,1}(3-2\eta) + \frac{h^2}{6}\frac{(1+2\eta)(2+2\eta)}{(dM_1/dM_2)_2} \tag{3-37b}$$

Then the drug solubility in the second layer is given by:

$$C_2 = \frac{(1-3\tau+2\eta\tau)}{(1+2\eta)(1-\eta)}\frac{6t_{lag,2}}{l_2}\left(\frac{dM_t}{dt}\right)_2 \tag{3-38}$$

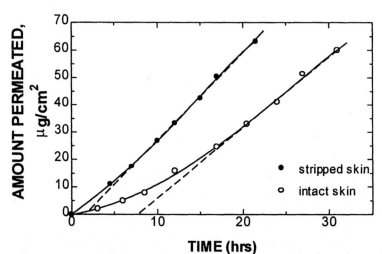

Figure III-21. Diffusion of progesterone through intact skin and stripped skin. (Graph reconstructed from data by Tojo et al. [20].)

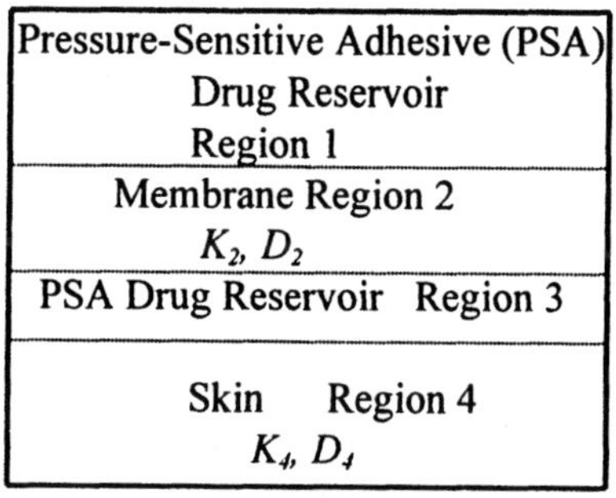

```
┌─────────────────────────────────────┐
│ Pressure-Sensitive Adhesive (PSA)   │
│         Drug Reservoir              │
│          Region 1                   │
├─────────────────────────────────────┤
│       Membrane Region 2             │
│          $K_2, D_2$                 │
├─────────────────────────────────────┤
│ PSA Drug Reservoir   Region 3       │
├─────────────────────────────────────┤
│                                     │
│       Skin     Region 4             │
│          $K_4, D_4$                 │
└─────────────────────────────────────┘
```

Figure III-22. Schematic diagram of a multi-laminate transdermal system. (Graph reconstructed from figure by Peterson et al. [21].)

where $\tau = t_{lag,1} / t_{lag,2}$ and $t_{lag,1} = l_1^2 / 6D_1$. Fig. III-21 shows drug diffusion kinetics of progesterone across intact skin and stripped skin. From Fig. III-21 the time lag and the drug release rate for intact skin and stripped skin can be obtained. The drug diffusivity and drug solubility are then calculated by using equations (3-37) and (3-38).

Peterson et al. [21] studied the release characteristics of a multi-laminate transdermal system as shown in Fig. III-22. The system consists of two drug reservoirs in an adhesive separated by a membrane. When applied to skin, the system becomes a reservoir-membrane-reservoir-membrane (skin) system. Under the pseudo-steady state assumption, the following equations [(3-39a) to (3-39c)] describe the permeation of drug through the skin:

$$L_1 \frac{dC_1}{dt} = -\frac{K_2 D_2 (C_1 - C_3)}{L_2} \tag{3-39a}$$

$$L_2 \frac{dC_3}{dt} = -L_1 \frac{dC_1}{dt} + D_4 \frac{\partial C_4}{\partial x}\bigg)_{x=0} \tag{3-39b}$$

$$C_4(x,t) = K_4 C_1(0) f_4(x,t) + \int_0^t f_4(x,\tau) K_4 \frac{\partial C_3(t-\tau)}{\partial t} d\tau \tag{3-39c}$$

where $f_4(x,t)$ is the solution to a unit step applied at $t = 0$ and $x = 0$.

The fractional release of drug through the skin is obtained by Laplace transform method as [21]:

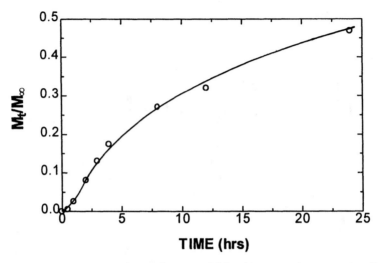

Figure III-23. Drug release from multi-laminate patch system. (Graph reconstructed from data by Peterson et al. [21].)

$$\frac{M_t}{M_\infty} = 1 - 2\sum_{n=1}^{\infty} \frac{\exp(-\frac{\beta_n^2 D_4 t}{L_4^2})\kappa(\frac{L_3}{L_1+L_3})(\xi_T - \beta_n^2)}{\cos\beta_n \left[\begin{array}{c}\kappa^2(\xi_3 - \beta_n^2)^2 + \kappa\{(\xi_T - \beta_n^2)(\beta_3 - \beta_n^2) + \\ 2\beta_n^2(\xi_T - \xi_3)\} + \beta_n^2(\beta_T - \beta_n^2)^2\end{array}\right]} \tag{3-40}$$

where $\xi_\tau = \frac{L_4^2}{D_4}\eta_\tau$, $\xi_3 = \frac{L_4^2}{D_4}\eta_3$, $\kappa = \frac{K_4 L_4}{L_3}$, $\eta_T = \frac{K_2 D_2(L_1 + L_3)}{L_1 L_2 L_3}$,

$\eta_3 = \frac{K_2 D_2 L_3}{L_1 L_2 L_3}$ and $\beta_n \tan(\beta_n)(\xi_\tau - \beta_n^2) = \kappa(\xi_3 - \beta_n^2)$. The error involved in

calculating the fractional release by using the first term (i.e. $n=1$) of equation (3-40) is small so that the equation can be simplified.

The time at which approximately 36.8% ($1/e$) of the initial drug amount remains in the system, T (i.e. "decay time"), can be estimated by the following approximation [21]:

$$T = L_1\left(\frac{1}{K_p(2)} + \frac{1}{K_p(4)}\right) + L_3\left(\frac{1}{K_p(4)}\right) \tag{3-41}$$

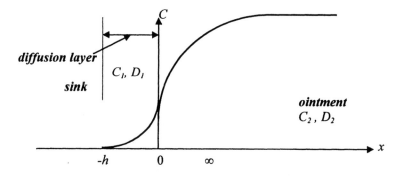

Figure III-24. Concentration profile in a matrix and a membrane.

where $K_p(2) = K_2 D_2 / L_2$ and $K_p(4) = K_4 D_4 / L_4$. Fig. III-23 shows the total drug diffusion through cadaver skin as a function of time along with the profile predicted by the simplified model ($n=1$).

III.6.   Drug Release from Membrane-Matrix Systems

III.6.1. *Dissolved drug*

Equations (3-27) and (3-28) and the equations presented in Table III-3 were derived for the case of constant drug concentration in the reservoir. However, a dosage form designer puts an additional coating onto the matrix to further control drug release. The above mentioned reservoir systems are not easy to fabricate when compared to the matrix systems. Fujiwara et al. [22] derived an explicit expression for the lag time of drug release through a membrane from a non-constant drug concentration in a matrix. The diffusion of a drug through the membrane from the matrix (*semi-infinite*), as illustrated in Fig. III-24, can be expressed by:

$$\frac{\partial C_1}{\partial t} = D_1 \frac{\partial^2 C_1}{\partial x^2}, \qquad -h < x < 0 \qquad (3\text{-}42)$$

$$\frac{\partial C_2}{\partial t} = D_2 \frac{\partial^2 C_2}{\partial x^2} \qquad 0 < x \qquad (3\text{-}43)$$

$$D_1 \frac{\partial C_1}{\partial x} = D_2 \frac{\partial C_2}{\partial x} \qquad x = 0 \qquad (3\text{-}44)$$

$$C_1 = 0 \qquad\qquad -h \le x < 0, \qquad t=0 \qquad\qquad (3\text{-}45a)$$

$$C_1 = C_o \qquad\qquad 0 \le x, \qquad\qquad t=0 \qquad\qquad (3\text{-}45b)$$

$$C_1 = KC_1 \qquad\qquad x = 0 \qquad\qquad\qquad (3\text{-}45c)$$

$$C_1 = 0 \qquad\qquad x = -h \qquad\qquad\qquad (3\text{-}45d)$$

where K is the partition coefficient of the drug at the interface between the membrane and the drug.

The following equations for drug concentrations in the vehicle and membrane can be given by [23]:

$$\frac{C_2}{C_s} = 1 - \frac{1}{1+\gamma} \sum_{n=1}^{\infty} \left(\frac{\gamma-1}{\gamma+1}\right)^n \left[erfc\left(2n + \frac{x/h}{\gamma K / 2\sqrt{\tau}} \right) + erfc\left(\frac{2n+2+x/h\big/_{\gamma K}}{2\sqrt{\tau}} \right) \right],$$
$$x > 0 \qquad (3\text{-}46)$$

$$\frac{C_1}{KC_o} = \left(\frac{\gamma}{\gamma+1}\right) \sum_{n=1}^{\infty} \left(\frac{\gamma-1}{\gamma+1}\right)^n \left[erf\left(\frac{2n+2+x/h}{2\sqrt{\tau}} \right) - erf\left(\frac{2n-x/h}{2\sqrt{\tau}} \right) \right], -h \le x \le 0$$
$$(3\text{-}47)$$

where $\tau = \dfrac{D_1 t}{h^2}$ and $\gamma = \dfrac{1}{K}\sqrt{\dfrac{D_2}{D_1}}$.

The cumulative amount of drug released from the system, M_t, can be expressed by [22,23]:

$$\frac{M_t}{S} = \frac{4C_o}{K+\sqrt{D_1/D_2}} \sqrt{\frac{D_1 t}{\pi}} \sum_{n=0}^{\infty} \left(\frac{K-\sqrt{D_1/D_2}}{K+\sqrt{D_1/D_2}} \right)^n \exp\left(-\frac{(2n+1)^2 h^2}{4D_1 t} \right)$$

$$- \frac{2C_o h}{K+\sqrt{D_1/D_2}} \sum_{n=0}^{\infty} \left(\frac{K-\sqrt{D_1/D_2}}{K+\sqrt{D_1/D_2}} \right)^n (2n+1)\, erfc\left(\frac{(2n+1)h}{2\sqrt{D_1 t}} \right) \quad (3\text{-}48)$$

For long times, equation (3-48) yields [22]:

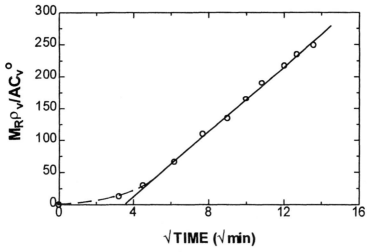

Figure III-25. Drug release from a membrane-matrix system. (Graph reconstructed from Parks et al. [23].)

$$M_t = 2C_o\sqrt{\frac{D_2 t}{\pi}} - \left(\frac{D_2}{D_1}\right)KC_o h = 2C_2^o S\sqrt{\frac{D_2}{\pi}}\left(\sqrt{t} - \frac{\gamma}{2}\sqrt{\frac{\pi h^2}{D_1}}\right) \quad (3\text{-}49)$$

The time lag for this system is given by:

$$t_{lag} = \left(\frac{D_2}{D_1}\right)^2 \frac{K^2 h^2 \pi}{4 D_2} \quad (3\text{-}50a)$$

$$slope = 2\sqrt{\frac{D_2}{\pi}} \quad (3\text{-}50b)$$

Fig. III-25 shows the permeation of ethyl salicylate from an unstirred 0.01% (w/w) Carbopol® gel vehicle through a silastic membrane. A time lag of 3.5 √min was observed. From the slope, one can determine the diffusion coefficient in the matrix. The diffusion coefficient of drug in the membrane can then be calculated from the time lag equation (3-50a) if K is known beforehand.

Guy and Hadgraft [24] and Addicts et al. [25] derived expressions for the percutaneous diffusion of a drug from an applied vehicle for a *finite* slab as shown in Fig. III-26. The diffusion equations and initial and boundary

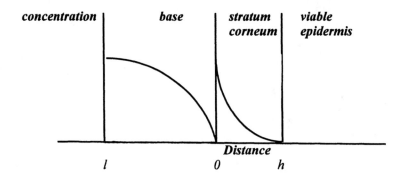

Figure III-26. Drug concentration of drug in matrix and membrane (a) and the effect of ointment base thickness on release profiles (b) [24].

conditions [(4-42) to (4-45d)] can be used except in the case of equations (3-43) and (3-45b) which are modified to:

$$\frac{\partial C_2}{\partial t} = D_2 \frac{\partial^2 C}{\partial x^2}, \qquad 0 < x < l \qquad (3\text{-}43a)$$

$$C_2 = C_o, \qquad 0 \le x \le l \qquad (3\text{-}45e)$$

respectively.

Taking Laplace transforms of equations (3-43) to (3-45e) and simplifying the resulting equations, Guy and Hadgraft [24] obtained the total amount of drug which diffuses through the membrane at time t:
for the short-time approximation [24]:

$$\frac{M_t}{M_\infty} = \frac{8\lambda p \tau^{3/2}}{(K + \lambda\sqrt{p})\sqrt{\pi}} \exp(-1/4\tau) \qquad (3\text{-}51)$$

where $K = \dfrac{C_{o,o}}{C_{s,o}}$, $\lambda = \dfrac{D_s l_o}{D_o l_s}$, $p = \dfrac{D_o l_s^2}{D_s l_o^2}$, and $\tau = \dfrac{D_s t}{l_s^2}$

and for the long-time approximation [24]:

$$\frac{M_t}{M_\infty} = 1 - \exp(-\lambda p \tau / K) \qquad (3\text{-}52)$$

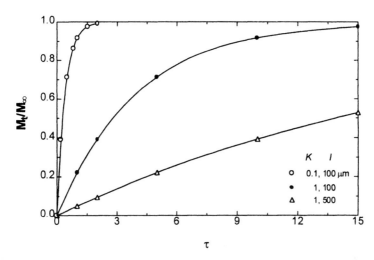

Figure III-27.   Drug release calculated by equation (3-52) with different K and base thickness values. (Graph reconstructed from data by Guy and Hadgraft [24].)

Fig. III-27 shows the effect of ointment base thickness on release profiles predicted by equation (3-52). The thickness of applied ointment base becomes important after the steady-state condition has been established.

III.6.2. *Dispersed drug*

The system described above is a membrane controlled matrix in which a drug is completely dissolved in a matrix material (dissolved state of drug). A rate-controlling membrane can be incorporated into dispersed drug matrices. Fig. III-28 shows a schematic diagram of a cylindrical coated matrix. At a given release time, t, a drug-depleted layer $r_o - r$ forms between the drug dissolution front and the outer membrane. For perfect sink conditions, the analysis of Roseman and Higuchi [26] for the boundary layer problem of dispersed monolithic matrices, can be adapted to this system.

The release rate of a drug under the pseudo-steady state approximation is given by:

$$\frac{dM_t}{dt} = -2\pi r D_e \frac{dC}{dr} \tag{3-56}$$

where r is the radius of the area under consideration and D_e is the diffusion coefficient of the drug. Integrating equation (3-56) yields:

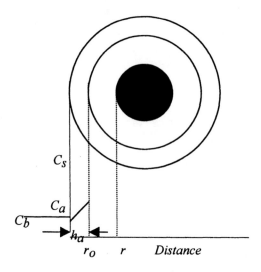

C_s

C_a

C_b

h_a

r_o r *Distance*

Figure III-28. Schematic diagram of a coated cylindrical matrix (dispersed drug).

$$\frac{dM_t}{dt} = -\frac{2\pi l D_e (C_o - C_s)}{\ln(r/r_o)} \qquad (3\text{-}57)$$

Assuming $C_b = 0$ (perfect sink), the rate of release through the membrane thickness, h_a, is given by:

$$\frac{dM_t}{dt} = \frac{2\pi l a_o D_a C_o}{h_a} \qquad (3\text{-}58)$$

where l and D_a are the length of the cylinder and the diffusivity of drug in the membrane, respectively. After rearranging equations (3-57) and (3-58) the drug release rate becomes:

$$\frac{dM_t}{dt} = \frac{2\pi l r_o K D_a}{h_a} \left(\frac{D_e C_s h_a}{- K D_a r_o \ln(r/r_o) + D_e h_a} \right) \qquad (3\text{-}59)$$

If drug loading is much higher than the drug's solubility ($A \gg C_s$), the release rate is given by:

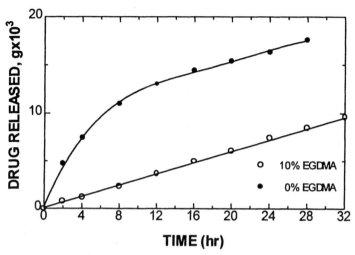

Figure III-29. The release of progesterone from membrane coated hydrogel cylinders. (Graph reconstructed from data by Lee et al. [27].)

$$\frac{dM_t}{dt} = -2\pi l r A \frac{dr}{dt} \tag{3-60}$$

Combining equations (3-59) and (3-60) and integrating the resulting equation yields:

$$\frac{r^2}{2}\ln\left(\frac{r}{r_o}\right) - \frac{1}{4}(r^2 - r_o^2) + \frac{D_e h_a}{2KD_a r_o}(r_o^2 - r^2) = \frac{C_s D_e t}{A} \tag{3-61}$$

The equations for other geometries (slab and sphere) can be obtained by a similar approach.

Fig. III-29 shows the release profiles of progesterone from membrane coated hydrogel cylinders. These devices were prepared by depleting the drug from the outer layer of the drug loaded hydrogel cylinder in alcohol and then soaking them in an ethanolic cross-linking [ethyleneglycol dimethacrylate (EGDMA)] solution. After drying, the device is exposed to UV light. As the amount of cross-linking agent is increased, the drug release slows down and follows a zero-order rate while that from a simple matrix follows first-order kinetics. If the membrane contains more than 10% EGDMA, the drug release is controlled primarily by the rate-controlling membrane with a negligible diffusion resistance in the matrix.

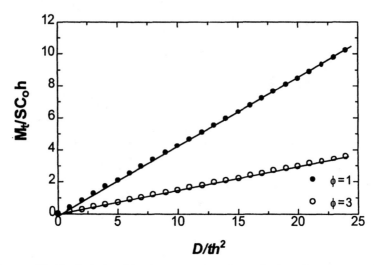

Figure III-30. Relationship between the dimensionless lag time and the dimensionless modulus.

III.7. Membrane Transport with Bioconversion

III.7.1. *Single layer systems*

If a drug is metabolized in a membrane (e.g. skin) while diffusing through it and the bioconversion is a first-order irreversible reaction, the following equation can be written for steady-state conditions:

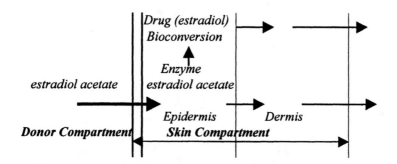

Figure III-31. Schematic illustration of the skin permeation/metabolism of estradiol prodrug [29].

$$\frac{\partial C}{\partial t} = D\frac{\partial^2 C}{\partial x^2} - kC \tag{3-62}$$

with the initial and boundary conditions:

$$C = C_o \qquad\qquad x = 0 \tag{3-63a}$$

$$C = 0 \qquad\qquad x = h \text{ and } t = 0 \tag{3-63b}$$

The solution of equation (3-62) can be found in Leypolt and Gogh [28] given by:

$$\frac{M_t}{SC_o h} = \frac{\phi}{\sinh(\phi)}\left(\frac{Dt}{h^2}\right) - 2\sum_{n=1}^{\infty}\frac{n^2\pi^2(-1)^{n+1}}{(n^2\pi^2 + \phi^2)^2}e^{-(n^2\pi^2+\phi^2)Dt\big/h^2} \tag{3-64}$$

The dimensionless time lag becomes:

$$\tau_{lag} = \frac{t_{lag}D}{h^2} = \frac{1}{2}\left[\frac{\coth(\phi)}{\phi} - \frac{1}{\phi^2}\right] \tag{3-65}$$

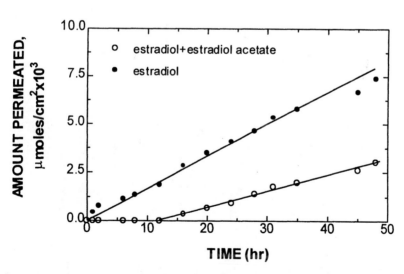

Figure III-32. Drug permeation profile of estradiol acetate (EA) and formation of estradiol (E) by metabolism in the skin. (Graph reconstructed from data by Tojo et al. [29].)

where DC_o/h is the steady-state flux through the membrane without metabolic reaction, ϕ is $h\sqrt{k/D}$, and η is $\phi/\sinh(\phi)$, a reduction factor due to the membrane metabolism.

Tojo et al. [29] investigated the dermal uptake and metabolism of an estradiol ester (Fig. III-31). The prodrug estradiol acetate is metabolized to estradiol in the epidermis during the transient diffusion as shown in Fig III-31.

The experimental and predicted amount of drug that permeates the skin at time t for EA $\rightarrow$ E in the skin is shown in Fig. III-32. The rate constant k for EA $\rightarrow$ E (first-order assumption) (0.51 hr^{-1}) and the diffusivity (2.06x10^{-8} cm^2/sec) were used in calculating the predicted values based on equation (3-64). The experimental data are well explained by the theoretical equation (3-64) during the early time of diffusion. A deviation occurs at later times possibly due to the decrease in enzyme activity caused by skin aging [29].

III.7.2. *Double layer systems*

The mathematical expressions for simultaneous diffusion and bioconversion of prodrug and the sequential enzyme reaction (prodrug $\rightarrow$ drug $\rightarrow$ metabolite), as shown in Fig. III-33, can be described by [30,31]:

$$D_p \frac{d^2 C_p}{dx^2} - k_1 C_p = 0 \tag{3-62a}$$

$$D_d \frac{d^2 C_d}{dx^2} + k_1 C_p - k_2 C_d = 0 \tag{3-67a}$$

$$D_m \frac{d^2 C_m}{dx^2} + k_2 C_d = 0 \tag{3-67b}$$

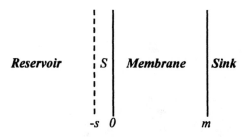

Figure III-33. Two-layer system with bioconversion.

where D_m is the diffusivity of metabolite, C_m is the concentration of metabolite, and k_2 is the bioconversion rate constant of drug to metabolite. The subscripts (p, d, and m) are the prodrug, drug, and metabolite, respectively. The subscripts (1 and 2) denote the bioconversion from the prodrug to drug and drug to metabolite, respectively. Here it is assumed that the diffusion of prodrug (and drug and metabolite) through the first membrane is expressed by Fick's first law and the diffusion through the second membrane is under steady-state conditions. The bioconversion by enzyme takes place only in the second membrane.
The boundary conditions are:

$$k'(C_{p(x=-s)} - C_{p(x=0)}) = -D_p \frac{dC_p}{dx}\bigg|_{x=0} \tag{3-68a}$$

where k' is the mass transfer coefficient.

$$D_d \frac{dC_d}{dx}\bigg|_{x=0} = 0 \tag{3-68b}$$

$$D_m \frac{dC_m}{dx}\bigg|_{x=0} = 0 \tag{3-68c}$$

$$C_{p(x=m)} = C_{d(x=m)} = C_{m(x=m)} = 0 \tag{3-68d}$$

The analytical solutions for equations (3-62a), (3-67a), and (3-67b) with respect to the concentration of prodrug, drug, and metabolite with these boundary conditions are given by [30,31]:

$$C_p = -\psi \sinh K_1(m-x) \tag{3-69a}$$

$$C_d = \varepsilon \sinh K_2(m-x) + \left(\frac{\psi}{K_1^2 - K_2^2}\right)\left(\frac{k_1}{D_d}\right)(\sinh K_1(m-x)) \tag{3-69b}$$

$$C_m = \left(\frac{k_2}{D_m}\right)\left[\frac{\varepsilon}{K_2}\cosh K_2 m + \left(\frac{\psi}{(K_1^2 - K_2^2)K_1}\right)\left(\frac{k_1}{D_d}\right)\cosh K_1 m\right](m-x)$$
$$-\frac{k_2}{D_m}\left[\frac{\varepsilon}{K_2^2}\sinh K_2(m-x) + \frac{\psi}{(K_1^2 - K_2^2)K_1^2}\left(\frac{k_1}{D_d}\right)\sinh K_1(m-x)\right] \tag{3-69c}$$

where $\quad K_2 = \sqrt{k_2 / D_d}$ $\qquad\qquad$ (3-70a)

$$\psi = \frac{-C_{p(x=-s)}k'}{D_p K_1 \cosh K_1 m + k'\sinh K_1 m} \qquad\qquad (3\text{-}70b)$$

$$\varepsilon = \left(\frac{-\psi K_1}{(K_1^2 - K_2^2)K_2}\right)\left(\frac{k_1}{D_d}\right)\left(\frac{\cosh K_1 m}{\cosh K_2 m}\right) \qquad\qquad (3\text{-}70c)$$

References

1. A. S. Michael, P. S. L. Wong, R. Prather, and R. M. Gale, "A Thermodynamic Method of Predicting the Transport of Steroids in Polymer Matrices," *AIChEJ*, 21, 1073 (1975).

2. G. Kallstrand and B. Ekmano, "Membrane Coated Tablets: A System for the Controlled Release of Drugs," *J. Pharm. Sci.*, 72, 772 (1983).

3. K. L. Smith, R. W. Baker, and Y. Ninomiya, "Development of BioLure Controlled Release Pheromone Products," in Controlled Delivery Systems, T. J. Roseman and S. C. Mansdorf (Eds.), Marcel Dekker, New York, 1983, p325.

4. S. Watano, H. Takaya, I. Wada, and K. Miyanami, "Modeling Drug Release from Granules Coated with an Aqueous Based System of Acrylate Membrane: Effect of Moisture Content on the Kinetics of Drug Release," *Chem. Pharm. Bull.*, 42, 238 (1994).

5. S. M. Lu and S. F. Lee, "Slow Release of Urea through Latex Film," *J. Control. Rel.*, 18, 171 (1992).

6. J. Crank, The Mathematics of Diffusion, 2nd Ed., Clarendon Press, Oxford, 1975.

7. W. R. Good and P. I. Lee, "Membrane-Controlled Reservoir Drug Delivery Systems," in Medical Applications of Controlled Release, Vol. I, R. S. Langer and D. L. Wise (Eds.), CRC Press, Baton Rouge, Fl, 1984, p1.

8. M. Bari and C. J. Kim, Unpublished data.

9. J. Shaw, "Development of Transdermal Therapeutic Systems," *Drug Dev. Ind. Pharm.*, 9, 959 (1983).

10. W. A. Rogers, R. S. Buritz, and D. Alpert, *J. Appl. Phys.*, 25, 868 (1954).

11. P. M. Short, E. T. Abbs, and C. T. Rhodes, "Effect of Nonionic Surfactants on the Transport of Testosterone across a Cellulose Acetate Membrane," *J. Pharm. Sci.*, 59, 995 (1970).

12. C. Barnes, *Physics*, 5, 4 (1934).

13. M. F. Armaly and K. R. Rao, *Invest. Ophthamol.*, 12, 491 (1973).

14. Y. W. Chien, Novel Drug Delivery Systems, 2nd Ed., Marcel Dekker, New York, 1992, p622.

15. V. P. Shah, N. W. Tymes, and J. P. Skelly, "Comparative In-Vitro Release Profiles of Marketed Nitroglycerin Patches by Different Dissolution Methods," *J. Control. Rel.*, 7, 79 (1988).
16. B. J. M. Hannoun and G. Stephanopoulos, "Diffusion Coefficients of Glucose and Ethanol in Cell-Free and Cell-Occupied Calcium Alginate Membranes," *Biotech. Bioeng.*, 28, 829 (1986).
17. W. R. Good, "Transderm-Nitro® Controlled Delivery of Nitroglycerin via the Transdermal Route," *Drug Dev. Ind. Pharm.*, 9, 647 (1983).
18. J. A. Barrie, J. D. Levine, A. S. Michaels, and P. Wang, "Diffusion and Solution of Gases in Composite Rubber Membranes," *Trans. Faraday Soc.*, 59, 869 (1963).
19. R. A. Siegal, "Permeation, Lag Times and Solute Consupmtion by Membranes in Series," *Proceed. Int. Symp. Control. Re. Bioact. Mater.*, 17, 75 (1990).
20. K. Tojo, C. C. Chiang, and Y. W. Chien, "Drug Permeation across the Skin: Effect of Penetrant Hydrophilicity," *J. Pharm. Sci.*, 76, 123 (1987).
21. T. A. Peterson, J. C. Hedenstrom, S. J. Dreyer, and J. C. Keister, "A Mathematical Model for the Skin Penetration Characteristics of a Multilaminate TDD Patch," *Pharm. Res.*, S-158 (1995).
22. K. Fujwara, M. Ueda, and T. Koizumi, "Lag Time Involved in the Experiments on the Drug Release from Ointments," *Chem. Pharm. Bull.*, 23, 3286 (1975).
23. J. M. Parks, R. L. Cleek, and A. L. Bunge, "Chemical Release from Topical Formulations across Synthetic Membranes: Infinite Dose," *J. Pharm. Sci.*, 86, 187 (1997).
24. R. H. Guy and J. Hadgraft, "A Theoretical Description Relating Skin Penetration to the Thickness of the Applied Medicament," *Int. J. Pharm.*, 6, 321 (1980).
25. W. J. Addicts, G. Flynn, N. Weiner, and R. Curl, "A Mathematical Model to Describe Drug Release from Thin Topical Applications," *Int. J. Pharm.*, 56, 243 (1989).
26. T. J. Roseman and W. I. Higuchi, "Release of Mrdroxyprogesterone Acetate from a Silicone Matrix," *J. Pharm. Sci.*, 59, 353 (1970).
27. E. S. Lee, S. W. Kim, S. H. Kim, J. R. Cardinal, and H. Jacobs, "Drug Release from Hydrogel Devices with Rate Controlling Barriers," *J. Membr. Sci.*, 7, 293 (1980).
28. J. K. Leypoldt and D. A. Gough, "Comments on the Penetrant Time Lag in a Diffusion-Reaction Systems," *J Phys. Chem.*, 84, 1058 (1980).
29. K. Tojo, K. H. Valia, G. Chotani, and Y. W. Chien, "Long Term Permeation Kinetics of Estradiol: (IV) A Theoretical Approach to the Simultaneous Skin Permeation and Bioconversion of Estradiol Esters," *Drug. Dev. Ind. Pharm.*, 11, 1175 (1985).
30. C. D. Yu, J. L. Fox, N. F. H. Ho, and W. I. Higuchi, "Physical Model Evaluation of Topical Prodrug Delivery–Simultaneous Transport and Bioconversion of Vidarabine-5'-Valerate II: Parameter Determinations," *J. Pharm. Sci.*, 68, 1347 (1979).

31. C. D. Yu, J. L. Fox, N. F. H. Ho, and W. I. Higuchi, "Physical Model Evaluation of Topical Prodrug Delivery–Simultaneous Transport and Bioconversion of Vidarabine-5'-Valerate I: Physical Model Development," *J. Pharm. Sci.*, 68, 1341 (1979)

Chapter IV

Swelling Controlled Systems

IV.1. Mathematical Expressions

IV.1.1. *Solvent diffusion*

The theoretical discussions of the previous chapters are based on Fick's first and second laws of diffusion. Fickian diffusion applies to rubbery polymers, which easily adapt to changes in their surrounding environment. For example, when rubbery polymers are immersed in swelling solvent and the temperature is raised, they respond rapidly to the temperature change to reach a new equilibrium condition. In this case the Fickian equation describes the diffusion of penetrant well. However, glassy polymers do not respond to their new environment as rapidly as rubbery polymers and their response is time-dependent. When glassy polymers come in contact with a solvent, they slowly react to their new environment with slow rearrangement of their polymer chains (polymer relaxation). In this case the relative magnitude of the diffusion of solvent and polymer relaxation determine the diffusional transport process [1]:

Case I (Fickian): the transport of molecules in the polymer matrix is dominated by the Fickian diffusion mechanism with negligible polymer relaxation.

Case II: the polymer relaxation predominantly controls the movement of molecules with negligible diffusion of the molecules.

Non-Fickian: both the diffusion process and polymer relaxation control (Anomalous) the transport of molecules.

In particular, when the polymer is highly swellable, the transport of molecules deviates from the Fickian diffusion mechanism. Upon contact with solvent, the glassy polymer' glass transition temperature is lowered below the experimental temperature and they revert to the rubbery gel state [2]. The concentration distribution of penetrant in the rubbery gel layer is dependent upon the activity of solvent in the surrounding environment. Fig. IV-1 shows the diffusion of a methanol molecule in poly(methyl methacrylate) beads. Optical observation reveals that a steady increase in the activity of solvent furnishes a constant concentration distribution across the gel layer. At the interface between the rubbery gel layer and unswollen glassy polymer, a steep concentration gradient is observed, as shown in Fig. IV-2.

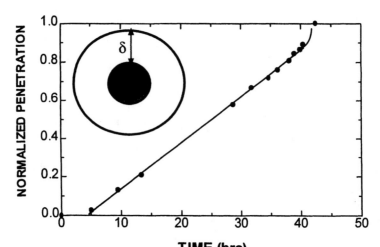

Figure IV-1. The penetration of methanol into a poly(methyl methacrylate) bead at 25°C. (Graph reconstructed from data by Lee and Kim [3].)

Case I diffusion has been discussed in the previous sections. In this section Case II will be studied. In this situation the diffusion process of solvent through the pre-swollen gel layer is rapid and negligible in the overall transport compared with swelling-induced polymer relaxation. For a slab, if the moving boundary front between the glassy core and the swollen gel layer advances with a constant velocity, the weight gain of solvent is proportional to time. When this takes place (rapid diffusion of penetrant and slow relaxation of polymer), the diffusion of a drug trapped in the matrix is relatively rapid. A constant release rate is obtained, which is governed by constant absorption rate of the penetrating solvent and the constant rate of polymer relaxation. This situation is similar to drug delivery systems controlled by polymer erosion (see Chapter V). The fractional amount of

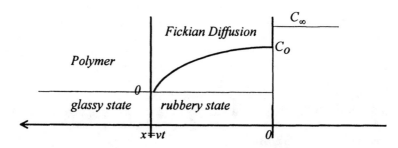

Figure IV-2. Concentration profile for Case II sorption [4].

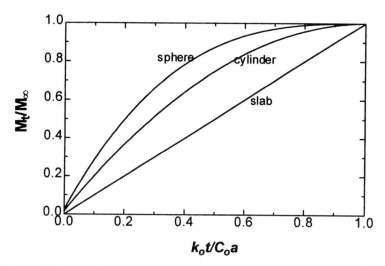

Figure IV-3. Fractional release for Case II transport in slabs, cylinders, and spheres.

molecules absorbed and de-sorbed can be expressed by:

$$\frac{M_t}{M_\infty} = 1 - \left[1 - \frac{k_o t}{C_o a}\right]^n \tag{4-1}$$

where k_o is the polymer relaxation constant, C_o is the equilibrium concentration of penetrant in the polymer matrix, a is the radius of the sphere (or cylinder or the half-thickness of a slab), and n is the geometry factor (for a slab, $n=1$, for a cylinder $n=2$, for a sphere $n=3$). Release profiles describing Case II kinetics in slabs, cylinders, and spheres are shown in Fig. IV-3. If swelling-induced relaxation controls the absorption of the penetrant, a constant relaxation rate results in a constant absorption rate for the slab geometry. In Fig. IV-4 dye from the polystyrene film is released in n-hexane at a constant rate. Under the same conditions, however, absorption of penetrant in a cylinder or sphere results in a continuous decrease in the absorption rate due to the continuous decrease in the area at the moving front separating the swollen and glassy polymer. This suggests that the constant rate of absorption of n-hexane controls the release of the dye in the slab geometry.

Both Case I and Case II are extreme cases describing the transport of molecules in a polymer matrix. When penetrant diffusion and polymer relaxation due to swelling both control drug release, anomalous diffusion

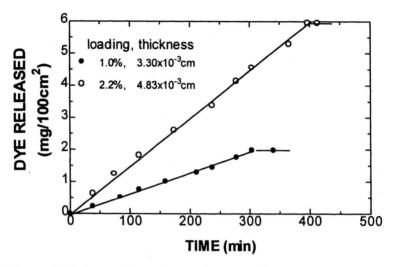

Figure IV-4. Dye release from polystyrene films in n-hexane. (Graph reconstructed from data by Hophenberg and Hsu [5].)

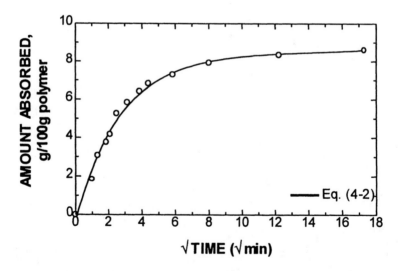

Figure IV-5. n-Hexane absorption in polystyrene microspheres and the coupled diffusion/relaxation model. (Graph reconstructed from data by Hopfenberg [4].)

results. A proposed model, which combines Fickian diffusion with a first-order relaxation process, is described by [4]:

$$\frac{M_t}{M_\infty} = 1 - \phi_F \left[\frac{6}{\pi^2} \sum_{n=1}^{\infty} \frac{1}{n^2} e^{-n^2 \pi^2 Dt/l^2} \right] + \phi_R e^{-kt} \tag{4-2a}$$

$$\phi_F + \phi_R = 1 \tag{4-3}$$

where ϕ_F and ϕ_R are the fractions contributed by diffusion and relaxation, respectively. Hopfenberg [5] reported that there is a critical sample dimension above which Case II kinetics do not occur. After initial Case II penetration, diffusional resistance develops in the swollen gel layer as the swollen gel shell becomes thicker. Fig. IV-5 shows experimental data and the diffusion-relaxation model [equation (4-2)]. Fickian diffusion or Case II kinetics individually cannot accurately predict experimental data.

The above approach can be applied to release kinetics of tablet matrices for moderately swelling systems. Drug release from the tablet by drug diffusion and polymer relaxation may be described by equations (4-2b) and (4-2c) for short time and long time approximations, respectively [6]:

$$\frac{M_t}{M_\infty} = 1 + \phi_R \left[\left(1 - \frac{kt}{a} \right)^2 \left(1 - \frac{2kt}{b} \right) \right]$$

$$- \phi_F \left\{ 4\sqrt{\frac{\tau_a}{\pi}} - \pi\tau - \frac{\pi}{3}\tau^{3/2} + 4\sqrt{\frac{\tau_b}{\pi}} - \frac{2a}{b} \left[8\frac{\tau_a}{\pi} - 2\pi\tau^{3/2} - \frac{2\pi}{3}\tau_a^2 \right] \right\} \tag{4-2b}$$

$$\frac{M_t}{M_\infty} = 1 - \phi_F \frac{32}{(2.4048)^2 \pi^2} e^{-D(\alpha_1^2 + \beta_0^2)t} + \phi_R \left(1 - \frac{kt}{a} \right)^2 \left(1 - \frac{2kt}{b} \right) \tag{4-2c}$$

where $\quad \tau_a = \dfrac{Dt}{a^2}, \tau_a = \dfrac{Dt}{b^2}, \alpha_1 = \dfrac{2.4048}{a}, \quad \beta_0 = \dfrac{\pi}{2b}$

and a and b are the radius and thickness of the tablet, respectively.

Neogi [7] derived an analytical expression for the non-Fickian absorption of vapors in polymeric membranes. A time and memory dependent diffusion coefficient together with a time-dependent solubility is applied to obtain the solution:

$$D(t) = D_i + \beta(D_o - D_i)e^{-\beta t} \tag{4-4}$$

$$C(t) = C_i + (C_f - C_i)(1 - e^{-\beta t}) \tag{4-5}$$

where β is the polymer relaxation constant, D_i the initial diffusivity, D_f the final diffusivity, C_i the initial concentration, and C_f the final concentration.

Depending upon the relative contributions of penetrant diffusion and polymer relaxation, solutions for the fractional absorption in a slab are given for the following cases:

(1) when $\beta = \infty$:

$$\frac{M_t}{M_\infty} = 1 - \frac{8}{\pi^2} \sum_{k=1}^{\infty} \frac{e^{-(2k+1)^2 \pi^2 D_o t / l^2}}{(2k+1)^2} \tag{4-6}$$

(2) when the relaxation time is not very small:

$$\frac{M_t}{M_\infty} = 1 - e^{-\beta t} - \frac{8}{\pi^2} \sum_{k=1}^{\infty} \frac{e^{-\frac{(2k+1)^2 \pi^2 D_o t / l^2}{1+(2k+1)^2 \pi^2 D_i / \beta l^2}}}{\left[1 - \frac{(2k+1)^2 \pi^2 (D_o - D_i)}{\beta l^2}\right](2k+1)^2} \tag{4-7}$$

(3) when the relaxation time is very large (i.e. $\beta = 0$):

$$\frac{M_t}{M_\infty} = 1 - \frac{8}{\pi^2} \sum_{k=1}^{\infty} \frac{e^{-(2k+1)^2 \pi^2 D_i t / l^2}}{(2k+1)^2} \tag{4-8}$$

(4) when the relaxation time is large (β is small) and D_i is negligible:

$$\frac{M_t}{M_\infty} = \frac{2\sqrt{\beta D_o}}{l} \qquad t < \frac{l}{2\sqrt{\beta D_o}} \tag{4-8a}$$

$$\frac{M_t}{M_\infty} = 1 \qquad t \geq \frac{l}{2\sqrt{\beta D_o}} \tag{4-8b}$$

IV.1.2. *Swollen gel thickness*

Lee and Lee [8] solved Fick's second law for the penetration of solvent into a polymer to predict the swollen rubbery gel layer thickness to be:

$$\frac{\partial C}{\partial t} = D \frac{\partial^2 C}{\partial x^2} \tag{4-9}$$

The boundary conditions are given by:

$$C = \overline{C}_d \qquad x = 0 \qquad t > 0 \tag{4-10a}$$

$$C = \overline{C}^* \qquad x = \delta(t) \tag{4-10b}$$

$$\overline{C}^* \overline{C}_d \frac{\partial \delta}{\partial t} = -D \left(\overline{C}_d \frac{\partial C}{\partial x}\Big|_{x=\delta} + \overline{C}^* \frac{\partial C}{\partial x}\Big|_{x=0} \right) \tag{4-10c}$$

where C is the penetrant volume fraction, C^* is the threshold solvent volume fraction at which a glassy polymer becomes rubbery, and C_d is the solvent volume fraction for polymer disentanglement, and $\delta(t)$ is the swollen gel thickness having a general form of [9]:

$$\frac{d\delta(t)}{dt} = K(\overline{C}_d - \overline{C}^*)^n \tag{4-11}$$

where K and n are constants.

The concentration profile of the penetrant and the thickness of the swollen gel layer [$\delta(t)$] can be obtained from equations (4-12) and (4-13):

$$\frac{C - \overline{C}^*}{\overline{C}_d - \overline{C}^*} = 1 - \frac{erf(\xi / 2\sqrt{\tau})}{erf(m)} \tag{4-12}$$

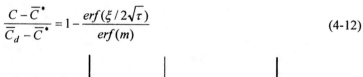

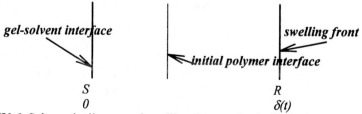

Figure IV-6. Schematic diagram of swelling front and gel-solvent interface.

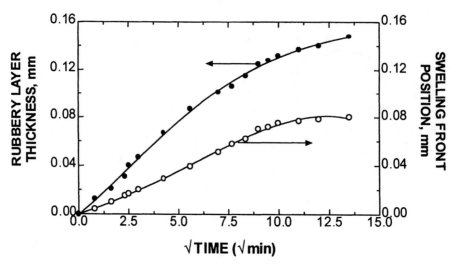

Figure IV-7. Moving boundaries of gel layer thickness and swelling front. (Graph reconstructed from data by Lee and Lee [8].)

$$\frac{\delta(t)K(\overline{C}_d - \overline{C}^*)^n}{D} = 2m\sqrt{\tau} \tag{4-13}$$

where

$$\xi = \frac{xK(\overline{C}_d - \overline{C}^*)^n}{D}, \qquad \tau = \frac{tK^2(\overline{C}_d - \overline{C}^*)^{2n}}{D}, \qquad \delta(t) = S(t) - R(t)$$

And m is subject to the following equation:

$$e^{m^2}\left[\sqrt{\pi}\,merf(m) - \frac{\overline{C}_d - \overline{C}^*}{\overline{C}_d}\right] = \frac{\overline{C}_d - \overline{C}^*}{\overline{C}^*} \tag{4-14}$$

Fig. IV-7 shows the experimental and predicted gel thickness of a polyimide film in N-methyl pyrrolidone with a swelling front position.

Koizumi et al. [10] presented mathematical expressions to estimate the maximum swelling parameter and the diffusivity of a solvent for long time and short time values. Fig. V-8 shows a schematic presentation of dimensional changes of a polymer during swelling. Equations (4-15) and (4-16) describe the thickness of the polymer matrix during swelling as:

$$dx = \frac{dx_o}{1 - \nu C} \tag{4-15}$$

$$\Delta H = H - H_o = \int_0^{H_o} dx - \int_0^{H_o} dx_o = \int_0^{H_o} \frac{vC}{1 - vC} dx_o = (H_\infty - H_o)(1 - e^{-kt}) \ (4\text{-}16)$$

where C is the water concentration in the film (relative to the equilibrium concentration), v is a parameter governed by the maximum swelling thickness, H is the thickness of swelling film, H_o is the initial thickness of dry film, and k is the first-order swelling rate constant.

For large values of time t, the concentration of the solvent is given by:

$$C = 1 - \frac{4}{\pi} \cos\left(\frac{\pi x_o}{2H_o}\right) \exp\left(-\frac{\pi^2 Dt}{4H_o^2 \tau_o}\right) \tag{4-17}$$

where τ_o is the tortuosity of the dry matrix and is assumed to decrease with the progress of swelling as:

$$\tau = (1 - vC)^2 \tau_o \tag{4-18}$$

$$\tau dx^2 = \tau_o dx_o^2 \tag{4-19}$$

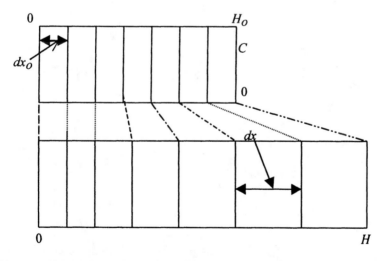

Figure IV-8. Schematic representation of the swelling model. (Graph adapted from figure by Koizumi et al. [10].)

Substituting equation (4-17) into (4-16) and integrating the resulting equation gives [10]:

$$\Delta H = \frac{vH_o}{1-v}\left[1 - \frac{8}{(1-v)\pi^2}\exp\left(-\frac{\pi^2 Dt}{4H_o^2\tau_o}\right)\right] \tag{4-20}$$

For short value of time, t, assuming diffusion in a semi-infinite medium, the concentration of solvent is given by:

$$C = 1 - erf\left(\frac{H_o - x_o}{2\sqrt{Dt/\tau_o}}\right) \cong 1 - \tanh\left(\frac{H_o - x_o}{\sqrt{\pi Dt/\tau_o}}\right) \tag{4-21}$$

Substituting equations (4-21) into (4-16) and integrating yields [10]:

$$\Delta H = \frac{v\log(2-2v)}{1-2v}\sqrt{\pi Dt/\tau_o} \tag{4-22}$$

Fig. IV-9 compares observed swelling profiles of hydroxypropyl cellulose film with the simulated values of equations (4-20) and (4-22).

IV.1.3. *Drug release*

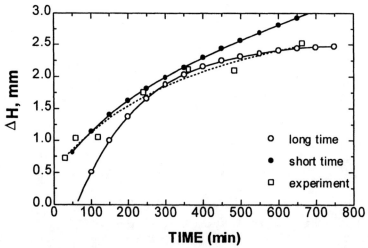

Figure IV-9. Swelling of HPC140-IM matrix. (Graph reconstructed from data by Koizumi et al. [10].)

Lee [11] used a time-dependent diffusion coefficient description of drug release from a hydrogel system similar to equation (4-4). The time-dependent diffusion coefficient is defined as:

$$D(t) = D_i + (D_\infty - D_i)(1 - e^{-kt}) \tag{4-23}$$

where D_∞ and k are the diffusion coefficient of drug and polymer relaxation constant, respectively.

Substituting $D(t)$ into equation (2-1) for the dissolved drug concentration, equation (2-87) for the dispersed drug, and redefining the time variable yields:

$$dT = D(t)dt \tag{4-24}$$

where

$$T = D_\infty \left[t - (1 - \frac{D_i}{D_\infty}) \frac{1}{k} (1 - e^{-kt}) \right] \tag{4-25}$$

Then the unsteady-state diffusion equation is identical to the original equation except for the time variable (T). The exact solutions for the swellable system of dissolved drug and dispersed drug can be expressed by replacing τ ($D_\infty t / a^2$) in equations (2-13a) and (2-104) with the following expression (4-26):

$$\tau - \left\{ (1 - \frac{D_i}{D_\infty}) \frac{D_\infty}{kl^2} \left[1 - e^{-kl^2 \tau / D_\infty} \right] \right\} \tag{4-26}$$

For example, the fraction of dissolved drug in spherical geometry is given by:

$$\frac{M_t}{M_\infty} = 1 - \sum_{n=1}^{\infty} \frac{6}{n^2 \pi^2} \exp\{-n^2 \pi^2 \{\tau - (1 - \frac{D_i}{D_\infty}) \frac{D_\infty}{ka^2} [1 - \exp(-\frac{ka^2}{D_\infty} \tau)]\} \tag{4-27}$$

For short times:

$$\frac{M_t}{M_\infty} = 6 \left(\frac{1}{\pi^2} \left\{ \tau - (1 - \frac{D_i}{D_\infty}) \frac{D_\infty}{ka^2} \left[1 - \exp\left(-\frac{ka^2}{D_\infty} \tau \right) \right] \right\} \right)^{1/2}$$
$$- 3 \left\{ \tau - (1 - \frac{D_i}{D_\infty}) \frac{D_\infty}{ka^2} \left[1 - \exp\left(-\frac{ka^2}{D_\infty} \tau \right) \right] \right\} \tag{4-28}$$

For long times:

$$\frac{M_t}{M_\infty} = 1 - \frac{6}{\pi^2}\left\{\tau - (1 - \frac{D_i}{D_\infty})\frac{D_\infty}{kl^2}[1 - \exp(-\frac{kl^2}{D_\infty}\tau)]\right\} \tag{4-29}$$

For a dispersed drug, M_t is the same as equation (2-103). However, equation (2-104) is modified to give:

$$\tau - (1 - \frac{D_i}{D_\infty})\frac{D_\infty}{ka^2}[1 - \exp(-\frac{ka^2}{D_\infty}\tau)] = \frac{1}{12}\left[6(\frac{A}{C_s}) - 4 - a_3\right] - \frac{1}{3}(\frac{A}{C_s} - 1)\delta^3 \tag{4-30}$$

To illustrate the usefulness of equation (4-27), Lee [11] analyzed the release data of thiamine HCl from a dehydrated polyHEMA sheet. The Debora number (release) concept was introduced to describe the drug release behavior of a hydrogel matrix as:

$$De_r = \frac{D_\infty}{ka^2} \tag{4-31}$$

The Debora number (release) describes the relative contribution of the drug diffusion time (a^2/D_∞) to the polymer relaxation time $(1/k)$. The dependence of drug release kinetics on De_r is illustrated in Table IV-1. Fickian diffusion takes place for $De_r \ll 1$ and $De_r \gg 1$ while anomalous or Case II diffusion takes place when De_r is on the order of 1. Lee and Lum [12] demonstrated that it is necessary to maintain $D_i/D_\infty \to 0$ to obtain zero order release kinetics for both dissolved and dispersed drug.

The ratio, D_i / D_∞, has a significant effect on the drug release behavior as illustrated in Fig. IV-10. As the ratio approaches 1, the drug release behavior becomes close to Fickian; whereas the drug release behavior becomes Case II (or zero-order kinetics) as the ratio approaches zero. Drug release from most common hydrogels shows an intermediate release behavior, indicating that the initial drug diffusion coefficient plays an important part in the drug release kinetics. However, as drug loading increases, the release behavior becomes Fickian [11].

Table IV-1. General Dependence of Release Behavior on Debora Number [11].

$De_r \Rightarrow 0$,	$D \Rightarrow D_\infty$	Fickian diffusion
$De_r \approx 1$ or > 1		Anomalous diffusion (including Case II)
$De_r \Rightarrow \infty$	$D \Rightarrow D_i$	Fickian diffusion (glassy-state)

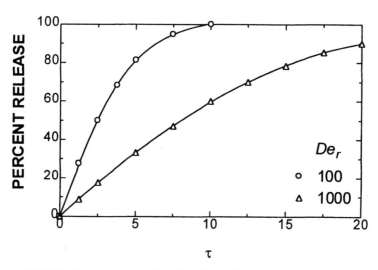

Figure IV-10. Drug release behavior of swellable polymer beads. (Graph reconstructed from data by Lee and Lum [12].)

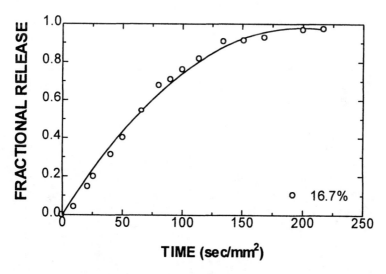

Figure IV-11. Drug release from a silicone polymer bead in n-hexane. (Graph reconstructed with data by Lee and Lum [12].)

Peppas and Franson [13] introduced the swelling interface number, S_W given by:

$$S_w = \frac{v\delta(t)}{D_{ai}}$$
(4-32)

where $\delta(t)$ is the time dependent thickness of the device's gel layer, D_{ai} is the diffusion coefficient of the active ingredient from the swollen layer, and v is the moving velocity of the glassy-rubbery interface. Drug release kinetics can be evaluated using S_W [13]:

$S_W \ll 1$ (0.01)	zero-order release
$S_W \gg 1$	Fickian release
$S_W \approx 1$	non-Fickian release

Analysis by Lee [11] and Peppas and Franson [13] allows one to screen polymer candidate materials in order to develop swelling controlled systems with zero-order kinetics.

Problem IV-1: Lee [11] studied the release of thiamine HCl from a poly(HEMA) film (Fig. IV-12). Due to the swelling of the polymer, release kinetics of the drug deviated from Fickian diffusion. Calculate the polymer relaxation rate constant of the polymer during drug release.

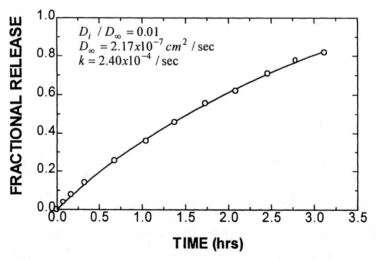

Figure IV-12. Release of thiamine HCl from poly(HEMA) film. (Graph reconstructed from data by Lee [11].)

Solution: First of all, one can calculate D_∞ from the late release portion because there is no polymer relaxation after the polymer has been fully swollen. Then D_i and k can be calculated from the release profile by non-linear regression analysis with equation in Table II-1 (1a). As shown in Fig. IV-12, the drug release kinetics is linear with time.

Kim [14] investigated the effect of the degree of polymer swelling on drug release kinetics from drug-polymer complex beads. It was found that it is necessary to have high swelling to achieve linear release kinetics from the swellable matrix. However, linear release kinetics also depends on the combination of the solvent and polymer. Kim [14] reported minimum degree of swelling of 2.8 (the ratio of equilibrium to initial diameter) for drug-polymer complex beads in water; whereas, Lee and Lum [12] obtained a value of 2.1 for poly(dimethylsiloxane) beads in pentane.

Shah et al. [15] reported Case II transport for drug-polymer conjugates (glassy polymer) of various substituted benzoates. The release kinetics is dependent on the relative rate of polymer relaxation, hydrolysis and drug diffusion. It was noted that Case II release kinetics resulted from a gradual increase of diffusion in the swollen gel layer. If polymer relaxation plays an important role in the drug release from drug-polymer conjugates via bond cleavage, equation (2-41) can be modified to give:

$$\frac{M_t}{M_\infty} = \frac{8kD_\infty}{L^2} \sum_{n=1}^{\infty} \frac{(1/\alpha_n)(1 - e^{-\alpha_n \tau}) - (1/k)(1 - e^{-k\tau})}{k - \alpha_n} \tag{4-33}$$

where

$$\tau = \frac{D_\infty t}{L^2} - \left[\left(1 - \frac{D_i}{D_\infty}\right) \frac{D_\infty}{k_r L^2} \left(1 - e^{-k_r t}\right) \right] \tag{4-34}$$

where k_r is the polymer relaxation constant and k is the hydrolysis rate constant.

Pitt and Shah [16] reported the release of nitrobenzoate from a copolymer of 2-p-nitrobenzoxyethyl methacrylate and methoxydiethoxyethyl methacrylate. The simulated drug release profiles were not in good agreement with the experimental data using equation (2-41) alone without taking into account the degree of hydration (swelling). Using an empirical relationship for the water content of the hydrolyzing gel given the residual ester content one can predict the drug release kinetics from side chains, cleavage, and polymer systems as shown in Fig. IV-13.

Bari and Kim [17] extended Lee's approach to the diffusion of a drug through swellable membrane reservoir systems. The diffusion of theophylline through water-insoluble/alcohol-soluble poly(HEMA) film was carried out in a diffusion cell. The transient diffusion of a drug through a fully swollen polymer membrane can be evaluated by:

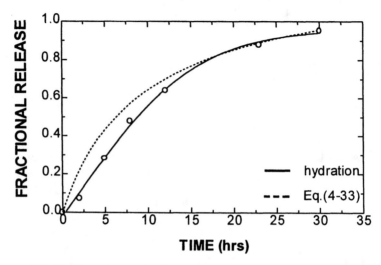

Figure IV-13. The release nitrobenzoate from drug-polymer conjugate with and without incorporation of hydration. (Graph reconstructed from data by Pitt and Shah [16].)

$$M_t = \frac{SD_\infty KC_s}{l}\left[t - \frac{l^2}{6D_\infty}\right] - \frac{2SD_\infty KlC_s}{\pi^2}\sum_{n=1}^{\infty}\frac{(-1)^n}{n^2}e^{-n^2\pi^2 D_\infty t/l^2} \quad (4\text{-}35)$$

The transient diffusion of drug through a dry membrane can be expressed by:

$$M_t = \frac{SKlC_s}{l}\left[\tau - \frac{1}{6}\right] - \frac{2SD_\infty KlC_s}{\pi^2}\sum_{n=1}^{\infty}\frac{(-1)^n}{n^2}e^{-n^2\pi^2\tau} \quad (4\text{-}36)$$

where τ is expressed by equation (4-26).

Fig. IV-14 shows the permeation of theophylline through swollen and dry poly(HEMA) films. From separate experiments with the swollen and dry membranes, one can independently calculate D_∞ and k.

The equations described so far deal with the diffusion process as through particular drug/polymer systems. Peppas et al. [18] examined Fickian diffusion and drug release with countercurrent solvent/drug diffusion and polymer swelling, and its effect on the concentration profiles in a swollen polymer matrix. Diffusion equations for counter-current drug/solvent diffusion and polymer swelling can be written as:

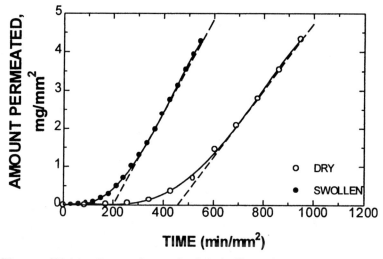

Figure IV-14. Permeation of theophylline from swollen and dry Poly(HEMA) film [17].

$$\frac{\partial C_A}{\partial t} = D_A \frac{\partial^2 C_A}{\partial x^2} \tag{4-37a}$$

$$\frac{\partial C_B}{\partial t} = D_B \frac{\partial^2 C_B}{\partial x^2} \tag{4-37b}$$

$$\frac{\partial C_S}{\partial t} = D_S \frac{\partial^2 C_S}{\partial x^2} \tag{4-37c}$$

where the subscripts *A, B,* and *S* are the drug in the (solvent-free) polymer, the drug in the gel layer, and the solvent in the gel layer, respectively.

Initial and boundary conditions are given by:

$$\frac{\partial C_A}{\partial x} = 0 \qquad\qquad x = 0 \tag{4-38a}$$

$$D_A \frac{\partial C_A}{\partial x} = D_B \frac{\partial C_B^*}{\partial x} \tag{4-38b}$$

$$\frac{\partial C_S^*}{\partial x} = 0 \qquad\qquad x = x^* \qquad\qquad\qquad (4\text{-}38\text{c})$$

$$C_S = C_S^o \qquad\qquad x = L \qquad\qquad\qquad (4\text{-}38\text{d})$$

$$C_B = C_B^o \qquad\qquad x = L \qquad\qquad\qquad (4\text{-}38\text{e})$$

$$C_A^* = C_B^* = C^* \qquad\qquad x = x^* \qquad\qquad\qquad (4\text{-}38\text{f})$$

$$\frac{\pi^2 d^2 (L - L_o)}{4} = \int_{x^*}^{L} \frac{\pi d^2}{4} \frac{M_s}{\rho} C_S dx \qquad\qquad (4\text{-}38\text{g})$$

where L is the position at the interface between the gel surface and water, x^* is the position at the moving swelling front, M_S is the molecular weight of the swelling solvent, ρ is the density of the swelling solvent, d is the diameter of the tablet, and L_o is the initial thickness of the tablet.

Under the condition of $D_A / D_B \cong 0$ and long time approximation [18]:

$$\overline{C}_B = \overline{C}_B^* - \frac{\overline{C}^*(\xi - \xi^*)}{1 - \xi^*} = \overline{C}^* \frac{1 - \xi}{1 - \xi^*} \qquad\qquad (4\text{-}39\text{a})$$

$$\frac{1 - \xi^*}{\xi^*} = \frac{\overline{C}^*(1 - \beta)}{2\varepsilon(1 - \overline{C}^*)} \frac{1}{\sum\limits_{n=1}^{\infty} e^{-\lambda_n^2 \tau}} \qquad\qquad (4\text{-}39\text{b})$$

$$1 - \xi^* = \frac{1 - \xi^*}{1 - \beta} \qquad\qquad (4\text{-}39\text{c})$$

where $\quad \xi = \dfrac{x}{L}, \quad \beta = \dfrac{M_s C_s^o}{\rho}, \quad \overline{C}_B = \dfrac{C_B}{C_B^o}, \quad \xi = \dfrac{D_A}{D_B}, \quad l = \dfrac{L}{L_o}, \quad \xi^* = \dfrac{x^*}{L_o},$

$\lambda_n = \dfrac{(2n-1)\pi}{2\xi^*}$, and $\tau = \dfrac{D_A t}{L_o^2}$.

Equations (4-39a) and (4-39c) give the drug concentration profile in the gel layer and the thickness of the gel layer, respectively. Equation (4-39b) can be used to calculate the position of the swelling interface. A similar solution for the concentration of the swelling solvent can be obtained using equation (4-37c).

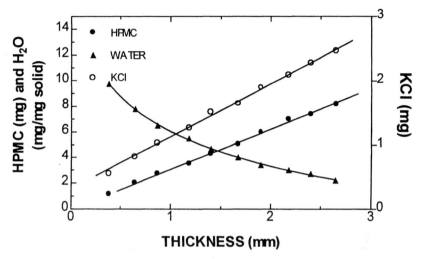

Figure IV-15. Concentration profiles of polymer (HPMC), water, and KCl in the HPMC gel layer. (Graph reconstructed from data by Peppas et al. [18].)

The amount of drug released at time t can be calculated from $\int D_B (\partial C_B / \partial x) \big|_{\xi=1}$ Fig. IV-15 shows the counter-current profiles of a solute and HPMC in the swollen rubbery gel layer.

Ritger and Peppas [6] introduced a simple phenomenological exponential relationship to describe the general solute release behavior of non-swellable and swellable polymeric devices, as follows:

$$\frac{M_t}{M_\infty} = kt^n \tag{4-40}$$

where k is a constant and n is the release exponent characteristic of the release mechanism. The release exponent n was determined based upon the theoretical equations for Fickian and Case II kinetics with equation (4-40) as

Table IV-2. Release Exponent of a Non-Swellable matrix [6].

slab	cylinder	sphere	Mechanism
0.5	0.45	0.43	Fickian
0.5<n<1.0	0.45<n<1.0	0.43<n<1.0	Anomalous
1.0	1.0	1.0	Zero-order or Case II

Table IV-3.   Release Exponent of a Swellable Matrix [6].

Slab	cylinder	sphere	Mechanism
0.5	0.45	0.43	Fickian
0.5<n<1.0	0.45<n<0.89	0.43<n<0.85	Anomalous
1.0	0.89	0.85	Zero-order or Case II

given in the Tables IV-2 and IV-3. Anomalous release kinetics may also be expressed by:

$$\frac{M_t}{M_\infty} = k_1 \sqrt{t} + k_2 t \qquad\qquad (4\text{-}41)$$

where k_1 and k_2 are constants.

IV.2. Hydrogel Systems

Polymer matrix systems, which maintain their original shape throughout the entire release time, except for those exhibiting non-Fickian and Case II kinetics, have been dealt. In preceding sections, polymeric materials, which are glassy in their dry state but rubbery-gel like when placed in contact with water, are commonly referred to as hydrogels, even though there is no exact definition of hydrogel. Water absorption into the polymer is induced by capillary, osmotic and hydration forces. Because hydrogels are prepared by cross-linking during or after the polymerization process, the polymer does not disintegrate in water. When a dry, cross-linked polymer network is brought in contact with water, the macromolecular chains swell to form a solvated network structure (Fig. IV-16). The swelling of the hydrogel network is constrained by the cross-linked structure. Equilibrium is reached when the thermodynamic swelling force is equal to the contractive force of the cross-linked network,. The rate at which the equilibrium swelling volume is reached is highly dependent upon polymer relaxation.

Release of drugs held in the space of the hydrogel is dependent upon the diffusion of solvent into the matrix and the diffusion of drug through the rubbery-gel layer. The swelling of the rubbery-gel layer is also time-dependent as discussed before. Therefore, controlling the swelling rate as well as its equilibrium swelling of the glassy hydrogel matrix is critical. Basically, for the hydrogel to be thermodynamically compatible with swelling solvent, the glassy transition temperature, T_g , must fall below the experimental temperature upon contact with swelling solvent (water). The

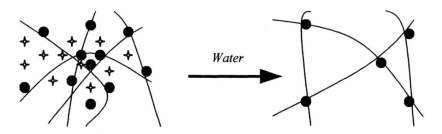

Figure IV-16. When water swells the hydrogel, the drug imbibed within the polymer network is released (+: drug) [14].

hydrogel, upon contact with the solvent, transforms from the glassy state to rubbery state. However, depending upon the response of glassy polymer to swelling solvent at the interface separating the glassy core and rubbery layer, the release kinetics of the drug can be interpreted differently ranging from Fickian to Case II. Theoretical expressions have been presented in the previous sections to describe drug release from these systems.

IV.2.1. *Method of hydrogel preparation*

Common hydrogels are synthesized via addition polymerization (free-radical polymerization). Here, a brief description of hydrogel synthesis is given. Those wishing to obtain in-depth knowledge of polymerization processes and kinetics should consult polymerization textbooks. There are several routes to synthesize hydrogel materials depending on how cross-linking is introduced: during the polymerization process or afterwards. For the introduction of cross-linking during the polymerization process, e.g. the polymerization of 2-hydroxyethyl methacrylate (HEMA), the HEMA monomer, and cross-linking agent, ethylene glycol dimethacrylate (EGDMA), are mixed and the initiator is added before the polymerization commences. EGDMA has vinyl groups on both ends, and therefore acts as a cross-linker to form a three-dimensional network. Common monomers used to obtain hydrogels are vinyl monomers as shown in Table IV-4 along with cross-linking agents. Cross-linking may also be introduced after the polymerization; e.g. the reactive functional groups of water-soluble linear polymers such as poly(vinyl alcohol) cross-linked with glutaraldehyde [19].

Common hydrogels are prepared by bulk or solution polymerization. In this process all chemical components are mixed and polymerized in a confined shape, usually a cylinder or sheet. In oral drug delivery systems, a bead form is preferred. The suspension polymerization process has been used to produce polymer beads from materials such as polystyrene, poly(methyl methacrylate), and poly(vinyl acetate). The suspension process has been well adapted to produce ion exchange resins and chromatography packing materials. Unlike polymer beads, which are usually 10-300 μm, hydrogel beads larger than 800 μm in diameter are needed to deliver water-soluble drugs over an extended period.

The most important step in the development of a suspension polymerization process is the choice of suitable suspending agents. If one attempts to carry out the suspension polymerization in the absence of such agents (or improper agents), the monomer droplets pass through a sticky viscous state and then coalesce into an agglomerated chunk during the polymerization [20]. There are two types of suspending agents: water-soluble organic polymers and finely divided gelatinous, insoluble inorganic materials. Inorganic suspending agents are favored over water-soluble polymers because of their ease of removal and tendency to produce beads with smooth surfaces. Suspending agents should be made in the reactor immediately before the

Table IV-4. Neutral Hydrophilic, Ionic, Neutral Hydrophobic, and Polyfunctional Cross-Linking Monomers for Hydrogel Systems [19].

Monomer Groups	Examples
Neutral (hydrophilic)	hydroxyalkylacrylates, hydroxyalkylmethacrylates, N-substituted acrylamides, N-substituted methacrylamides, N-vinyl-2-pyrrolidone
	Ex: $CH_2 = C(H) - C = O \qquad CH_2 = C(H) - C = O$ $\qquad\quad CH_3 \quad O-alkyl-OH \qquad\qquad CH_3 \quad NH_2$
Anionic (hydrophilic)	acrylic acid, methacrylic acid, crotonic acid, sulfopropyl methacrylate, sulfoethyl methacrylate, styrenesulfonate, AMPS*
	Ex: $CH_2 = C(H) - C = O \qquad CH_2 = C - C = O$ $\qquad\quad CH_3 \quad OH \qquad\qquad CH_3 \ O-(CH_2)_{2-3}SO_3^-$
Cationic (hydrophilic)	vinylpyridine, dimethylaminoethyl methacrylates, trimethyl aminoethyl (meth)acrylate, MAPTAC*
	Ex: $CH_2 = C - C = O \qquad\qquad CH_2 = C - C = O$ $\qquad\quad CH_3 \ O-(CH_2)_2 N^+(CH_3)_3 \quad CH_3 \ O-(CH_2)_2 NH(CH_3)_2$
Neutral (hydrophobic)	acrylics, methacrylics, vinyl acetate, styrene
	Ex: $CH_2 = C(H) - C = O \ \ CH_2 = CH - O - C - CH_3 \ CH_2 = CH - phenyl$ $\qquad\quad CH_3 \quad O-alkyl \qquad\qquad\quad O$
Crosslinking Agents	N,N-methylenebisacrylamide, ethylene glycol dimethacrylates, divinyl benzene, methylenebis(4-phenyl-isocyanate)
	Ex: $CH_2 = CH - X - CH = CH_2$

*AMPS: 2-acrylamido-2-methyl-1-propanesulfonic acid
MAPTC:[3-(methacryloylamino)propyl]trimethylammonium chloride

polymerization is carried out. Anchor-type stirrers operated at low stirring rates (50-150 rpm) are best for producing the large beads (>800 μm) needed for drug delivery systems.

A typical process to produce hydrogel beads is shown in Fig. IV-17. $MgCl_2 \cdot 6H_2O$ is dissolved in water in a batch reactor, followed by the dropwise addition of an aqueous solution of NaOH with slow stirring (50 rpm) to form a finely divided gelatinous precipitate of $Mg(OH)_2$ [21]. The monomer phase is then added, consisting of monomer, initiator, and cross-linking agent. The polymerization is carried out at a high temperature for several hours. After the polymerization is complete, the suspending agent is removed by adding a concentrated HCl solution. The beads are obtained by filtration and impurities are removed by Soxhlet extraction with ethanol before the beads are dried and sieved.

Next, the drug is loaded into the hydrogel beads by simply equilibrating them in a concentrated drug solution in water and/or ethanol. The equilibrium degree of swelling of the hydrogel in the drug loading solvent is an important parameter [22], as shown in Fig. IV-18. It determines both the size of the beads and the amount of drug that will be delivered by the beads. This parameter has to be controlled to accommodate both the smallest and the largest controlled-release dosage unit that patients can tolerate.

In order to use hydrogels as drug delivery systems, the hydrogels should provide a high degree of swelling and slow rate of swelling because one has to deliver drugs with favorable release kinetics for a long release time. The high degree of swelling furnishes the desired release kinetics, which are close to zero-order or anomalous due to the increase of drug diffusivity. However, in most cases, it results in short release duration. To extend the release time, hydrogels have been prepared consisting of hydrophilic and hydrophobic segments such as poly(hydroxyethyl methacrylate-co-methyl methacrylate). In this way, the hydrogels are highly swellable in the drug loading solvent (such as alcohol) and low to moderately swellable in water [22]. Drug diffusion through the polymer matrix is the rate–controlling step, resulting in Fickian release kinetics. Other procedures

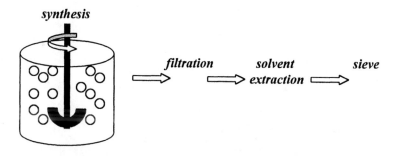

Figure IV-17. Suspension polymerization process [14].

have been proposed to achieve zero-order release kinetics from low swellable hydrogels in water, e.g. non-uniform concentration distributions (see Chapter VII).

IV.2.2. *Characterization of hydrogels*

The swelling and network characteristics of hydrogels can be evaluated by a Flory-Rehner type equation developed by Lucht and Peppas [23] for a highly cross-linked hydrogel:

$$\frac{1}{M_c} = \frac{2}{\overline{M}_n} - \frac{v[\ln(1-v_2)+v_2+\chi v_2^2](1-v_2^{2/3}N)^3}{v_1(v_2^{1/3}-v_2/2)(1+v_2^{1/3}/N)^2} \qquad (4\text{-}42)$$

where M_c is the number average molecular weight between cross-links, M_n the number average molecular weight of uncross-linked hydrogel, χ the Flory interaction parameter of the water-hydrogel system, $\overline{v}$ the specific volume of hydrogel, v_2 the hydrogel volume fraction, and $_1$ the molar volume of the swelling solvent. The parameter N is the number of cross-links in the chain expressed by:

$$N = 2\frac{\overline{M}_c}{M_r} \qquad (4\text{-}43)$$

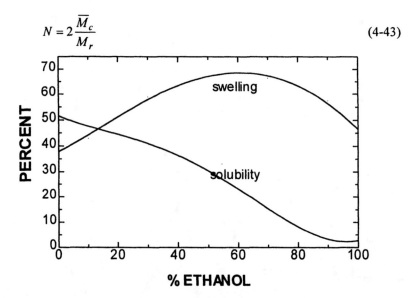

Figure IV-18. Degree of polymer swelling and the composition of the swelling solvents. (Graphs reconstructed from data by Lee [23].)

where M_r is the molecular weight of the monomer unit. The mesh size, ξ, which represents the maximum size of drug molecule that can diffuse through the polymer network, is calculated by:

$$\xi = v_2^{-\frac{1}{3}} \varphi N^{\frac{1}{2}} C_n^{\frac{1}{2}} \tag{4-44}$$

where C_n is the hydrogel rigidity factor and φ (=1.54$A°$) the C-C bond length. The value of χ can be calculated with the solubility parameter δ:

$$\chi = \frac{1}{x} + \frac{V_m(\delta_1 - \delta_2)}{RT} \tag{4-45}$$

where V_m is the molar volume and δ_1 and δ_2 are the solubility parameters of the polymer and the solvent, respectively. The polymer-solvent interaction parameter χ is at a minimum when δ_1 and δ_2 are equal, resulting in maximum swelling. The value of δ for a solvent can be calculated by:

$$\delta = \left(\frac{\Delta H_v - RT}{V_m} \right) \tag{4-46}$$

where ΔH_v is the heat of vaporization. δ and χ can be found in the literature [24].

The polymer volume fraction is be determined by:

$$v_2 = \frac{v_p}{v_s} = \frac{w_{p,d} / \rho_p}{w_{p,d} / \rho_p + (w_s - w_{p,d}) / \rho_w} \tag{4-47}$$

where v_s is the swollen gel volume, v_p the polymer volume, $w_{p,d}$ the dry polymer weight, w_s the swollen gel weight, ρ_p the polymer density, and ρ_s the solvent weight.

Fig. IV-19 illustrates the effect of the degree of cross-linking on the hydrogel network structure.

IV.2.3. *Dimensional changes during drug release*

During drug release and swelling solvent influx, dimensional size changes of drug-loaded hydrogels occur in which the matrix dimension reaches a maximum followed by a gradual decline to an equilibrium size. On the other hand, the swelling dimension of a drug free matrix increases monotonically to its equilibrium size. This maximum dimension occurs because the dissolved drug in the hydrogel matrix generates an osmotic force.

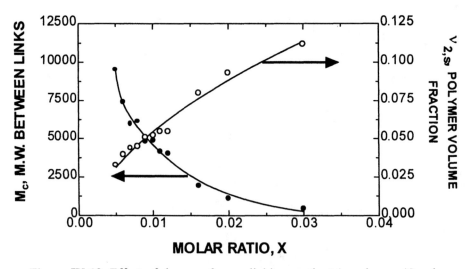

Figure IV-19. Effect of degree of cross-linking on the M_c and $v_{2,s}$. (Graph reconstructed from data by Peppas and Benner [25].)

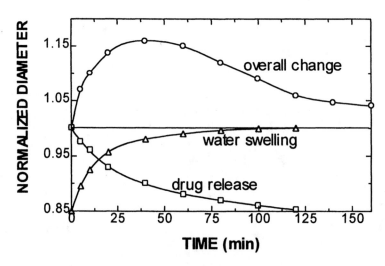

Figure IV-20. Dimensional change during drug release due to the effect of water swelling, drug release, and osmotic pressure. (Graph reconstructed from data by Lee and Kim [27].)

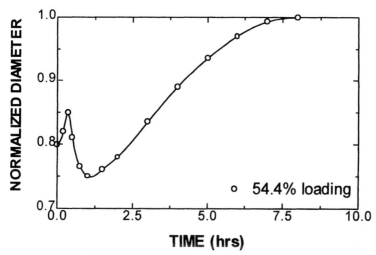

Figure V-21.   Experimental observation of dimensional changes during drug release. (Graph reconstructed from data by Kim and Lee [26].).

During early time of drug release, the swelling contribution from the osmotic force is much greater than the polymer swelling. The swelling of polymer increases slowly to equilibrium while the osmotic force decreases due to the release of drug. The combination of these two processes gives rise to a maximum dimension as shown in Fig. VI-20.

The dimensional changes of hydrogel matrices are highly dependent upon the hydrogel's degree of swelling. If the degree of swelling is much greater than that created by an osmotic force, a maximum peak will not be observed during drug release. Fig. IV-21 shows that as drug loading increases, the first peak appears due to the high swelling from the osmotic force at the early stage of drug release and then falls down a little bit before increasing monotonically to its equilibrium swelling due to polymer swelling.

Owing to the non-monotonic changes of a hydrogel's dimension, the release rate of a drug from a hydrogel matrix is surprisingly slow especially at late release times. High swelling (or large dimensional changes) at early release times allows for a high drug diffusion coefficient in the matrix while the diffusion of drug from the contracted matrix is slower. In extreme cases, the drug release from a low-water swellable hydrogel matrix (degree of swelling < 5%) with high alcohol swelling reaches 80% very rapidly, after which it falls off very slowly to completion. However, the release of a drug from the hydrogel system furnishes much higher polymer swelling than the contribution of osmotic force generated by dissolved drug avoiding the tailing problem in drug release as shown in Fig. IV-21.

References

1. J. Crank and G. S. Park, Diffusion in Polymers, Academic Press, New York, 1968.
2. P. I. Lee, "Kinetics of Drug Release from Hydrogel Matrices," *J. Control. Rel.*, 2, 277 (1985).
3. P. I. Lee and C. J. Kim, "Effect of Geometry on the Swelling Front Penetration in Glassy Polymers," *J. Membr. Sci.*, 65, 77 (1992).
4. H. B. Hopfenberg, "The Effect of Film Thickness and Sample History on the Parameters Describing Transport in Glassy Polymers," *J. Membr. Sci.*, 3, 215 (1978).
5. H. B. Hopfenberg and K. C. Hsu, "Swelling-Controlled, Constant Rate Delivery Systems," *Polym. Eng. Sci.*, 18, 1186 (1978).
6. P. L. Ritger and N. A. Peppas, "A Simple Equation for Description of Solute Release II. Fickian and Anomalous Release from Swellable Devices," *J. Control. Rel.*, 5, 37 (1987).
7. P. Neogi, "Anomalous Diffusion of Vapors through Solid Polymers," *AIChE J.*, 29, 829 (1983).
8. H-R Lee and Y-D Lee, "Mathematical Models and Experiments for Swelling Phenomena before Dissolution of a Polymer Film," *Chem. Eng. Sci.*, 46, 1771 (1991).
9. G. Astari and G. C. Sartl, "A Class of Mathematical Models for Sorption of Swelling Solvent in Glassy Polymers," *Polym. Eng. Sci.*, 18, 388 (1978).
10. T. Koizumi, S. P. Panomsuk, T. Hatanaka, and K. Katayama, "Kinetics of Swelling of Compressed Cellulose Matrices: A Mathematical Model," *Pharm. Res.*, 13, 329 (1996).
11. P. I. Lee, "Interpretation of Drug-release Kinetics from Hydrogel Matrices in terms of Time-Dependent Diffusion Coefficients," in Controlled Release Technology: Pharmaceutical Applications, W. R. Good and P. I. Lee (Eds.), Americal Chemical Society Symposium Series No. 348, American Chemical Society, Washington, DC, 1987, p71.
12. P. I. Lee and S. K. Lum, "Swelling-Induced Zero-Order Release from Rubbery Polydimethylsiloxane Beads," *J. Control. Rel*, 18, 19 (1992).
13. N. A. Peppas and N. M. Franson, "The Swelling Interface Number as a Criterion for Prediction of Diffusional Solute Release Mechanisms in Swellable Polymers," *J. Polym. Sci. Polym. Phys. Ed.*, 21, 983 (1983).
14. C. J. Kim, "Hydrogel Beads for Oral Drug Delivery," Chemtech, 24 (8), 36, (1994).
15. S. S. Shah, M. G. Kulkari and R. A. Mashelkar, "pH Dependent Zero Order Release from Glassy Hydrogels: Penetration vs. Diffusion Control," *J. Control. Rel.*, 15, 121 (1991).
16. C. G. Pitt and S. S. Shah, "Manipulation of the Rate of Hydrolysis of Polymer-Drug Conjugates: The Degree of Hydration," *J. Control. Rel.*, 33, 397 (1995).
17. M. Bari and C. J. Kim, Unpublished data.

18. N. A. Peppas, R. Gurny, E. Doelker, and P. Buri, "Modelling of Drug through Swellable Polymeric Systems," *J. Membr. Sci.*, 7, 241 (1980).

19. S. H. Gehrke and P. I. Lee, In <u>Special Drug Delivery Systems, Manufacturing and Production Technology</u>, Tyle, P. Ed., Marcel Dekker, New York, NY, 1990, pp333.

20. C. J. Kim and P. I. Lee, "Synthesis and Characterization of Suspension Polymerized Poly(vinyl-alcohol) beads with Core-Shell Structure," *J. Appli. Polym. Sci.*, 46, 2147 (1992).

21. N. Friis and A. E. Hamielec, "Heterophase Polymerization," in <u>Polymer Reaction Engineering: An Intensive Short Course on Polymer Production Technology</u>, McMaster University, Hamilton, Canada, 1980.

22. K. F. Mueller, S. J. Heiker, and W. L. Plankl, U.S. Patent 4,224,427 (1980).

23. P. I. Lee, Synthetic Hydrogels for Drug Delivery: Preparation, Characterization, and Release Kinetics, In <u>Controlled release Systems: Fabrication Technology</u> Vol. II, D. S. T. Hsieh, Ed., CRC Press, Boca Raton, Fl, 1988, pp61.

24. L. M. Lucht and P. A. Peppas, "Cross-linked Structures in Coals: Models and Preliminary Experimental Data," in <u>Chemistry and Physics of Coal Utilization</u>, B. S. Cooper and L. Petrakis (Eds.), American Institute of Physics, New York, 1981, pp28.

25. N. A. Peppas and R. E. Benner, Jr., "Proposed Method of Intracordal Injection and Gelation of Poly(vinyl alcohol) Solution in Vocal Cords: Polymer Considerations," *Biometerials*, 1, 158 (1980).

26. C. J. Kim and P. I. Lee, "Effect of Loading on Swelling-Controlled Drug Release from Hydrophobic Polyelectrolyte Gel Beads," *Pharm. Res.*, 9, 1268 (1992).

27. P. I. Lee and C. J. Kim, "Probing Mechanisms of Drug Release from Hydrogels," *J. Control. Rel.*, 16, 229 (1991).

Chapter V

Polymer Dissolution Controlled Systems

V.1.   Classification of Polymer Degradation and Erosion

The drug delivery systems described in the previous chapters are based on polymeric materials, which may swell but do not disintegrate (dissolve) during or after the release. This poses no problems for oral delivery systems or for the cases where a non-degradable drug carrier does not matter to the receptor environment. However, there are some situations in which it is beneficial for the polymer to degrade naturally during or after drug release. Otherwise, the polymeric carrier needs to be removed from the body after completing the drug. Table V-1 shows several classifications for biodegradable/erodible polymer delivery systems. The degradation mechanism varies among chemical classification [1].

In general, drug release from a matrix controlled system does not furnish zero-order kinetics unless intricate fabrication processes used in manufacturing e.g. ununiform concentration distribution, modification of geometry, etc. If the matrix polymer is highly swellable, which may provide zero-order kinetics, the total release time is often too short to apply to extended release dosage forms. However, drug release from biodegradable/erodible polymer matrices may easily give zero-order (linear) release kinetics as long as a constant surface area of the dosage form is maintained during drug release. This will be discussed in a later section. Biodegradable polymers play an important role in the administration of many potent bio-macromolecules. When nonbio-degradable polymers are used, bio-macromolecules may aggregate or precipitate within pores and channels of the matrix before being released [2]. If the degradation of the matrix controls the release, especially below a threshold level of drug concentration, the release rate may be manipulated by drug loading level and geometry and complete release can be obtained. In this chapter, the process of degradation designates the cleavage of large polymer chains to smaller chains and eventually to single monomers. An erosion process describes the slow dissolution of polymer without molecular changes.

In type I degradation, first the polymer chain of water-insoluble polymers is broken down to smaller, water-soluble molecules primarily by hydrolysis of labile ester bonds in the polymer backbone. Then drug dispersed physically in the interstices of the polymer matrix releases. Linear polyesters such as poly(lactic acid), poly(glycolic acid), or copolymers of lactic acid and glycolic acid (Fig. V-1) have been used for medical applications (suture) without significant toxic effects [3]. The by-products of homopolymer or copolymer degradation are lactic acid and glycolic acid,

$$-[-O-CH_2-\overset{\overset{O}{\|}}{C}-]_n-$$

A

$$-[-O-\overset{CH_3}{\underset{|}{CH}}-\overset{\overset{O}{\|}}{C}-]_n-$$

B

Figure V-1.   Chemical   structure   of   biodegradable   polymers   A: poly(glycolic acid); B: poly(lactic acid).

which are commonly found in metabolic cycles in the body.   Other biodegradable polymers which follow type I degradation are poly(ortho ester)s which have the structure shown in Fig. V-2.   Unlike poly(lactic acid) and poly(glycolic acid), poly(ortho ester)s were developed specifically for controlled drug delivery systems and degraded via polymer surface erosion [4].

Table V.1. Classification of Chemical Bio-degradation [1].

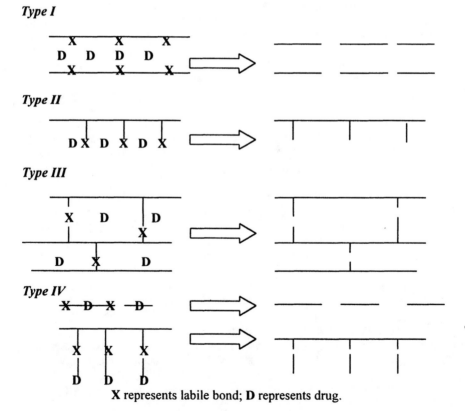

Type I

Type II

Type III

Type IV

X represents labile bond; **D** represents drug.

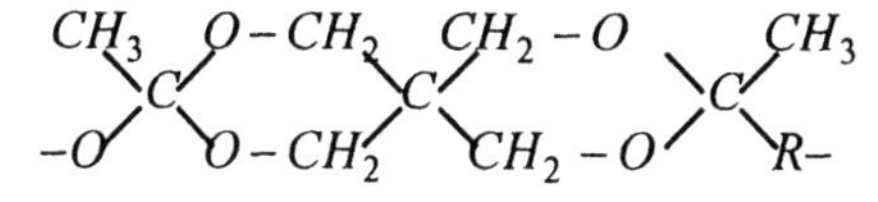

$$\underset{-O^{\diagdown}}{\overset{CH_3}{\diagdown}}\underset{O-CH_2^{\diagup}}{\overset{O-CH_2}{\diagdown}}\underset{CH_2-O^{\diagup}}{\overset{CH_2-O}{\diagdown}}\underset{R-}{\overset{CH_3}{\diagup}}$$

Figure V-2. Chemical structure of biodegradable poly(ortho ester)

      In systems based on type II erosion, the drugs dispersed physically in the polymer are released as the side chain groups of the water-insoluble polymer are broken and polymer becomes hydrophilic due to side chain cleavage. The resulting hydrophilic polymer dissolves (erosion). Unlike systems based on type I degradation, the polymer backbone structure remains intact and there are no byproducts formed (no reduction in the molecular weight of the polymer). In most cases, these polymers are formed with two monomers. One monomer has labile groups (ester, anhydride, or acid) which are hydrolyzed in a high pH environment (Fig. V-3). An example of type II erosion is a copolymer of glutamic acid and ethyl glutamate. The ester group in ethyl glutamate is hydrolyzed to glutamic acid, which increases the total concentration of glutamic acid in the polymer, resulting in solubilization (or erosion). Other examples include polyanhydrides and polyacids in which carboxy anhydride and carboxylic acid functional groups are hydrolyzed, respectively [5,6].

      In type III degradation systems, the polymer chains are cross-linked with linear polymer or short chain molecules. Then the main polymer chain contains a hydrolyzable bond (e.g. esters) or the cross-linked molecule contains the hydrolyzable group (e.g. amide). When the labile group is hydrolyzed, the drug is released from the matrix, leaving the skeleton behind. Polyvinylpyrrolidone is cross-linked with bisacrylamide or low molecular weight polyethylene glycol reacts with vinyl pyrrolidone forming the polymer structure shown in Fig. V-4. Cleavage takes place by hydrolysis of amide or ester links [6,7].

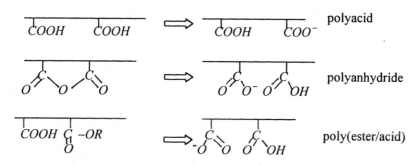

Figure V-3. Solubilization of polycarboxylic acid and polyanhydride.

$-[-CH_2 - \underset{R}{CH-}]_n - CH_2 - \underset{C=O}{CH} - [-CH_2 - \underset{R}{CH-}]_m -$ $-[-CH_2 - \underset{R}{CH-}]_n - CH_2 - \underset{C=O}{CH} - [-CH_2 - \underset{R}{CH-}]_m -$

with vertical chain:

$\begin{array}{c} C=O \\ NH \\ CH_2 \\ C=O \end{array} \Longrightarrow \begin{array}{c} C=O \\ NH_2 \\ + \\ HCH \\ O \end{array}$

$-[-CH_2 - \underset{R}{CH-}]_n - CH_2 - \underset{R}{CH} - [-CH_2 - CH-]_m -$

$-[-CH_2 - \underset{R}{CH-}]_n - CH_2 - \underset{C=O}{CH} - [-CH_2 - \underset{R}{CH-}]_m -$
NH_2

Figure V-4. Cleavage of cross-linked polyvinylpyrrolidone.

In type IV degradation systems, the drug molecules to be released are an integral part of the polymer chain. The drug is located in the linear polymer chain or attached to the side chain of the polymer structure. The bond between drug and polymer chain is labile so that the bond is hydrolyzed before the drug is released. This can be achieved by reacting a monomer and the drug, and then polymerizing them, or conjugating a polymer with the drug at a reactive sight.

From a physical point of view, one can classify erosion/degradation: either heterogeneous or homogeneous erosions regardless of the chemical pathway of degradation and erosion.

V.2. Heterogeneous Degradation and Erosion

For a heterogeneous eroding system in which the polymer degrades from the surface, the release kinetics will be the same as for polymer degradation. As the polymer segments degrade and the boundary moves, the drug occupied in the segments is released into the dissolution medium.

For a spherical bead having a radius a and a uniformly dispersed drug concentration C_o, the amount of drug released at time t, as shown in Fig. V-6, is:

$-[-CH_2 - \underset{C=O}{CH-}]_n - [-CH_2 - \underset{COOH}{\overset{CH_3}{C}-}]_m -$ $\Longrightarrow$ $-[-CH_2 - \underset{C=O}{CH-}]_n - [-CH_2 - \underset{COOH}{\overset{CH_3}{C}-}]_m -$

O
$CH_2 - CH_2 - O - \underset{O}{C} - CH_2O - C_6H_4Cl_2$ O
CH_2CH_2OH
$+$

$HO - \underset{O}{C} - CH_2O - C_6H_4Cl_2$

Figure V-5. Hydrolysis of polyagent based on methacrylate polymers.

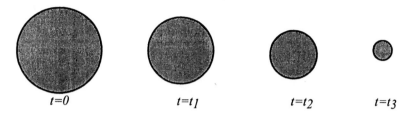

$t=0$ $\quad\quad\quad\quad t=t_1$ $\quad\quad\quad\quad t=t_2$ $\quad\quad\quad t=t_3$

Figure V-6. Heterogeneous erosion process.

$$\frac{dM_t}{dt} = k_o 4\pi R^2 \tag{5-1}$$

where k_o is the surface degradation rate. The amount of active material released in time t, M_t will be given by the material balance equation:

$$M_t = \frac{4\pi}{3} C_o [a^3 - R^3] \tag{5-2}$$

The total mass released at time t_∞, the time for total erosion, is:

$$M_\infty = \frac{4\pi C_o a^3}{3} \tag{5-3}$$

Taking the derivative of equation (5-2) with respect to time and substituting the result into equation (5-1) yields R as a function of time as:

$$R = a - \left(\frac{k_o}{C_o}\right)t \tag{5-4}$$

The expression for the fractional drug release is:

$$\frac{M_t}{M_\infty} = 1 - \left[1 - \frac{k_o t}{C_o a}\right]^3 \tag{5-5}$$

One can generalize the expression for fractional release as follows:

$$\frac{M_t}{M_\infty} = 1 - \left[1 - \frac{k_o t}{C_o a}\right]^n \tag{5-6}$$

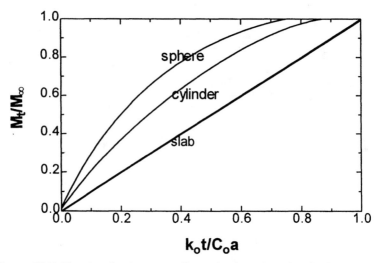

Figure V-7. Fractional release vs. dimensionless time for the heterogeneous erosion medium.

where n is 1 for a slab, 2 for a cylinder and 3 for a sphere. Theoretical release kinetics is presented in Fig. V-7. Note that zero-order release kinetics can be obtained only by slab geometry as predicted by equation (5-6). Release of hydrocortisone from the n-butyl half-ester of methyl vinyl ether maleic anhydride (n-BMVEMA) copolymer and its degradation is shown in Fig. V-8 [5]. The n-BMVEMA polymer is synthesized from the esterification of MVEMA copolymer (Gantranzes®) with n-butyl alcohol by the following reaction:

$$-CH_2 - CH - O - CH - CH - \quad \quad \quad -CH_2 - CH - O - CH - CH -$$

The n-BMVEMA is hydrolyzed easily by the ionization of carboxylic acid groups (Type II) because the anhydride group of the MVEMA is partially esterified. As illustrated in Fig. V-8, the completion of drug release coincides with complete hydrolysis of the polymer, indicating that the diffusion of drug from the matrix is negligible for controlling the release rate and that the surface erosion rate of polymer dominates the release process. As mentioned earlier, the erosion rate is highly influenced by the pH of the dissolution medium due to the ionization of carboxylic acid groups. It may be expected that the ionization of carboxylic acids is dependent upon ionic strength of the dissolution medium, which effects the release of drug. Erosion controlled release systems based on hydrolysis of the carboxylic acid labile groups of the polymer chain can be used in environments maintaining constant pH and ionic strength.

Fig. V-9 shows the release of p-nitroaniline from poly(fumaric acid-sebasic acid) 50/50 in 0.1 M pH 7.4 phosphate buffer at 37°C. Drug release coincides with polymer erosion [10]. Fumaric acid (FA) and sebasic acid (SA) segments of the copolymer provide hydrophilicity and hydrophobicity of the copolymer, respectively. As SA content in the copolymer increases, the polymer erosion time is extended [11].

$$HO-\overset{O}{\underset{}{C}}-(CH_2)_8-\overset{O}{\underset{}{C}}-OH \; + \qquad HO-\overset{O}{\underset{}{C}}-C-CH=CH-\overset{}{\underset{O}{C}}-OH \quad \Longrightarrow$$

$$-[-\overset{O}{\underset{}{C}}-(CH_2)_8-\overset{O}{\underset{}{C}}-O-]_x-O-[-\overset{O}{\underset{}{C}}-CH=CH-\overset{O}{\underset{}{C}}-O-]_y-$$

Zhang et al. [12] presented a theoretical model to describe the drug release from an erodible tablet. As discussed in Chapter II, the tablet may be considered to be the combined geometry of slab and cylinder. Drug release and surface erosion occur from both the flat surfaces and the radial side. Equation (5-6), for a single shape, is appropriate to demonstrate the drug release and erosion from the combined shape. The mathematical expression proposed for this configuration is given by:

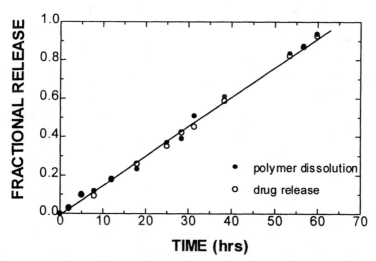

Figure V-8. Release of hydrocortisone from n-BMVEMA matrix. (Graph reconstructed from data by Heller et al. [5].)

$$\frac{dM_t}{dt} = 2\pi k_o r(r+l) \tag{5-7a}$$

where r and l are the radius and thickness of the eroding tablet at time t, respectively. The time dependent radius and thickness of the tablet can be expressed by:

$$l = l_o - \frac{k_o}{C_o}t \qquad\qquad r = r_o - \frac{k_o}{C_o}t \tag{5-7b}$$

where r_o and l_o are the initial radius and thickness of the tablet, respectively.

Integrating equation (5-7a) after substituting equation (5-7b) yields:

$$\frac{M_t}{M_\infty} = 1 - \left[1 - \frac{k_o t}{C_o r_o}\right]^2 \left[1 - \frac{2k_o t}{C_o l_o}\right] \tag{5-8}$$

Fig. V-10a demonstrates that complete release of diclofenac Na coincides with complete dissolution of hydroxypropylmethylcellulose polymer (HPMC E5), implying that the erosion process controls the drug release mechanism. It is interesting to note that drug release in an erodible matrix is independent of drug solubility at low drug loading level or may be inferred from Fig. V-10. This is not common in other diffusion-controlled systems when greater drug solubility implies faster drug diffusion. However, the drug release kinetics may change as the loading increases because the

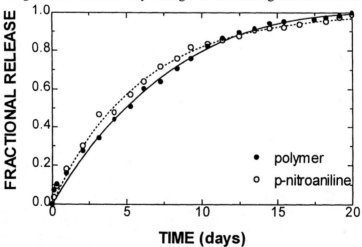

Figure V-9. Release of p-nitroaniline from poly(fumaric acid-sebasic acid). (Graph reconstructed from data by Domb et al. [10].)

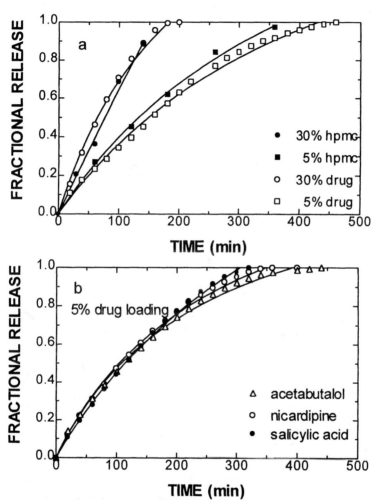

Figure V-10. Effect of drug loading (a) and drug solubility (b) on the drug release from HPMC E5 tablets [13].

contribution of drug diffusion to the overall release plays an important role. The contribution of the erosion of polymer on the drug release becomes smaller. Kim [13] found that drug release kinetics from HPMC E5 (erosion controlled) depend on drug solubility [Fig. 10(b)]. As drug solubility increases, drug release becomes faster due to faster influx of water. This results in faster erosion of the polymer. If the drug solubility is less than 0.5%, the dissolution of the drug becomes the rate-controlling step, giving rise to Fickian kinetics. However, the release of nicardipine HCl from HPMC

E5 tablets is not influenced by drug loading ranging from 5% to 30% [13]. In this case, one may postulate that the increase of the drug in the matrix does not increase the influx of water.

V.3.   Homogeneous Degradation and Erosion

The release of drug, from a homogeneous erosion matrix, in which the polymer materials are degraded or eroded throughout the entire matrix (any position in the matrix), is more complicated due to a combination of drug diffusion and polymer erosion. First, we will deal with the dispersed drug system. As described in the Higuchi model (Chapter II-2), the release rate of a drug from the matrix is expressed by:

$$\frac{dM_t}{dt} = \left(\frac{A^2 PC_o}{2t} \right)^{1/2} \tag{5-9}$$

where P is the permeability of the polymer, which is equal to DC_{sm}, and A is the surface area of both sides of the slab. For an eroding system, however, the permeability of drugs in the matrix increases with time due to the gradual cleavage of polymer chains via hydrolysis.

The permeability of the matrix can be estimated as follows [4]:

$$\frac{P}{P_0} = \frac{N_o}{N_o - Z} \tag{5-10}$$

where N_o is the initial number of bonds, Z is the number of cleaved bonds, and P_o is the initial permeability of the matrix. Assuming the rate of chain cleavage, dZ/dt, is first-order and proportional to the number of cleaved chains present, then

$$\frac{dZ}{dt} = K(N_o - Z) \tag{5-11}$$

where K is the first-order rate constant. Integration of equation (5-11) yields:

$$Kt = \ln\left(\frac{N_o}{N_o - Z} \right) \tag{5-12}$$

Equations (5-10) and (5-12) can be rearranged to yield:

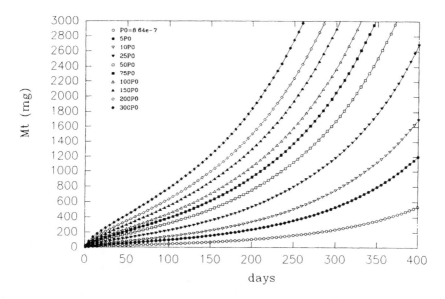

Figure V-11. Theoretical calculation of drug release from erosion controlled systems containing dispersed drug.

$$P = P_o e^{Kt}$$

(5-13)

Substituting equation (5-13) into equation (5-9) yields:

$$\frac{dM_t}{dt} = \left(\frac{A^2 P_o e^{Kt} C_o}{2t} \right)^{1/2}$$

(5-14)

A plot of the integrated form of equation (5-14) is given in Fig. V-11. Due to polymer erosion the permeability increases, and the release rate increases when the erosion rate exceeds the diffusion rate.

Heller et al. [14] studied the release of levonorgestrel from a poly(ortho ester) containing 30% drug and various amounts of calcium lactate, which is slightly acidic. This poly(ortho ester) does not erode fast enough to deliver the drug within a targeted period due to the acidic nature of the polymer. As a result, calcium lactate is added to the drug-loaded polymer matrix to enhance the erosion rate. Depending on the amount of calcium lactate, the rate of polymer erosion and drug release is changed. Due to the presence of calcium lactate within the matrix, homogeneous erosion occurs because the penetration of water into the matrix causes the whole matrix to be a weak acid. Polymer erosion takes place everywhere in the matrix

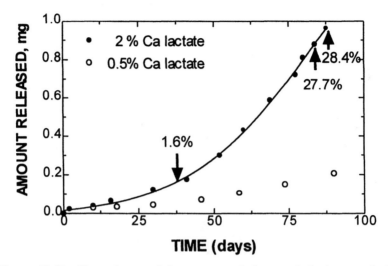

Figure V-12. The release of levonorgestrel from poly(ortho ester) film containing 30% drug and Ca lactate. (Graph reconstructed from data by Heller et al. [14].)

simultaneously. Basic excipients such as $Mg(OH)_2$ stabilize the polymer degradation and the rate of hydrolysis slows down [14]. As shown in Fig. V-12, the drug release kinetics from the poly(ortho ester) matrix qualitatively follows the pattern predicted by the theoretical model.

V.4.   Acid-Catalyzed Degradation and Erosion Systems

There are polymeric materials whose labile bonds are susceptible to acid catalyzed hydrolysis. Polymer erosion in these systems can be governed by the degree of acidic excipients incorporated in the matrix. For example, poly(ortho ester)s are stable in basic and neutral environment but are easily hydrolyzed in acidic media. The acceleration and retardation of polymer erosion is highly dependent upon excipient concentration in the polymer matrix. Another property of poly(orther ester) is its relative hydrophobicity, resulting in minimal water diffusion into the polymer matrix. One can design surface erosion controlled systems based on poly(ortho ester) if the erosion rate is fast enough to consume the water as it diffuses into the polymer matrix.

Fig. V-13 illustrates that the release of mitomycin C (1 wt%) in the poly(ortho ester) (M_w=29,600) matrix is a function of the amount of acidic and basic excipients [15]. Over a given concentration range, the release of the drug is linearly dependent upon the amount of the excipients. Above a certain concentration level, the amount of the excipients will not further accelerate or

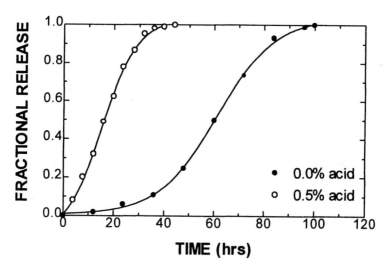

Figure V-13. The release of mitomycin C (1.0%) from poly(ortho ester) disks containing ascorbic acid. (Graph reconstructed from data by Merkl et al. [15].)

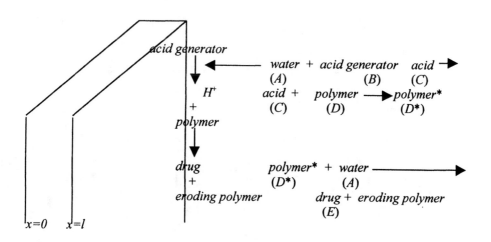

Figure V-14. Schematic diagram for acid catalyzed erosion system. (Graph reconstructed from figure by Joshi and Himmelstein [16].)

retard the release rate. This is most likely why drug release is governed by drug diffusion following water penetration into the polymer matrix. In particular, polymer erosion and drug release do not take place simultaneously. As the amount of $Mg(OH)_2$ increases, the polymer erosion still continues even after drug release is completed.

Joshi and Himmelstein [16] developed a mathematical model for drug release from acid catalyzed erosion systems, as depicted in Fig. V-14. The polymer matrix (denoted by D) contains a phthalic anhydride (B) as an acidic excipient and a drug (E). When the matrix is in contact with water, it diffuses into the matrix and hydrolyzes the anhydride to generate the catalytic acid (C) as follows:

$$A + B \Rightarrow C \qquad\qquad r_1 = k_1[A][B] \qquad\qquad (5\text{-}15)$$

The acid then catalyzes the polymer degradation:

$$C + D \Leftrightarrow D^* \qquad\qquad r_2 = k_2[C][D] - k_{-2}[D^*] \qquad\qquad (5\text{-}16)$$

The unstable intermediate ester (D^*) reacts with water to form degradation products:

$$D^* + A \Rightarrow C + products \quad r_3 = k_3[D^*][A] + k_4[D][A] \qquad\qquad (5\text{-}17)$$

The degradation products are water soluble and diffuse out of the matrix along with the drug and the catalyst into the surrounding environment as:

$$\frac{\partial C_i}{\partial t} = \frac{\partial}{\partial x} D_i(x,t) \frac{\partial C_i}{\partial x} + v_i \qquad\qquad (5\text{-}18)$$

where C_i is the concentration of diffusing species i, D_i is the diffusion coefficient of the species, x is the diffusion distance (total thickness $2a$), v_i is the net reaction rate of species i, and t is the time. The diffusion coefficient of the species i is assumed to be dependent on the concentration of polymer according to:

$$D_i = D_i^o e^{\frac{\mu(C_d^o - C_d)}{C_d^o}} \qquad\qquad i = A, B, C, E \qquad\qquad (5\text{-}19)$$

where D_i^o is the diffusion coefficient of the species i in the unhydrolyzed polymer, C_d^o is the initial polymer concentration, C_d is the polymer concentration at time t, and μ is a constant. Equation (5-18) is subject to the following initial and boundary conditions:

$$C_i(x,0) = 0 \qquad \text{for} \qquad 0 < x < a, i = A, C, D^* \tag{5-20a}$$

$$C_i(x,0) = C_i^o \qquad \text{for} \qquad 0 < x < a, i = B, D, E \tag{5-20b}$$

$$D_i(0,t)\frac{\partial C_i(0,t)}{\partial x} = 0, \qquad 0 < t, i = A, B, C, E \tag{5-20c}$$

$$D_i(0,t)\frac{\partial C_i(a,t)}{\partial t} = k_i\{C_{i,bulk} - C_i(a,t)\}, 0 < t, i = B, C, E \tag{5-20d}$$

where C_i^o and $C_{i,bulk}$ are the initial concentration of species i in the matrix and the bulk concentration of species in the medium, respectively. As shown in equations (5-18)-(5-20), drug release from acid catalyzed erosion processes relies on an interaction of the reaction and diffusion of multiple components in the matrix.

This model has been applied to the experimental data of Nguyen et al. [17]. Fig. V-15 shows the theoretical predictions and experimental data for a matrix containing 0.5% phthalic anhydride. The model predicts the experimental results qualitatively. The Thiele modulus, a dimensionless number, used to describe the relative contribution of diffusion process and reaction rate is given by:

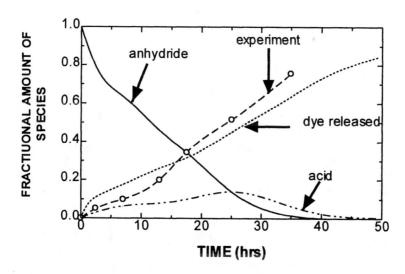

Figure V-15. Release of chemical species from poly(ortho ester) disc containing 0.5% anhydride. (Graph reconstructed from data by Joshi and Himmelstein [16].)

$$\phi^2 = \frac{a^2/D_{Ao}}{1/k_1 C_{Bo}} = \frac{\tau_d}{\tau_r} \tag{5-21}$$

where τ_d and τ_r are characteristic time constants for the diffusion process and reaction rate, respectively.

In Fig. V-15, a Thiele modulus of 1.06 was found for the matrix containing 0.5% phthalic anhydride, indicating that both the diffusion and the reaction mechanisms are similar controlling factors for drug release. However, other matrices containing 0.25% and 1.0% phthalic anhydride showed ϕ of 0.766 and 1.512, respectively, indicating that the governing release kinetics are reaction controlled (the rate of hydrolysis) and diffusion controlled, respectively.

V.5. Polymer Degradation via Autocatalysis

Polyesters [i.e. polylactic acid (PLA), polyglycolic acid (PGA), and poly(lactic acid-co-glycolic acid) (PLA/GA)] conform to a different degradation pattern. Fig. V-16 shows the *in vivo* degradation profiles of cylinders of different molecular weight PLA placed subcutaneously in the backs of rat [17]. The high molecular weight PLA showed a typical sigmoidal degradation curve characterized by a slow initial degradation followed by rapid degradation. A low molecular weight PLA, however, initially degraded rapidly. As investigated by GPC, a shift of the molecular weight distribution occurs during degradation in which the high molecular weight polymer is degraded to a lower molecular weight polymer. During the induction time (slow degradation), the high molecular weight polymer chains are split into low molecular weight polymer units. Then the intermediate molecular weight polymer degrades further to smaller oligomers or monomers. The smaller oligomers or monomers (lactic acid and glycolic acid) may contribute to the acid catalyzed degradation process of the polymer.

Vert and coworkers [19,20] investigated autocatalytic degradation mechanism of PLA and PLGA using various techniques such as weight loss, size exclusion chromatography (SEC), potentiometry, crystallinity, and water absorption. The degradation of PLA and PLGA is dependent on the chemical structures of the polymer and the change of the morphology of the polymer specimens. Himmelstein and George [21] modified the theoretical model of diffusing oligomers described in equation (5-18). Unlike poly(ortho ester) in which the degradation products do not participate in the polymer degradation process, the acidic species produced by the poly(lactide-glycolide) degradation catalyzed the hydrolysis of ester linkages [19,20]. These considerations are included in the modified model. However, it was assumed that only the smallest oligomers, ranging from monomer to tetramers, are able to catalyze the hydrolysis of the ester bond and diffuse through the polymer

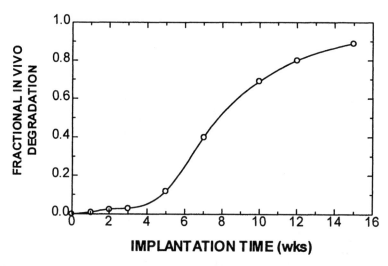

Figure V-16. *In vivo* drug release from cylindrical shapes of copolymer of l-LA and dl-HIVA. (Graph reconstructed from data by Fukuzaki et al. [17].)

matrix. In order to calculate the rate of oligomer production and the change in distribution of molecular weight, Grancher's random scission distribution calculation method [22] was used as follows:

$$f_p(i) = \frac{(1-p)^{i-1}}{1+p(M-1)}(f_i + p\sum(2+p(n-1-i)f(n)))$$ (5-22)

where f is the frequency distribution of the oligomer i and M is the number average degree of polymerization.

This model predicts the shift of the molecular weight distribution to lower molecular weights in the center of the matrix as release. This agrees with experimental observation [19,20]. Smaller oligomers are produced which catalyze the hydrolysis reaction and diffuse through the polymer matrix. However, near the surface of the matrix, the smaller oligomers escape from the matrix into the surrounding environment, resulting in the absence of catalyzed hydrolysis. Therefore, at the center of the matrix, the concentration of small oligomers is high and the rate of hydrolysis of the ester linkage is more rapid than near the surface. The molecular weight distribution throughout the matrix is shifted significantly and one may theoretically predict a non-normal distribution of molecular weight near the surface. This has been observed experimentally by Vert et al. [19,20].

V.6. Polymer Erosion/Drug Diffusion Controlled Systems

Drug release from a degradable or erodible matrix may occur through the drug diffusion layer. Lee [23] reported a theoretical expression for the drug diffusion/polymer dissolution controlled system. Upon contact with a dissolution medium, the dissolution medium diffuses into the polymer matrix and dissolved drug in the matrix is released. When the polymer concentration at the interface between the polymer and dissolution medium reaches a critical level, the polymer begins dissolving. When the diffusion rate of dissolution medium and the polymer dissolution rate are equal, or balanced, the drug-depleted layer is synchronized and constant until the dry polymer core completely dissolves as shown in Fig. V-18. At this point, the diffusion of drug through the synchronized gel layer reaches a pseudo-steady state. If the surface area at the swelling front is constant during the synchronized period in planar geometry, the release kinetics are zero-order.

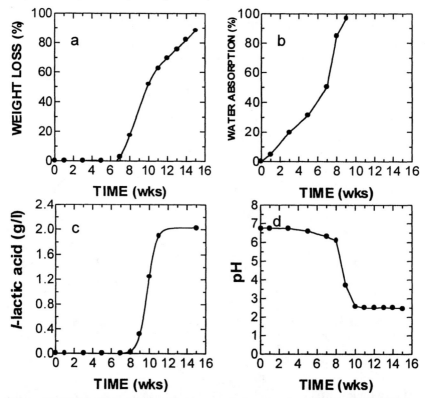

Figure V-17. Change of some parameters during the degradation of PLA50 in saline. (a) Weight loss, (b) water absorption, (c) l-lactic acid concentration, and pH. (Graph reconstructed from data by Li et al. [19].)

Lee [23] used a heat balance integral method to solve the diffusion and mass balance equations for non-swelling but erodible matrices in the form of planar slabs:

$$\frac{\partial C}{\partial C} = D\frac{\partial^2 C}{\partial x^2}$$

(5-23)

The initial and boundary conditions are:

$$D\frac{\partial C}{\partial t} = (A - C_s)\frac{\partial R}{\partial t} \qquad\qquad x = R \qquad\qquad (5\text{-}24\text{a})$$

$$\frac{\partial C}{\partial x} = (A - C_s)\left(\frac{\partial R}{\partial t} - \frac{\partial S}{\partial t}\right) \qquad x = S - R \qquad (5\text{-}24\text{b})$$

$$R = a \qquad\qquad\qquad t = 0 \qquad\qquad (5\text{-}24\text{c})$$

$$C = 0 \qquad\qquad\qquad x = S \qquad\qquad (5\text{-}24\text{d})$$

$$C = C_s \qquad\qquad\qquad x = R \qquad\qquad (5\text{-}24\text{e})$$

$$\left(D\frac{\partial C}{\partial x}\right)^2 + (A - C_s)\frac{\partial S}{\partial t}\frac{\partial C}{\partial x} + (A - C_s)D\frac{\partial^2 C}{\partial x^2} = 0 \qquad x = S - R \qquad (5\text{-}24\text{f})$$

The fractional release of a drug from this type matrix is given by:

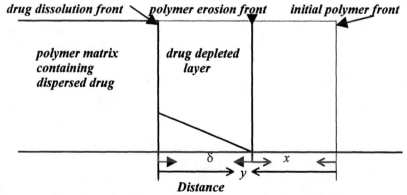

Figure V-18. Schematic diagram of an erosion/diffusion controlled system containing dispersed drug.

$$\frac{M_t}{M_\infty} = \delta + \left(\frac{Ba}{D}\right)\tau - \delta\left(\frac{C_s}{C_o}\right)\left(\frac{1}{2} + \frac{a_3}{6}\right) \tag{5-25}$$

$$\tau = \frac{1}{12}\left(6\left(\frac{C_o}{C_s}\right) - 4 - a_3\right)\left(\delta - \frac{1}{2h}\ln(1 + 2\delta h)\right) \tag{5-26a}$$

where B is the rate of surface erosion, D is the diffusion coefficient of the drug, τ is the dimensionless time (Dt/l^2), δ is the thickness of the diffusional layer, ($(S–R)/l$), l is the half of membrane thickness, C_o is the drug loading, C_s is the drug solubility, and a_3 is given by:

$$a_3 = \frac{C_o}{C_s} + \delta h - \sqrt{\left(\frac{C_o}{C_s} + \delta h\right)^2 - (1 + 2\delta h)} \tag{5-26b}$$

$$h = \frac{1}{2}\left(1 - \frac{C_o}{C_s}\right)\left(\frac{Bl}{D}\right) \tag{5-26c}$$

The fractional release initially obeys first-order kinetics followed by zero-order kinetics depending upon Bl/D, as shown in Fig. V-19. For a given value of Bl/D (i.e. 1), the fractional release from a planar erodible matrix obeys zero-order kinetics as the drug loading level, (A/C_s), is increased above the drug's solubility in the matrix. The diffusion front coincides with the erosion front as A/C_s increases [23]. The simultaneous completion of the diffusion front and erosion front is noticeable when Bl/D increases for a given drug loading level. One may postulate that at high loading levels ($A/C_s \approx 10$) and/or when the drug has low drug solubility in the polymer matrix, the drug release from a planar erodible polymer matrix may be zero order with an initial Fickian diffusion.

If there is no drug diffusion layer (i.e. $\delta=0$), then equation (5-25) reduces to equation (5-5). When $A<C_s$, the fractional release can be calculated from [23]:

$$\frac{M_t}{M_\infty} = \sqrt{\frac{4\tau}{3}} + \left(\frac{Ba}{D}\right)t \tag{5-27a}$$

However, if the swelling is involved in the drug release processes, the equation is complicated by many physical parameters characterizing polymer and solvent, which cannot be easily determined.

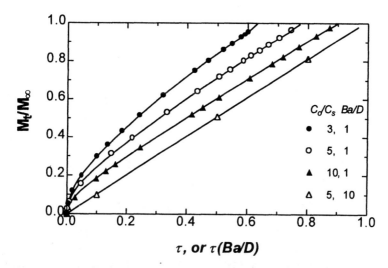

Figure V-19. Effect of drug loading, erosion, and drug diffusion on drug release kinetics from erosion/diffusion controlled matrices.

Fischel-Ghodsian and Newton [24] analyzed equation (5-23) under the pseudo-steady-state approximation in which the concentration gradient is linear. The rate of the diffusion front movement can be expressed by [24]:

$$\frac{dR}{dt} = \frac{D}{\left(\dfrac{A}{C_s} - 1\right)(R - S)}$$

(5-27b)

The release rate then becomes:

$$\frac{dM_t}{dt} = \frac{DSC_s}{R - S}$$

(5-27c)

At steady-state, $d(R-S)/dt=0$ and $R-S$ becomes:

$$(R - S)_{ss} = \frac{D}{aB(A/C_s - 1)}$$

(5-27d)

Then the steady-state release rate becomes:

$$\left(\frac{dM_t}{dt}\right)_{ss} = aBSC_s\left(\frac{A}{C_s} - 1\right) \tag{5-27e}$$

V.7.   Swelling/Erosion Controlled Systems

If the polymer material used to formulate controlled release dosage forms is swellable and erodible, drug release phenomenon is a little more complicated than that described for erosion/diffusion systems. When swellable/erodible polymer is in contact with water, the polymer swells in the early stage of release because the polymer concentration at the interface between the dissolution medium and the swollen gel is above the polymer's solubility. The erosion rate of the swollen gel provides a small contribution in the drug release from the matrix. However, as soon as the polymer concentration reaches a threshold level, the swollen polymer starts to erode. During these processes (swelling and erosion), drug release takes place through the swollen gel layer. At first, water diffuses in the polymer matrix and the polymer becomes a swollen gel and the drug dissolution (or polymer swelling front) is formed. When the swelling rate and erosion rate are equal, the moving fronts (swelling and erosion fronts) are synchronized so that the gel thickness between the erosion fronts and swelling front is constant until the swelling front disappears or meets at the core of matrix, as illustrated in Fig. V-20. Within the synchronized region (constant gel thickness), the linear concentration gradient is established such that the drug concentration at the swelling front is constant as an initial concentration and that at the erosion front assumed to be 0 under perfect sink conditions. The sooner the synchronized gel layer is established, the earlier the drug release becomes linear. However, the linear drug release can be achieved only from planar geometry in which the amount of drug at the swelling front is constant due to a constant surface area. For cylindrical or spherical geometry, nonlinear (non-Fickian) release is observed. This is attributed to the decreasing surface area at the swelling front as the front moves inwards.

Harland et al. [25], Lee [23], Lee and Peppas [26], and Narasimhan and Peppas [27] mathematically interpreted the drug release from a swelling/erosion controlled matrix system (planar geometry). The equations of solvent diffusion and drug release are

$$\frac{\partial C_{ss}}{\partial t} = D\frac{\partial^2 C_{ss}}{\partial x^2} \tag{5-28a}$$

$$\frac{\partial C_{dd}}{\partial t} = D\frac{\partial^2 C_{dd}}{\partial x^2} \tag{5-28b}$$

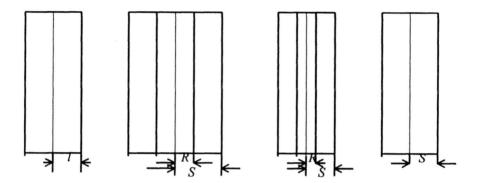

Figure V-20. Schematic presentation of the swelling/erosion controlled system.

$$\frac{\partial C_p}{\partial t} = D_p \frac{\partial^2 C_p}{\partial x^2} - \frac{dS}{dt}\frac{\partial C_p}{\partial x} \qquad (5\text{-}28c)$$

where the subscripts s, d, and p denote the swelling solvent, the drug, and the polymer, respectively. Equation (5-28c) describes the diffusion of the dissolved polymer through the swollen gel layer.

The initial and boundary conditions for equations (5-28a) -(5-28c) are:

$$t=0 \qquad\qquad C_s = C_d = 0 \qquad\qquad (5\text{-}29a)$$

$$(C_s + C_d)\frac{\partial R}{\partial t} = -(D\frac{\partial C_s}{\partial x} + D_d \frac{\partial C_d}{\partial x}) \qquad \text{at } x = R \qquad (5\text{-}29b)$$

$$C_s = C_s^*, \qquad C_d = C_d^* \qquad\qquad \text{at } x = R \qquad (5\text{-}29c)$$

$$C_s = C_{s,eq}, \qquad C_d = C_{d,eq} \qquad\qquad \text{at } x = S \qquad (5\text{-}29d)$$

$$S = l \qquad\qquad\qquad \text{at } t = 0 \qquad (5\text{-}29e)$$

$$C_s = C_{s,o} \qquad\qquad\qquad \text{at } t = 0 \qquad (5\text{-}29f)$$

The polymer and drug concentration at the interface R in terms of volume fraction are given as follows:

$$C_p^* = \frac{\dfrac{1}{\rho_p}}{\left(\dfrac{1}{\rho_p} + \dfrac{T_g - T}{\beta/\alpha_f}\dfrac{1}{\rho_s} + \dfrac{1}{\rho_d}\right)} , \; C_d^* = \frac{\dfrac{1}{\rho_d}}{\left(\dfrac{1}{\rho_p} + \dfrac{T_g - T}{\beta/\alpha_f}\dfrac{1}{\rho_s} + \dfrac{1}{\rho_d}\right)} \qquad (5\text{-}29\text{g})$$

where ρ, β, α_f, T_g, and T are the density, the expansion coefficient contribution of the solvent to the polymer, the linear expansion coefficient of the polymer, the glass transition temperature of the polymer, and the experimental temperature, respectively. The equilibrium concentration of polymer and drug at the rubbery/solvent interface S is given as follows:

$$\ln C_{s,eq} + (1 - \frac{1}{\varepsilon})(1 - C_{s,eq}) + \chi(1 - C_{s,eq})^2$$
$$+ \bar{V}_s \rho_p (\frac{2}{M_c} - \frac{1}{M_n})(\frac{2}{1 - C_{s,eq}} - (1 - C_{s,eq})) = 0 \qquad (5\text{-}29\text{h})$$

$$\ln C_{d,eq} + (1 - \frac{1}{\varepsilon})(1 - C_{d,eq}) + \chi_d(1 - C_{d,eq})^2$$
$$+ \bar{V}_d \rho_p (\frac{2}{M_c} - \frac{1}{M_n})(\frac{2}{1 - C_{d,eq}} - (1 - C_{d,eq})) = 0 \qquad (5\text{-}29\text{i})$$

where χ is the polymer-solvent, χ_d is the drug-polymer interaction parameter, M_n is the number average molecular weight of the polymer, M_c is the critical polymer molecular weight, $\bar{V}_s$ is the molar volume of the solvent, and $\bar{V}_d$ is the drug molar volume. x and x_d are defined as:

$$x = \frac{M_n v}{\bar{V}_s} , \qquad\qquad x_d = \frac{M_n v}{\bar{V}_d} \qquad (5\text{-}29\text{j})$$

where v is the specific volume of the polymer. At the end of the boundary layer,

$$-D_p \frac{\partial C_p}{\partial x} = 0, \qquad x = S^+(t), \qquad 0 < t < t_r \qquad (5\text{-}29\text{k})$$

$$-D_p \frac{\partial C_p}{\partial x} = k_d, \qquad x = S^+(t), \qquad t > t_r \qquad (5\text{-}29\text{l})$$

where k_d is the disentanglement rate and can be calculated by [27]:

$$k_d = \frac{r_g}{t_r} \qquad (5\text{-}29m)$$

where r_g is the radius of gyration of the polymer chains and t_r is the minimum time taken by the polymer chains to disentangle.

The solvent/rubbery interface, S, moves as:

$$\frac{\partial S}{\partial t} = \frac{D_s C_{s,eq}}{C_{s,eq} + C_{d,eq}} \frac{\partial C_s}{\partial x} + \frac{D_d C_{d,eq}}{C_{s,eq} + C_{d,eq}} \frac{\partial C_d}{\partial x} - \frac{D_p}{C_{s,eq} + C_{d,eq}} \frac{\partial C_p}{\partial x} \qquad (5\text{-}29n)$$

Pseudo-steady state solutions have been developed for these equations, assuming that the concentration profiles of the drug and the solvent in the swollen gel are linear [27]:

$$-\frac{S-R}{B} - \frac{A}{B^2}(S-R) = t \qquad (5\text{-}30a)$$

$$A = D_s(C_{s,eq} - C_s^*)\left(\frac{C_{s,eq}}{C_{s,eq} + C_{d,eq}} + \frac{1}{C_s^* + C_d^*} \right)$$
$$+ D_d(C_d^* - C_{d,eq})\left(\frac{C_{d,eq}}{C_{s,eq} + C_{d,eq}} + \frac{1}{C_s^* + C_d^*} \right) \qquad (5\text{-}30b)$$

$$B = \frac{k_d}{C_{s,eq} + C_{d,eq}} \qquad (5\text{-}30c)$$

The fractional release of the drug can be expressed by [27]:

$$\frac{M_t}{M_\infty} = \frac{C_{d,eq} + C_d^*}{2l}\left(\sqrt{2At} + Bt \right) \qquad (5\text{-}31)$$

When $B^2 / A \gg 1$, the contribution of drug diffusion to the overall drug release kinetics is minimal and the first term of the right-hand side of equation (5-31) can be neglected giving:

$$\frac{M_t}{M_\infty} = \frac{k_d(C_{d,eq} + C_d^*)}{2l(C_{s,eq} + C_{d,eq})} t , \qquad (5\text{-}32a)$$

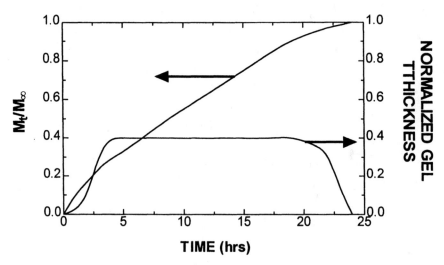

TIME (hrs)

Figure V-21. Theoretical profiles of swollen gel thickness and fractional release with time for a well-chosen swelling/erosion controlled system.

For $B^2 / A \ll 1$, the drug diffusion through the swollen gel layer governs drug release kinetics and then

$$\frac{M_t}{M_\infty} = \sqrt{\frac{A}{2}} \frac{C_{d,eq} + C_d^*}{l} \sqrt{t} \qquad (5\text{-}32b)$$

The glass/rubbery interface, R, and the rubbery/solvent interface, S, can be obtained under the pseudo-steady state approximation [27]:

$$(C_s^* + C_d^*)\frac{dR}{dt} = -\frac{D_s}{S-R}(C_{s,eq} - C_s^*) - \frac{D_d}{S-R}(C_{d,eq} - C_d^*) \qquad (5\text{-}33a)$$

$$\frac{dS}{dt} = \frac{C_{s,eq}}{C_{s,eq} + C_{d,eq}} \frac{D_s}{S-R}(C_{s,eq} - C_s^*)$$

$$+ \frac{C_{d,eq}}{C_{s,eq} + C_{d,eq}} \frac{D_d}{S-R}(C_{d,eq} - C_d^*) - \frac{k_d}{C_{s,eq} + C_{d,eq}} \qquad (5\text{-}33b)$$

The gel thickness during the synchronized period can be expressed by combining equations (5-33a) and (5-33b) and setting $d(S{-}R)/dt = 0$ [27]:

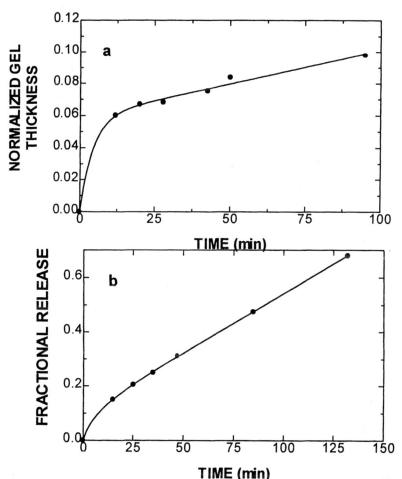

Figure V-22. Model prediction of normalized gel thickness (a) and fractional release (b) from PVA tablets. (Graph reconstructed from data by Narashinhan and Peppas [27].)

$$S-R=\frac{1}{k_d}\left\{\begin{array}{l} D_s(C_{s,eq}-C_s^*)\left(C_{s,eq}-\dfrac{C_{s,eq}+C_{d,eq}}{C_s^*+C_d^*}\right) \\[4mm] +D_d(C_{d,eq}-C_d^*)\left(C_{d,eq}-\dfrac{C_{s,eq}+C_{d,eq}}{C_s^*+C_d^*}\right) \end{array}\right\} \qquad (5\text{-}33c)$$

Equations (5-31) and (5-32) suggest that the selection of a polymer-solvent-drug system meeting the above condition could lead to a zero-order release system, as shown in Fig. V-21. This can be obtained by choosing the solvent, polymer, and drug with appropriate values for diffusivities of solvent and polymer, equilibrium concentrations of solvent and drug, polymer molecular weight, and solvent-polymer interaction parameter. Narashinhan and Peppas [27] demonstrated the validity of this model as shown in Figs. V-22a and V-22b. The predictions were made with parameters determined independently from various equations.

Some of parameters in equations (5-31)-(5-32) can be estimated or determined from physicochemical properties of the drug, drug release experiments, and swelling/erosion measurements [27]. In cases where some parameters are not known, the drug release kinetics from swelling/erosion controlled systems can be expressed semi-empirically by [25]:

$$\frac{M_t}{M_\infty} = \alpha\sqrt{t} + \beta t \tag{5-34}$$

where α and β are related to a drug diffusion and a polymer erosion term, respectively. In the overall drug release process, both swelling and polymer erosion occur simultaneously. However, when the two fronts (swelling and erosion) are synchronized, the diffusional term becomes negligible and the drug release rate is independent of time and drug solubility [25].

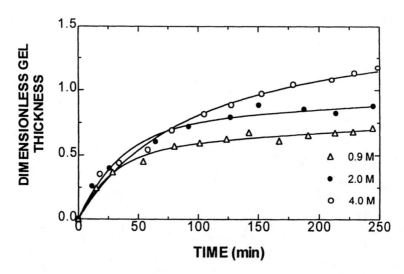

Figure V-23. Dimensionless gel thickness of different polyethylene oxide tablets. (Graph reconstructed from data by Kim [28].)

Recently Kim [28] studied drug release from polyethylene oxide (PEO) matrices including measurement of the swelling and erosion fronts. When the molecular weight of PEO is below 2×10^6, a synchronized gel layer was observed as shown in Fig. V-23. Apicella et al [29] also reported a constant gel thickness with polymer molecular weight of 0.6×10^6, although the matrices formulated with $M_w = 4 \times 10^6$ did not furnish constant gel thickness but an ever increasing gel layer. Kim [28] demonstrated that zero-order release kinetics might be maintained when using PEO of $M_w = 0.9 \times 10^6$ regardless of drug solubility and drug loading. A noted exception is diclofenac Na (solubility ≈ 25000 mg/l). For diclofenac Na, drug diffusion plays an important role in release kinetics, as shown in Fig. V-23 [28]. For highly water-soluble drugs (e.g. diclofenac Na), water penetration is much faster than the rate of swelling, leading to rapid diffusion of the drug through the unswollen polymer matrix.

Kim and Lee [30] observed the same phenomenon with the noncross-linked poly(methyl methacrylate-co-methacrylic acid) beads loaded with polypeptide. The PMMA/MAA has the same composition of commercially available polymer, Eudragit L & S, which is used for enteric coating. Because of the specific application of Eudragit L & S (enteric coating), its dissolution rate is too fast to be used for erosion-controlled delivery systems. Lowering the initiator concentration, resulting in the low polymerization rate, may increase the molecular weight of PMMA/MAA. However, high molecular weight PMMA/MAA is not dissolved, even at alkaline pH. The PMMA/MAA used in Fig. V-24 was made from polymer having an intermediate molecular weight, which dissolves at weak base or

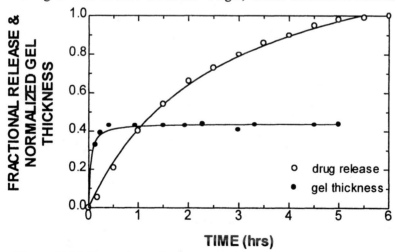

TIME (hrs)

Figure V-24. Dynamic swelling/erosion behavior and drug release of GHRH from erodible PMMA/MAA beads. (Graph reconstructed from data by Kim and Lee [30].)

neutral pH. The swelling/dissolution and fractional release profiles are shown in Fig. V-24. The swollen gel thickness initially increases followed by the constant gel thickness region (synchronization) before decreasing.   As observed for tablets, the synchronized gel layer (constant) is formed after swelling and dissolution rates are balanced.   As shown in Fig. V-24, the overall dimensional changes (dissolution front) reach a maximum the early stage of high swelling, drug release slowly decreases. After the dissolution front (or overall dimension) passes a maximum level, the dissolution front and swelling front move at the same rate until the core disappears.   The swelling front accelerates near the center of the core, as found commonly in spherical or cylindrical geometry. Due to the decrease of surface area at the swelling front, a linear release rate is not obtainable.

V.8. Preparation of Biodegradable Microparticles

Due to their bio-compatibility, cost, and regulatory approval, a major application of biodegradable polymers [poly(lactic acid), poly(glycolic acid), and poly(lactic acid-co-glycolic acid)] is the delivery of bioactive peptides, proteins, and vaccines. Bio-active peptides, proteins, and vaccines have very short half-lives so that the parenteral (injection and implant) route is the most suitable route of administration for these drugs. Several microencapsulation processes have been developed for the controlled release of the bioactive peptides, proteins, and vaccines; e.g., solvent evaporation (O/W, W/O, O/O, and W/O/W emulsions) and phase separation methods.

In solvent evaporation procedures (O/W, W/O, and O/O), drugs are dissolved or dispersed in a liquid phase which has a lower boiling temperature.   The solution or dispersion is then emulsified in another liquid phase with the aid of surfactants.   As soon as a homogeneous emulsion has been achieved, the resulting emulsion is heated to remove the dispersed solvent, resulting in the precipitation of biodegradable polymers as monolithic microparticles.   For example, injectable microparticles of poly(lactic acid) containing adriamycin have been prepared by the O/O solvent evaporation method [31].   Fig. V-25 illustrates the processes of the O/O solvent evaporation method. Adriamycin and poly(lactic acid) were dissolved in a small quantity of water and water-miscible acetonitrile at 40°C and the resulting solution was dispersed in paraffin oil containing Span 40 (2% w/w). The O/O emulsion was agitated for 24 hours under atmospheric pressure at room temperature and the dispersed medium (acetonitrile) was allowed to evaporate.   The solidified micro-particles were recovered by centrifugation followed by a purification process to remove the residual solvents and surfactant before drying under vacuum.

The O/W emulsion solvent evaporation method is not suitable for the preparation of micro-particles when water-soluble bio-active drugs are encapsulated due to high partitioning into the aqueous phase. This leads to

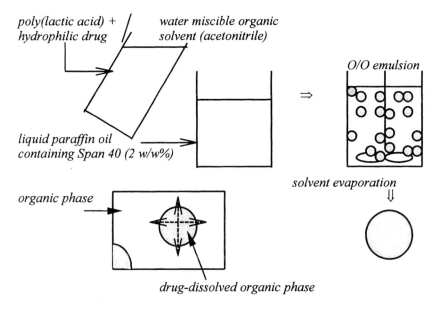

Figure V-25. Schematic procedure of an O/O emulsion solvent evaporation method for the preparation of poly(lactic acid) microparticles containing a bioactive drug. (Graph reconstructed from figure by Hyon [31].)

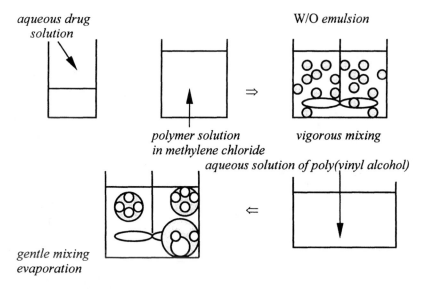

Figure V-26. Schematic diagram for W/O/W emulsion/evaporation processes.

poor encapsulation efficiency of the micro-particles. The O/W solvent evaporation process has been modified to overcome the problem by the addition of co-solvent to the oil phase and formation of reverse micelles [32,33].

The most commonly used micro-encapsulation of highly water-soluble bio-active drugs is the W/O/W double emulsion method shown in Fig. V-26. In this method [34, 35], a small volume of aqueous drug solution of drugs is dispersed in an organic solution of biodegradable polymers (primary emulsion). The primary W/O emulsion is subsequently dispersed again in water containing a surfactant to produce a double emulsion (W/O/W). The organic solvent diffuses into the water and evaporates. Then, the biodegradable polymers solidify and entrap the bio-active drugs. For example [36], a bio-active drug (Leuprolide acetate) and gelatin were dissolved in water at 60°C followed dispersion in a methylene chloride solution of poly(lactic acid-co-glycolic acid) with a homogenizer (W/O). The W/O emulsion was then re-emulsified in an aqueous solution of 0.25% poly(vinyl alcohol). The organic solvent (methylene chloride) was allowed to evaporate with stirring. The resulting micro-particles are washed and lyophilized. To optimize dosage form formulations, one has to consider the effect of polymer solution concentration, stabilizer concentration, and the mixing intensity on the morphology of the micro-particles. All these parameters are believed to affect drug release kinetics [36].

In a phase separation process [37], an aqueous solution of a bio-active drug (LHRH) is emulsified in a solution of poly(lactic acid-co-glycolic acid) in methylene chloride to form a W/O emulsion. A non-solvent for the copolymer is slowly added to the W/O emulsion and the copolymer is precipitated out around the aqueous phase. The micro-particles are then transferred to a large volume of non-solvent to remove residual solvent and surfactant and for further hardening.

References

1. J. Heller, "Controlled Release of Biologically Active Compounds from Bioerodible Polymers," *Biomaterials*, 1, 51 (1980).
2. K. W. Leong, "Synthetic Biodegradable Polymer Drug Delivery Systems," in Polymers for Controlled Drug Delivery, P. T. Tarcha (Ed.), CRC Press, Boca Raton, Fl., 1991, p127.
3. R. J. Kelly, *Rev. Surg.* (Mar. AP), 142 (1970).
4. J. Heller, "Development of Poly(ortho esters): A Historical Overview," *Biomaterials*, 11, 659 (1990).
5. J. Heller, R. W. Baker, R. M. Gall, and J. O. Rodin, "Controlled Drug release by Polymer Dissolution. I. Partial Esters of Maleic Anhydride Copolymers – Properties and Theory," *J. Appl. Polym. Sci.*, 22, 1991 (1978).

6. K. R. Sidman, A. D. Schwope, W. D. Steber, S. E. Rudolph, and S. B. Poulin, "Biodegradable, Implantable Sustained Release Systems Based on Glutamic Acid Copolymers," *J. Membr. Sci.*, 7, 277 (1980).

7. J. Heller, R. E. Helwing, R. W. Baker, and M. E. Tuttle, "Controlled Release of Water-Soluble Macromolecules from Bioerodible hydrogels," *Biomaterials*, 4, 262 (1983).

8. H. T. Dellicolli, "Pine Kraft Lignin as a Pesticide Delivery System," in Controlled Release Technologies: methods, Theory, and Applications, Vol. II, A. F. Kydonieus (Ed.), CRC Press, Boca Raton, Fl., 1980, p225.

9. L. A. Carpino, H. Ringsdorf, and H. R. Her, "Pharmacologically Active Polymers. 10. Preparation and Polymerization of 1-O-(4-Methacroylaminophenyl)- -givcopyranoside," *Markromol. Chem.*, 177, 635 (1976).

10. A. J. Domb, E. Mathiowitz, E. Ron, S. Giannos, and R. Langer, *J. Polym. Sci. Polm. Chem.*, 29, 571 (1991).

11. J. W. Leong, B. C. Brott, and R. Langer, *J. Biomed. Mater. Res.*, 19, 941 (1985).

12. G. H. Zhang, W. A. Vadimo, and I. Chaudy, "Drug Release from Erodible Tablets," *Proceed. Int. Symp. Control. Rel. Bioact. Mater.*, 17, 331 (1990).

13. C. J. Kim, Unpublished data.

14. J. Heller and R. W. Baker, "Theory and Practice of Controlled Drug Delivery from Bioerodible Polymers," in Controlled Release of Bioactive Materials, R. W. Baker (Ed.), Academic Press, New York, 1980, p1.

15. A. Merkl, J. Heller, C. Tabatabay, and R. Gurny, "The Use of Acidic and Basic Excipients in the Release of 5-Fluorouracil and Mitomycin C from a Semi-Solid Bioerodible Poly(orthoester)," *J. Control. Rel.*, 33, 415 (1995).

16. A. Joshi and K. J. Himmelstein, "Dynamics of Controlled Release from Bioerodible Matrices," *J. Control. Rel.*, 15, 95 (1991).

17. T. H. Nguyen, T. Miguchi , and K. J. Himmelstein, "Erosion Characteristics of Catalyzed Poly(orthoester) Matrices," *J. Contol. Rel.*, 5, 1 (1987).

18. H. Fukuzaki, M. Yoshida, M. Asano, M. Kumakura, T. Mashimo, H. Yuasa, K. Imai, and H. Yamanaka, "In Vivo Characteristics of Low Molecular Weight Copolymers Composed of L-lactic Acid and Various DL-Hydroxy Acids as Bio-degradable Carriers for Drug Delivery Systems," *Biomaterials*, 11, 441 (1990).

19. S. M. Li, H. Garreau, and M. Vert, "Structure-Property Relationships in the Case of the Degradation of Massive Aliphatic Poly-(-Hydroxy Acids) in Aqueous Media, Part 1: Poly(DL-Lactic Acid)," *J. Mat. Sci. Mat. Med.*, 1, 123 (1990).

20. S. M. Li, H. Garreau, and M. Vert, "Structure-Property Relationships in the Case of the Degradation of Massive Aliphatic Poly-(-Hydroxy Acids) in Aqueous Media, Part 2 Degradation of Lactide-Glycolide Copolymers: PLA37.5GA25 and PLA75GA25," *J. Mat. Sci. Mat. Med.*, 1, 131 (1990).

21. K. J. Himmelstein and J. George, "Erosion of Polymers with Autocatalysis," *Proceed. Int. Symp. Control. Rel. Bioact. Mater.*, 20, 53 (1993).

22. G. Grander, in Biodegradable Polymers and Plastics, Vert et al. (Eds.), 1991.

23. P. I. Lee, "Diffusional Release of a Solute from a Polymer Matrix – Approximate Analytical Solutions, *J. Membr. Sci.*, 7, 255 (1980).

24. F. Fischer-Ghodsian and J. M. Newton, "Analysis of Drug Release Kinetics from Degradable Polymeric Device," *J. Drug Targeting*, 1, 51 (1993).

25. R. S. Harland, A. Gazzaniga, M. E. Sanglli, P. Colombo, and N. A. Peppas, "Drug/Polymer Matrix Swelling and Dissolution," *Pharm. Res.*, 5, 488 (1988).

26. P. I. Lee and N. A. Peppas, "Prediction of Polymer Dissolution in Swellable Controlled-Release Systems," *J. Control. Rel.*, 6, 207 (1987).

27. B. Narashinhan and N. A. Peppas, "Molecular Analysis of Drug Delivery Systems Controlled by Dissolution of the Polymer Carrier," *J. Pharm. Sci.*, 86, 297 (1997).

28. C. J. Kim, "Drug Release from Compressed Hydrophilic POLYOX-WSR Tablets," *J. Pharm. Sci.*, 84, 303 (1995).

29. A. Apicella, B, Cappello, M. Del Nobile, M. I. La Rotonda, G. Mensitieri, and L. Nicolais, *Biomaterials*, 14, 83 (1993).

30. C. J. Kim and P. I. Lee, "Peptide Release from Erodible Hydrophobic Anionic Gel Beads," *Proceed. Int. Symp. Control. Rel. Bioact. Mater.*, 19, 208 (1992).

31. S.-H Hyon, "Ophthalmic Drug Delivery Systems using Biodegradable Polymers," *Polymer Preprint*, 37(2), 125 (1996).

32. L. R. Beck, D. R. Lewis, D. H. Cosgrove, C. T. Riddel, S. L. Lowry, and T. Epperly, "A New Long Injectable Microcapsule System for Administration of Progesterone," *Fertil. Steril.*, 31, 545 (1979).

33. J. H. Eldridge, J. K. Steas, J. A. Neulbrock, J. R. McGhee, T. R. Tice, and R. M. Gilley, "Biodegradable Microspheres as a Vaccine Delivery System," *Molec. Immun.*, 28, 287 (1991).

34. Y. Ogawa, M Yamamoto, H. Okada, T. Yashiki, and T. Shimamoto, "A New Technique of Efficiently Entrap Leuprolide Acetate into Microcapsules of Polylactic Acid or Copoly(lactic/glycolic Acid)," *Chem. Pharm. Bull.*, 36, 1095 (1989),

35. S. Cohen, T. Yoshioka, M. Lucaretti, L. H. Hwang, and R. Langer, "Controlled Delivery Systems for Proteins Based on Poly(lactic/glycolic acid) Microspheres," *Pharm. Res.*, 8, 713 (1991).

36. H. Rafati, A. G. A. Coombes, J. Adler, J. Holland, S. S. Davis, "Protein-Loaded Poly(DL-lactic-co-glycolide) Microparticles for Oral Administration: Formulation, Structural and Release Characteristics," *J. Control. Rel.* 43, 89 (1997).

37. L. M. Sanders, J. S. Kent, G. I. Mcrae, B. H. Vickery, T. R. Tice, and D. H. Lewis, "Controlled Release of Leutinizing Hormone Releasing Hormone Analogue from Poly(d,l-Lactide-co-Glycolide) Microspheres," *J. Pharm. Sci.*, 73, 1294 (1984).

Chapter VI

Ion Exchange Resin Drug Delivery Systems

VI.1. Exchange Processes and Equilibrium

Ion exchange resins have been developed for cation and anion removal from water. Ions to be exchanged, or removed, from water diffuse into the resin and replace counter ions in the polymeric resin chains. The exchanged ions diffuse out of the resin. The same principle has been applied to drug delivery systems. The use of ion exchange resins to deliver drugs is based on the principle that ionic drugs will bind to the functional groups of the resin [1]. For example:

$$R\text{-}SO_3^-Na^+ + Cl^{-\,+}NH_2 - A \implies R - SO_3^- -^+NH_2 - A$$

$$R\text{-}N^+Cl^- + Na^{+\,-}OOC - B \implies R - N^+ -^-OOC - B$$

where $Cl^{-\,+}NH_2 - A$ and $Na^{+\,-}OOC - B$ represent a basic and an acidic drug, respectively, and $R - SO_3^-Na^+$ and $R - N^+Cl^-$ represent cation and anion exchange resins, respectively. Oral administration of these resinates (drug/resin complexes) liberates the drug by an ion exchange reaction with counter ions present in the gastro-intestinal fluid.

In the stomach:
$$\overset{HCl}{R - SO_3^- -^+NH_2 - A \implies Cl^{-\,+}NH_2 - A + R - SO_3^-H}$$

$$R - N^+ -^-OOC - B \implies HOOC - B + R - N^+Cl^-$$

In the intestine:
$$\overset{NaCl}{R - SO_3^- -^+ NH_2 - A \implies Cl^{-\,+}NH_2 - A + R - SO_3^-Na^+}$$

$$R - N^+ -^-OOC - B \implies Na^{+\,-}OOC - B + R - N^+Cl^-$$

The major advantage of using an ion exchange resin system for drug delivery is that the number of available functional charge groups limits the amount of drug that can be loaded onto the resin. Many of the problems

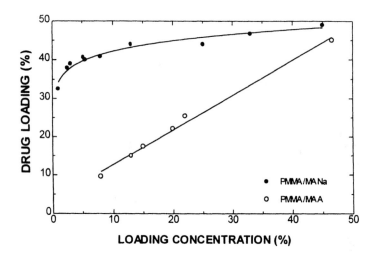

Figure VI-1. Comparative drug loading in nonionic beads and ionic beads. (Graph reconstructed from data by Kim and Lee [2].)

experienced with other monolithic matrix systems are not observed, e.g., faster drug release due to high loading. One can load poorly water-soluble drugs (less than 2%) to a loading level higher than 30%. Fig. VI-1 illustrates most the effect of the polymer type (nonionic and ionic) on drug loading. At high loading levels, most of the drug is bound to the ion exchange resin matrix, resulting in a long drug release. The pH and ionic strength of the dissolution medium do not affect the kinetics of drug release from strong cation exchange resins (i.e. sulfonic acid) [3]. However, drug release from weak cation exchange resins is retarded in weak acidic conditions. In general, sulfonic acid groups form stronger complexes than carboxylic acid groups.

In contrast, the disadvantages are that micro-porous ion exchange resins furnish faster drug diffusion and that the kinetics of drug release from gel type resins (tightly cross-linked) are controlled purely by drug-diffusion through the gel, resulting in a prolonged tailing-off of release until drug exhaustion.

It has been reported that the kinetics of drug release from drug/resin complexes are dependent upon the amine moieties of the drugs used, e.g. -NH_2, -NH-, -N-, and -N^+- [1]. The order of decreasing complex strength among the amine drugs follows -N- > -NH- > -NH_2. Quaternary amine drugs do not form complexes.

The law of mass action may be applied to describe the ion exchange phenomenon. If the exchange is treated as a simple stoichiometric reaction, this ion exchange reaction can be expressed as follows:

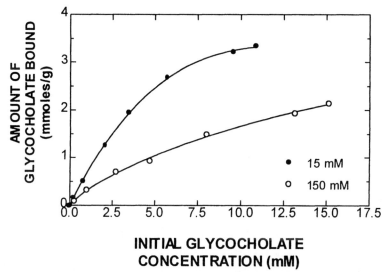

**INITIAL GLYCOCHOLATE
CONCENTRATION (mM)**

Figure VI-2. Binding isotherm of glycocholate into cholestyramine resins.
(Graph reconstructed from data by Polli and Amidon [4].)

$$A^+ \quad + \quad (R^-)B^+ \quad \Leftrightarrow \quad B^+ \quad +(R^-)A^+$$

where (R^-) is the cation ion exchange resin, A^+ is the incoming counter ion,
and B^+ is the drug to be released. According to the fundamental law of mass
action, the selectivity coefficient, K_B^A, has the form

$$K_B^A = \frac{[A^+]_r[B^+]}{[A^+][B^+]_r}$$

where $[A^+]_r$ is the concentration of bounded counter ion in the resin, $[B^+]$
is the concentration of free drug, $[A^+]$ is the concentration of free counter
ion, and $[B^+]_r$ is the concentration of bounded drug in the resin. Fig. VI-2
shows an equilibrium binding isotherm of glycocholate on cholestyramine
(anionic ion exchange resin) [4]. The amount of glycocholate complexation
to the resin increases as the glycocholate concentration increases. As
expected from the law of mass action for ion exchange, lower concentration
of ion exchange resin binding site and higher concentration of bile salt
(glycocholate ion) favor complex formation [4].

An important characteristic of ion exchange reactions is the
preferential binding of one ion over another. In ion exchange resin delivery
systems, (R^-) preferentially binds with A^+ rather than B^+. A selectivity

coefficient of equation (7-1) greater than one implies that the ion exchange resin prefers to bind with A^+.

VI.2. Commercial Ion Exchange Resin Materials

Commonly used ion exchange resins are classified as cation exchange or anion exchange resins depending upon whether the labile counter ion is a cation or anion. The matrix possesses ionic functional groups such as $-SO_3^-$ – and -COO$^-$ in cation exchangers and -N$^+$- in anion exchangers. Polymeric ion exchange resins are generally synthesized via a cross-linking reaction with the appropriate vinyl monomers. Sulfonic polystyrene resins are cross-linked with styrene and divinylbenzene (DVB) to which the sulfonic acid groups are introduced by treatment with sulfuric acid as shown in Fig. VI-3.

The major anion exchange resins are prepared by the same process as that for sulfonated polystyrene cross-linked with DVB. However, instead of sulfonation with sulfuric acid, the cross-linked polystyrene is chloromethylated and then further treated with a tertiary amine to obtain a quaternary amine binding site as shown in Fig. VI-4.

Carboxylic acid type cation exchange resins are directly prepared by the cross-linking polymerization of carboxylic acids (methacrylic acid or acrylic acid) with divinylbenzene as shown in Fig. VI-5. Ion exchange resins are able to swell due to the substitution of ionic groups. The degree of swelling of these resins depends on the degree of substitution of the ionic groups and the degree of cross-linking.

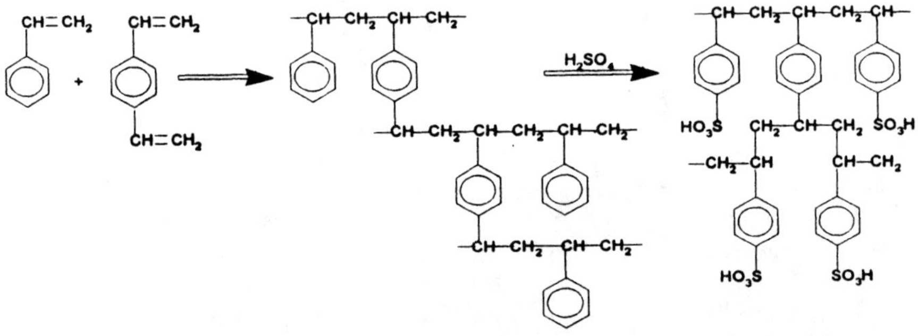

Figure VI-3. Synthetic process of sulfonated poly(styrene-co-divinylbenzene) (PS/DVB).

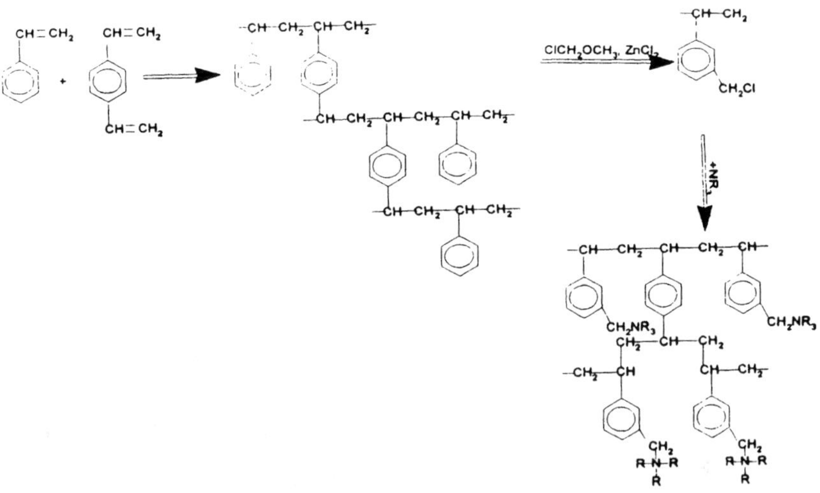

Figure VI-4. Synthetic process of quaternary amine poly(styrene-co-divinylbenzene).

Ion exchange resins containing sulfonic acid have a pK_a range near 1 and carboxylic acid has a pK_a range of 4-6. Carboxylic acid containing functional groups will be poorly dissociated in an acidic medium. Unlike strong cation exchange resins, the resins containing carboxylic acid have little complex formation with salt forms of drug other than HCl salt.

The two types of ion exchange resins are divided according to their morphological structures: gel or microporous. The gel-type resins are produced by the suspension polymerization of styrene or carboxylic acids with a cross-linking agent (i.e. DVB). In order to minimize the degree of swelling for use of ion exchange process for water treatment, the polymer beads are highly cross-linked, resulting in the slow diffusion of ions. Fast

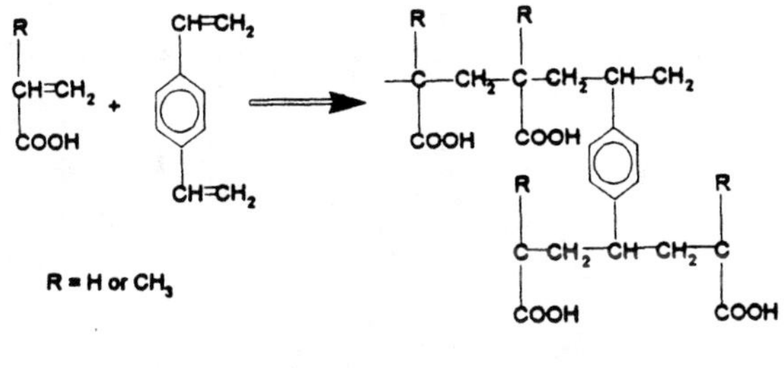

Figure VI-5. Synthetic process of cross-linked poly(methacrylic acid).

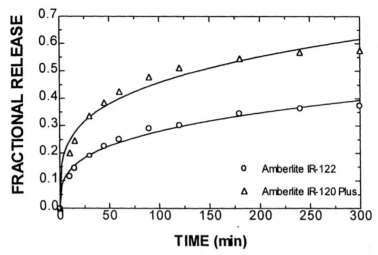

Figure VI-6. Release profiles of Amberlite Resins. (Graph reconstructed from data by Burke et al. [5].)

exchange reactions can be facilitated by a modification of the polymerization process before polymerization by adding a porogen, which is extracted after polymerization, to create the microporous resin structure.

VI.3. Drug Release from Commercial Ion Exchange Resins

Strongly acidic resins (sulfonic acid) are ionized at all pHs, whereas weakly acidic resins (carboxylic acid) are ionized in neutral and alkaline pH. Similarly, strongly basic resins (quaternary amine) remain ionized at all pHs, and weakly basic resins (tertiary amine) are ionized in acidic media. Strongly acidic resins produce stronger drug-resin complexes than weakly acidic resins, resulting in a slower release of drug from these resins. Weakly acidic resins are not ionized at gastric pH and do not release the bound drug. The particle size, percent cross-linking, exchange capacity, porosity, and acid-base strength of the functional groups are some of the important physicochemical properties on the performance of the CRDF [1]. Typical release profiles are shown in Fig. VI-6. The drug releases via square-root-of-time kinetics followed by a severe tailing without providing a complete release. However, there are several advantages to using ion exchange resins for sustained release dosage forms:

(1) The preparation of ion exchange dosage forms is simple.

(2) Drug loading is only limited by the exchanging capacity of the resin.

(3) No uncontrolled burst effect is experienced with drug-resin complex dosage forms even at high drug loading.

(4) Ion exchange resins provide designing different dosage forms (suspension, tablet, or capsule) and different route of administration (oral, ocular, or chewable).

However, there are some limitations using ion exchange resins for CRDF:

(1) Drug release kinetics follows the square-root-of-time because tightly cross-linked gel-type resins are used in drug resinate preparations, leading to a significant tailing.

(2) Complete drug release is not achieved.

Microencapsulation processes have been applied in order to modify or extend the release kinetics of ion exchange resin systems, e.g., hot melt [6], coacervation [7], interfacial polymerization [8], and solvent evaporation [9]. One of the commercial products is based on the Pennkinetic® system in which the drug-resinate beads are impregnated with a water-soluble substance and coating with ethylcellulose via the Wurster process. In this system, the drug-resin complex is impregnated with polyethylene glycol to reduce the swelling of resin particles in water. Ethylcellulose acts as a rate-controlling membrane barrier to control the movement of counter ions and drugs, resulting in a reduced drug release rate [10].

Fig. VI-7 shows the *in vitro* release and blood concentration level of dextromethorphan by the Pennkinetic® system. These suspensions are composed of syrup, granulated sugar, starch, gum etc. and a combination of uncoated and coated resinates. The coated resinates retard drug release as

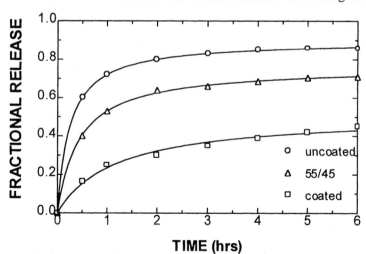

TIME (hrs)

Figure VI-7. *In vitro* release profile of dextromethorphan by the Pennkinetic® system containing coated and uncoated drug resins. (Graph reconstructed from data by Amsel et al. [10].)

Table VI-1. Drug-Resin Products [32].

Product	Active Ingredient	Manufacturer
Tussionex®	Hydrocodone, Chlorpheniramine	Medeva Pharmaceuticals
Ionamin®	Phenteramine	Medeva Pharmaceuticals
Nicorette®	Nicotine	SmithKline Beecham
Betoptic® S Ophthalmic Suspension	Betaxolol	Alcon Laboratories

shown in Fig. VI-8. The release of drug from uncoated resin particles, which act as the immediate release portion of drug release, reaches 80% in a short time and then tails off due to the slow diffusion of drug from the deep core of the tight gel. The 80% release indicates that 65% of bead radius is exhausted. Kim [11], however, reported that highly swellable polyelectrolyte gels consisting of sulfopropyl methacrylate potassium in polymer chain provide for complete release of drug without tailing during long release time. This resin containing sulfonate is independent of pH and ionic strength like commercial strong cation exchange resins.

Garcia et al. [8] encapsulated diclofenac Na loaded resin particles by the interfacial polymerization of hexamethylenediamine and sebacoyl chloride in the organic phase (chloroform/cyclohexane 1:4) containing 15 v/v% of Span 55. Others [7,12] have used coacervation in which two oppositely charged polymers react to form a polymeric complex layer around the drug-resinate particles, encapsulating the drug loaded resins. These encapsulation processes, however, do not improve drug release kinetics or achieve complete drug release because the core drug-resinate is the same. Microencapsulated systems simply extend the release of the drug from the drug-resinates.

Commercial dosage forms based on ion exchange resins are listed in Table VI-1.

VI.4. Swellable Polyelectrolyte Gels

Recently, ion exchange resin delivery systems based on swellable polyelectrolyte gels have been reexamined for further refinements. Due to the minimal swelling of commercial resins (strong cation exchange resins), the kinetics of drug release are controlled by drug diffusion. As discussed earlier for non-Fickian diffusion and hydrogel systems, the swelling of the polymer can be modified in order to achieve more favorable release kinetics. When a highly swellable ion exchange polyelectrolyte gel is used, the release kinetics changes from square-root-of-time behavior to anomalous (or close to zero-order) kinetics as shown in Fig. VI-9. The anomalous behavior of the systems depends upon the degree of swelling of the polyelectrolyte. This polyelectrolyte gel is synthesized by copolymerizing ethyl acrylate and methyl methacrylate or homopolymerizing ethyl acrylate via a suspension process, followed by saponification in a KOH-ethylene glycol solution. This process was developed to obtain spherical beads of polymer containing acrylate functional groups. It has been reported that polyelectrolytes based on acrylic acid are less susceptible to the pH effect than those based on methacrylic acid [13]. Acrylic acid-based polyelectrolytes may deliver drug reasonably well, even below a pH of 6. This is not the case with the methacrylic acid-based one. The release of propranolol HCl from drug-poly(acrylate potassium) beads follows zero order kinetics as shown in Fig. VI-8. As discussed under the time dependent diffusion analysis in Chapter IV, the swelling of polymer increases as drug is released, leading to an increase of the diffusion coefficient. The increasing diffusivity leading to $D_i / D_\infty \ll 1$ is due to the time dependent increase in the swelling of the matrix and the surface area. The equilibrium degree of swelling was about 3.45 ($= d_\infty / d_i$, where d_∞ and d_i are the equilibrium and initial diameter of the bead, respectively) in loosely cross-linked poly(potassium acrylate) and 2.8 in poly(methyl methacrylate-co-acrylate potassium). However, the ionic beads consisting of methacrylic acid and methyl methacrylate provided an equilibrium degree of swelling of 1.6, giving the release kinetics close to square-root-of-time.

The complex formation during drug loading of polyelectrolyte gels and the dissociation of the drug/resin complex during drug release can be observed. When the drug dissociates from the drug/resin complex, a clear

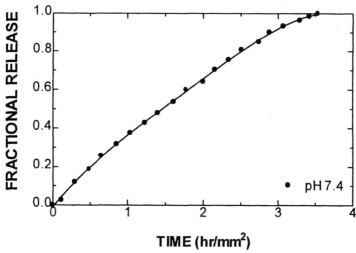

Figure VI-8. Release of propranol HCl from PA-K beads.   (Graph reconstructed from data by Kim [13].)

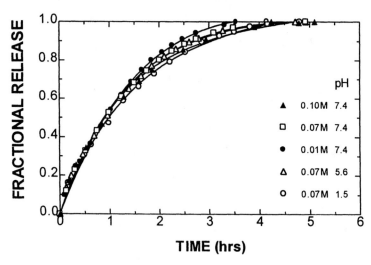

Figure VI-9. Effect of pH and ionic strength on the release of oxprenolol HCl from PSMK/HEMA gels at pH 7.4. (Graph reconstructed from data by Kim [11].)

dissociation front, in most cases white in color due to precipitation of drug around the undissociated core, moves toward the core leaving a transparent drug depleted gel layer. Finally, the moving front disappears when it meets the center of the core. The polyelectrolyte gels consisting of carboxylate moieties are very sensitive to pH variation. In particular, in acidic environment (pH < 5) the carboxylate ion converts to carboxylic acid which does not swell at that pH, resulting in unfavorable release kinetics. Kim [11] demonstrated that swellable polyelectrolyte gels containing sulfonate groups provide release kinetics, which are independent of pH and ionic strength of the dissolution medium. Fig. VII-9 shows pH and buffer concentration-independent release kinetics from poly(sulfopropyl methacrylate potassium-co-2-hydroxyethyl methacrylate) (PSPMK/HEMA) gel matrices. The drug release from PSPMK/HEMA is controlled by the diffusion of the drug through the drug depleted gel layer because drug release from erodible polyelectrolyte gels consisting of sulfopropyl methacrylate is slightly dependent on pH and ionic strength [11]. Drug diffusion through the gel layer masks the effects of pH and buffer concentration of dissolution medium.

VI.5. Erodible Polyelectrolyte Gels

As discussed for the polymer/erosion controlled systems in Chapter V, the synchronized movement of the eroding front and the swelling front may lead to zero-order release kinetics. These swelling/erosion controlled systems can be made with polyelectrolyte polymers. Water-soluble polyelectrolytes in water form complexes between the hydrochloride salt of the cationic drug and the anionic carboxylate chain of the polyelectrolyte. During drug release, the drug-polyelectrolyte complex is dissociated by incoming counter ions from the dissolution medium, as observed in ion exchange resins and highly swellable polyelectrolyte gels. The dissociated drug diffuses out of the matrix while the drug-free polyelectrolyte begins swelling. When the polymer concentration reaches a threshold, the swollen gel begins to erode, as found in the swelling/erosion controlled systems. Kim and Nujoma [14] have demonstrated that the synchronization of two fronts is achieved during drug release from noncross-linked poly(methyl methacrylate-co-methacrylate sodium) (PMMA/MANa) beads as shown in Fig. VI-10. This erodible PMMA/MANa has 37.5 mole% MAA and a molecular weight of 600,000. It dissolves at pH above 9.0 but does not dissolve below pH 8.0. As a result, one can obtain noncross-linked PMMA/MANa beads. The initial swelling rate is greater than the erosion rate due to the higher polymer concentration at the erosion front. As soon as the polymer concentration reaches a low enough level to erode, a balanced rate of swelling and erosion is obtained, giving rise to the synchronized gel layer. As soon as a critical concentration of polymer at the erosion front is reached, the polymer begins to dissolve and the system establishes a constant gel thickness due to the balanced swelling and erosion processes as illustrated in Fig. VI-10. A linear release of drug is expected. However, a linear release profile is not observed

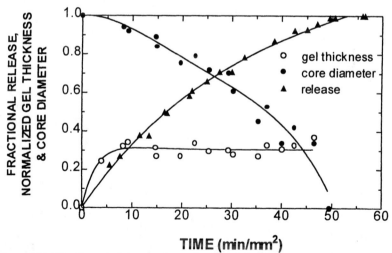

Figure VI-10. Drug release and synchronized fronts of swelling and erosion of uncross-linked PMMA/MANa beads at pH 7.4. (Graph reconstructed from data by Kim and Nujoma [14].).

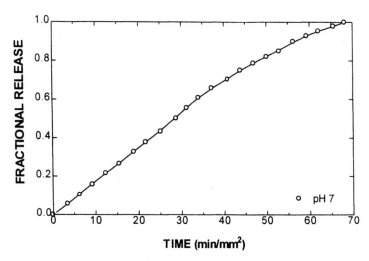

Figure VI-11. The release of diphenhydramine HCl from erodible PMMA/A-Na (38 mol% A-Na) gel film. (Graph reconstructed from data by Kim [15].)

due to diminishing release surface area of drug-PMMA/MANa beads with time [14]. This study led to an investigation of the linear release of drugs from erodible films.

Fig. VI-11 shows the release profile of diphenhydramine HCl from erodible drug-poly(methyl methacrylate-co-acrylate sodium) (PMMA/A-Na) film [15]. The release of diphenhydramine HCl from erodible drug-PMMA/A-Na complexes is independent of the buffer concentration and pH at pH higher than 7.0. These observations suggest that erodible drug-resin complex systems exhibit more promising characteristics compared to the release of drug from the unionized carboxylic acid polymer and swellable polyelectrolyte gels. The release of drug from unionized poly(carboxylic acid) is strongly dependent upon the hydrolysis of carboxylic acid. On the other hand, the dissociation of the drug/resin complex is not greatly dependent upon pH and buffer concentration, because of the fully ionized carboxylate chain. A drug loading level of greater than 40% can be achieved in erodible drug-resin systems. These systems are substantially different from swelling/erosion controlled systems consisting of only nonionic polymer where, at such high loading, drug release is controlled by diffusion of drug (Fickian) rather than the swelling/erosion of the polymer. Due to pH dependent swelling and/or erosion characteristics of polymers containing carboxylate pendant groups, it is not feasible for these ionic gels to be employed as oral drug delivery systems. pH conditions change as a dosage form travels along the gastro-intestinal (GI) tract. Nujoma and Kim [16] demonstrated a (pseudo) zero-order release of water-soluble drugs from

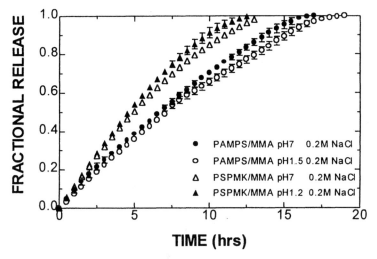

TIME (hrs)

Figure VI-12. Effect of simulated intestinal/gastric fluids on the release of verapamil HCl from drug-PSPMK/MMA and drug-PAMPS/MMA tablets. (Graph reconstructed from data by Nujoma and Kim [17] and Konar and Kim [18].)

erodible, drug/resin complex, tablets using noncross-linked poly(sulfopropyl methacrylate potassium-co-alkyl methacrylate).

As shown in Fig. VII-12, drug release from drug-noncross-linked poly(sulfopropyl methacrylate potassium-co-methyl methacrylate) (PSPMK/MMA) maintains zero-order release kinetics for a long period of time. This is because the drug in the matrices is bound to the polymer side chain until the complex is dissociated by incoming counter ions. The complex has a drug loading of greater than 40 wt%. The complexation between sulfonate groups and secondary amines is much stronger than that between carboxylate groups and secondary amines. It has been found that drug release is independent of the pH of the disssolution medium as long as the ionic strength is higher than 0.1 M, which is commonly observed in GI fluid [17]. Swelling phenomenon during drug release from drug-resinate matrices has not been observed (i.e. purely dissociation/erosion controlled system). Konar and Kim [18] applied this approach to obtain erodible poly(acrylamidomethylpropanesulfonic acid sodium-co-methyl methacrylate) (PAMPS/MMA). The release of verapamil HCl from drug-PAMPS/MMA tablets is slightly slower than that from drug-PSPMK/MMA tablets [16]. It has been observed that drug release from PAMPS/MMA is less sensitive to the type of amine of the drug than that from SPMK/MMA and is more dependent upon drug solubility.

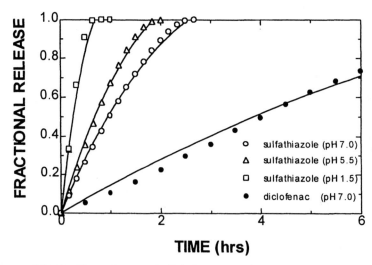

Figure VI-13. The release of diclofenac Na from drug-PTMAEM/MMA tablets. (Graph reconstructed from data by Konar and Kim [19].)

Konar and Kim [19] applied water-soluble polyelectrolytes to anionic drugs. In order to prevent the pH dependence of drug release due to tertiary amine groups in the cationic polymer, fully ionized quaternary amine monomer has been used. Water soluble, cationic polymers based on trimethylaminoethyl methacrylate chloride were developed. As shown in Fig. VII-13, drug release is linear from the beginning to approximately 80% release before tailing toward completion. Drug release kinetics of drug-resinate tablets tested in 0.05 M, 0.1 M, and 0.2 M NaCl is superimposable. However, the release of diclofenac Na from drug-PTMAEMC/MMA tablets tested in 0.05 M NaCl at pH 5.5 slows down slightly [18,19]. At lower pH, drug release is stopped due to negligible solubility of diclofenac in its acid form. Insoluble diclofenac acid stays within the tablets, preventing the dissolution of water soluble PTMAEMC/MMA. The release of sulfathiazole Na (24% solubility in water) increases drastically compared to that of diclofenac Na (2.6% solubility in water). The faster release of sulfathiazole Na from drug-resinates is presumably due to the increase of hydrophilicity of sulfathiazole-PTMAEMC/MMA. The hydrophilicity of drug-PTMAEMC/ MMA is dependent on the solubility of anionic drugs in the acid form. Attempt has been made to form drug-PTMAEMC/MMA based on Na salicylate. Salicylate-PTMAEMC/MMA formed was dissolved back into water when stirring was enforced. Solubilities of diclofenac (acid), sulfathiazole, and salicylic acid are nil, 0.06%, and 0.2%, respectively. Copolymers containing sulfopropyl methacrylate are more hydrophobic than those containing trimethylaminaoethyl methacrylate. Nujoma and Kim [16]

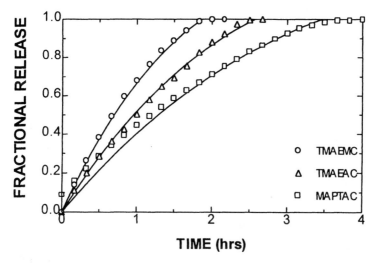

Figure VI-14. The effect of type of quaternary amine on the release of sulfathiazole. (Graph reconstructed from data by Konar and Kim [20].)

formed water insoluble complex with PSPMK/MMA and diltiazem HCl whose solubility in water is about 60%. As shown in Fig VII-12 for anionic polymers, drug release from cationic polymers was dependent on the type of quaternary amine incorporated in the polymers as shown in Fig. VII-14. It seems that for a given polymer composition (50 mole% MMA), polymers consisting of MAPTAC yield longer release times [20].

VI.6. Principle of Diffusion in the Ion Exchange Resin Matrix (Shrinking-Core Model)

Many researchers have presented theoretical expressions for drug release kinetics. These equations are based on the diffusion of a dissolved drug in a matrix [21-24] and the diffusion of drug across a thin liquid film at the periphery of the resin particle. They failed to take into account the moving boundary layer occurring when the ions in the solution come in contact with the fixed ions of the resin [25-27]. Kim [28] presented a pseudo-steady state shrinking-core model, which is based on a non-catalytic gas-solid reaction, or chemical leaching process [29,30], within nonporous particles describing the ionization of hydrophobic ionic beads. This model can be applied to drug release from ion exchange resins.

During drug release from an ion exchange resinate a five step sequence can be visualized [31]:

(1)   Diffusion of counter ions through the film surrounding the resin particle to the surface of the resin,

(2)   Penetration and diffusion of counter ions through the drug depleted layer to the surface of the undissociated core,

(3)   Dissociation of drug from the drug-resin complex at this reaction surface,

(4)   Diffusion of liberated drug through the drug depleted layer to the exterior surface of the resin,

(5)   Diffusion of liberated drug through the film surrounding the particle into the dissolution medium.

This process is depicted in Fig. VI-15 where Fig. VI-15a shows the concentration gradient of inward-moving counter ions, and Fig. VI-15b shows the concentration gradient of outwardly moving drug ions. This type of analysis can be found in other physical systems such as the gas-solid reaction and the chemical leaching process [29-31]. The kinetics of these two processes depend upon the film diffusion resistance, drug and counter ion diffusion resistance in the rubbery gel layer, and dissociation of drug-resinate at the interface of the resin. As the solution ions exchange with the resinate's

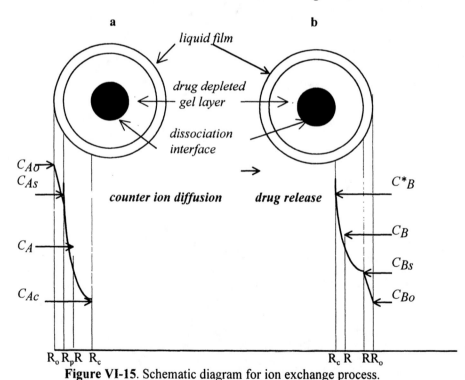

Figure VI-15. Schematic diagram for ion exchange process.

drug ions, a clear gel layer forms at the surface. Solution ions continue to be exchanged, forming a dissociated, rubbery gel layer of increasing thickness and a decreasing, or shrinking, unionized drug-resin core.

Fig. VI-16 clearly shows a photograph of the moving front of the shrinking core during drug release from drug-PMMA/MANa. The dark core is the un-dissociated drug-resin, at the surface of which dissociated drug diffuses out through the clear drug depleted layer. This shrinking core is not commonly observed during drug release from commercial ion exchange resins due to the refractive index difference. However, the moving front has been observed in the ion exchange process of Cu^{++} and Co^{++} ions from weak acid exchange resins [25]. At times, some of these steps are negligible compared with others. For example, vigorous stirring can affect the minimization of mass transfer of drug in the boundary layer. The dissociation reaction of the drug/resin complex may be so fast compared with the diffusion of drug.

The processes of diffusion of counter ions and drug in the drug depleted layer can be expressed by the following differential equations (pseudo steady-state) in the case of first-order dissociation [30]:

$$D_A \frac{1}{r^2}\left(\frac{\partial}{\partial r} r^2 \frac{\partial C_A}{\partial r}\right) = 0 \quad R_c \leq r \leq R_p \tag{6-1}$$

$$D_B \frac{1}{r^2}\left(\frac{\partial}{\partial r} r^2 \frac{\partial C_B}{\partial r}\right) = 0 \quad R_c \leq r \leq R_p \tag{6-2}$$

with the following boundary conditions:

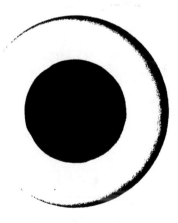

Figure VI-16. A photograph of the shrinking-core of a drug-resin complex bead.

$$\frac{\partial C_A}{\partial r}\bigg)_{r=R_p} = -\frac{k_{MA}}{D_A}(C_{AS} - C_{Ao}), \quad \frac{\partial C_B}{\partial r}\bigg)_{r=R_p} = \frac{k_{MB}}{D_B}C_{Bs} \qquad (6\text{-}3)$$

$$\frac{\partial C_A}{\partial r}\bigg)_{r=R_c} = \frac{k_s}{D_A}C_{Ac}, \qquad\qquad C_B(R_c,t) = C_B^* \qquad (6\text{-}4)$$

where

C_A	= counter ion concentration
C_B	= drug concentration
C_{Ao}	= counter ion concentration in the bulk solution
C_{As}, C_{Bs}	= counter ion concentration and drug concentration at the surface of the resin bead, respectively
R_p	= particle radius
R_c	= radius of the undissociated core
k_{MA}, k_{MB}	= mass transfer coefficients of the counter ions and the drug in the liquid boundary layer
k_s	= the first order irreversible dissociation rate constant
D_A, D_B	= diffusion coefficients of the counter ion and the drug in the drug depleted layer
C_B^*	= solubility of the drug

The rate of consumption of counter ion can be expressed in terms of the mass transfer of counter ion A from bulk solution to the surface of bead, or the diffusion through the shell layer, or the rate of reaction at the moving front as [30]:

$$t = \frac{R_p^2 \rho_M}{3C_{Ao}D_{eA}}\left[\frac{D_{eA}}{R_p k_{MA}}X + \frac{1+2(1-X)-3(1-X)^{2/3}}{2} + \frac{3D_{eA}}{R_p k_s}(1-(1-X)^{1/3})\right]$$

$$(6\text{-}5)$$

where $X = 1-(R_c/R_p)^3$ and ρ_M = concentration of the drug in the resinate.

It may be deduced from equation (6-5) that when mass transfer in the boundary film is the rate-limiting step, equation (6-5) reduces to:

$$t = \frac{R_p \rho_M}{3C_{Ao}k_{MA}}X \qquad (6\text{-}6)$$

Likewise, when diffusion in the drug-depleted layer is the limiting factor, equation (6-5) reduces to:

$$t = \frac{R_p^2 \rho_M}{6 C_{Ao} D_{eA}} [1 + 2(1 - X) - 3(1 - X)^{2/3}] \tag{6-7}$$

When the reaction at the moving boundary interface controls, equation (6-5) reduces to:

$$t = \frac{R_p \rho_M}{k_s C_{Ao}} [1 - (1 - X)^{1/3}] \tag{6-8}$$

Solutions for other reaction orders (zero, second, and fractional) and geometries can be found numerically [28].

    Steps (1)-(3) of the drug delivery process in systems of drug/resin complex matrices occurs quickly while steps (4) and (5) control the release of drug. For this case, the differential material balance equation is solved for the drug-depleted layer giving [30]:

$$t_p = \frac{\rho_M R_p^2}{6 D_{eB}(C_B^* - C_{Bo})} \left[1 + 2(1 - X) - 3(1 - X)^{2/3} + \frac{2}{N_{sh}} X \right] \tag{6-9}$$

When diffusion in the drug-depleted layer controls the release kinetics, equation (6-9) reduces to:

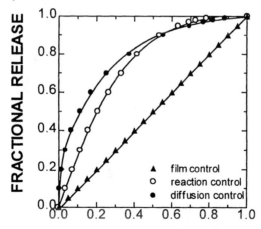

DIMENSIONLESS TIME

Figure VI-17. Fractional release [31].

$$t_p = \frac{\rho_M R_p^2}{6 D_{eB}(C_B^* - C_{Bo})}[1 + 2(1-X) - 3(1-X)^{2/3}] \qquad (6\text{-}10)$$

where C_{Bo} is the initial drug concentration in the dissolution medium. When external mass transfer in the boundary layer controls the release kinetics, equation (6-9) is further reduced to:

$$t_p = \frac{\rho_M R_p}{3 k_{mB}(C_B^* - C_{Bo})} X \qquad (6\text{-}11)$$

Throughout the aforementioned processes, the external mass transfer rate at the boundary layer is negligible for high stirring in the drug/resin delivery systems. In this case drug release kinetics can be written:

Table VI-2. Fractional Release-Time Expressions for Various Shaped Particles [31].

	slab	cylinder	sphere
	$X = 1 - l/L$	$X = 1 - (r/a)^2$	$X = 1 - (r/a)^3$
film diffusion	$\dfrac{t}{\tau} = X$	$\dfrac{t}{\tau} = X$	$\dfrac{t}{\tau} = X$
	$\tau = \dfrac{\rho_A L}{b k_s C_A}$	$\tau = \dfrac{\rho_A L}{b k_s C_A}$	$\tau = \dfrac{\rho_A R}{3 b k_s C_A}$
gel diffusion	$\dfrac{t}{\tau} = X^2$	$\dfrac{t}{\tau} = X + (1-X)\ln(1-X)$	$\dfrac{t}{\tau} = 1 - 3(1-X)^{2/3} + 2(1-X)$
	$\tau = \dfrac{\rho_A L^2}{2 b D_A C_A}$	$\tau = \dfrac{\rho_A R^2}{4 b D_A C_A}$	$\tau = \dfrac{\rho_A R^2}{6 b D_A C_A}$
reaction	$\dfrac{t}{\tau} = X$	$\dfrac{t}{\tau} = 1 - (1-X)^{1/2}$	$\dfrac{t}{\tau} = 1 - (1-X)^{1/3}$
	$\tau = \dfrac{\rho_A L}{b k_s C_A}$	$\tau = \dfrac{\rho_A R}{b k_s C_A}$	$\tau = \dfrac{\rho_A R}{b k_s C_A}$
drug diffusion	$\dfrac{t}{\tau} = X^2$	$\dfrac{t}{\tau} = X + (1-X)\ln(1-X)$	$\dfrac{t}{\tau} = 1 - 3(1-X)^{2/3} + 2(1-X)$
	$\tau = \dfrac{\rho_A L^2}{2 b D_B C_B}$	$\tau = \dfrac{\rho_A R^2}{4 b D_B C_B}$	$\tau = \dfrac{\rho_A R^2}{6 b D_B C_B}$
film diffusion	$\dfrac{t}{\tau} = X$	$\dfrac{t}{\tau} = X$	$\dfrac{t}{\tau} = X$
	$\tau = \dfrac{\rho_A L}{b k_s C_A}$	$\tau = \dfrac{\rho_A R}{2 b k_s C_A}$	$\tau = \dfrac{\rho_A R}{3 b k_s C_A}$

$$t = \frac{R_p^2 \rho_M}{3 C_{Ao} D_A} \left[\frac{1}{2} \left(1 + \frac{D_A C_{Ao}}{2 D_B C_B^*} \right) (1 + 2(1-X) - 3(1-X)^{2/3}) + \frac{3 D_A}{R_p k_s} \left(1 - (1-X)^{1/3} \right) \right]$$

(6-12)

If the rate of counter ion diffusion through the drug depleted layer is much faster than the rate of drug diffusion, equation (6-12) can be written as:

$$t = \frac{R_p^2 \rho_M}{6 C_B^* D_B} \left(1 + 2(1-X) - 3(1-X)^{2/3} \right) + \frac{R_p \rho_M}{C_{Ao} k_s} \left(1 - (1-X)^{1/3} \right) \quad (6-13)$$

Fig. VI-17 illustrates the fractional conversion (or release) of a single spherical particle with a boundary layer versus the fractional dimensionless time [31]. Beyond 80% drug release, it is difficult to differentiate between the release mechanisms for chemically controlled and diffusion controlled release. However, one may easily control the film mass transfer resistance by vigorously mixing the dissolution system in a batch system and providing for a high circulation rate over the column system. Although a spherical particle is a common geometry in ion exchange, other geometries, especially small disc pellets, can be produced. A similar mathematical interpretation for the pellet may be applied to the following fractional release vs. time as shown in Table VI-2 [31]. It is interesting to note that the theoretical expressions shown in Table VI-2 are very similar to the equations derived for the drug release from dispersed drug matrix systems discussed in Chapter II.

Nujoma [32] applied a kinetic model based on a pseudo-steady state shrinking core model on the release of drug (e.g., diltiazem HCl, propranolol HCl, and verapamil HCl) from drug-PMMA/MANa beads. The plot shown in Fig. VI-18 can be used to identify the controlling drug release mechanism. Fig. VI-18 shows that the dissociation reaction mechanism best describes for the release of diltiazem HCl from drug-PMMA/MA beads. In this analysis, the mass transfer coefficient has been determined independently by Tojo et al. [33]. At vigorous stirring conditions (>300 rpm), the mass transfer resistance through the stagnant boundary is negligible compared to the overall release kinetics. However, one can not justify the release kinetics based solely on a pure dissociation mechanism. It has been reported that drug release from erodible propranolol-PMMA/ANa films takes about 5-6 hrs. Drug release from propranolol-PMMA/MANa beads takes much longer (50 hrs). This indicates that drug diffusion through the swollen gel layer contributes significantly to the release kinetics in addition to the dissociation process. However, the combined dissociation and drug diffusion mechanism fails to describe the overall release kinetics, as shown in Fig. VI-18. This indicates that the dissociation reaction and drug diffusion in series do not describe adequately the release kinetics of drug-polyelectrolyte gel beads.

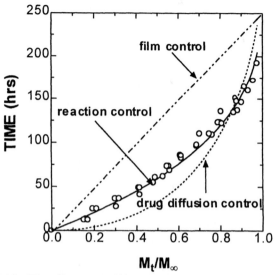

Figure VI-18. The release of diltiazem HCl from drug-PMMA/MANa beads along with drug release mechanisms. (Graph reconstructed from data by Nujoma [32].)

One may postulate that the drug release rate increases during drug release due to the swelling of the polymer. In this case, time-dependent diffusion coefficient methods discussed in Chapter IV, can be adapted for swellable polyelectrolytes. The following equation describes drug release kinetics governed by dissociation and drug diffusion in conjunction with the swelling of polymer:

$$\left(\frac{D_\infty t}{R_p^2} - \left(1 - \frac{D_i}{D_\infty}\right) \frac{D_\infty}{R_p^2 k_d} (1 - e^{-k_d t}) \right) = \frac{\rho_M}{6 C_B^*} \left(1 + 2(1 - X) - 3(1 - X)^{2/3}\right) \quad (6\text{-}14)$$

where k_d is the dissociation induced polymer relaxation rate constant and D_i and D_∞ are the initial and equilibrium diffusion coefficient, respectively.

Nujoma [32] applied this approach successfully to drug release from drug-PMMA/MANa beads. The equilibrium diffusion coefficient (D_∞) is determined from the later portion of drug release and equation (6-10), as suggested by Lee [34]. Then equation (6-14) with the determined value of D_∞ is applied to the entire experimental release data as shown in Fig. VI-18. As shown in Fig. VI-19, equation (6-14) expresses drug release kinetics well for drug-PMMA/MANa beads. It is interesting to note that the initial diffusion coefficient is very small compared to the equilibrium diffusion

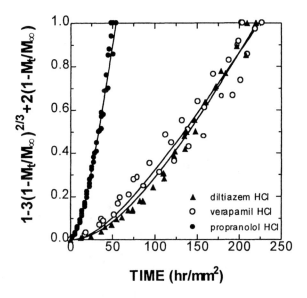

Figure VI-19. Application of time-dependent diffusion coefficient method to the release of diltiazem from drug-PMMA/MANa beads.

coefficient and that there is no difference in the predicted release profile by setting $D_i = 0$.

VI.7. Release Kinetics from Water Soluble Polyelectrolyte Complex

The drug release kinetics from erodible drug-polyelectrolyte resinate tablets can be explained by a heterogeneous dissociation/erosion mechanism. If the drug is bound to the polyelectrolyte, then the drug release rate at a time t from a tablet, having a radius r_o (cm), a thickness l (cm), and a drug concentration in a tablet C_o (mg/cm^3), is:

$$\frac{dM_t}{dt} = 2\pi k_e R(R + L) \tag{6-15}$$

where k_e is the drug-resinate dissociation/erosion rate constant (mg/cm^{2}h) and R and L are the radius and thickness of tablet at time t, respectively. However, the time dependent change of the radius and thickness of tablet can be expressed by equation (5-7b). Integrating equation (6-15) following substitution of equation (5-7b) yields:

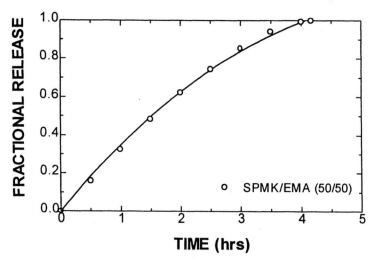

Figure VI-20. Application of heterogeneous dissociation/erosion method to the release of propranolol from drug-PSPMK/EMA tablets. (Graph reconstructed from data by Nujoma [32].)

$$\frac{M_t}{M_\infty} = 1 - \left[1 - \frac{k_e t}{C_o r_o}\right]^2 \left[1 - \frac{2k_e t}{C_o l}\right] \qquad (6\text{-}16)$$

where $M_\infty = \pi r_o^2 l C_o$.

One can easily see the relevant equations for a cylinder and a slab if r_o / l is smaller or larger, respectively. Nujoma [32] used equation (6-16) to characterize the release kinetics of labetalol HCl from drug-PAMPSNa/MMA tablets, as shown in Figure VI-20. The dissociation/erosion rate constant is reported to increase as the content of drug-resinate in the tablet decreased. This is attributed the greater influx of water into the tablet along with counter ions as more water-soluble excipient (dextrose) is incorporated into the tablet.

References

1.   E.H. Schacht, "Ionic Polymers as Drug Carriers", in Controlled Drug Delivery, Vol. I, Bruck, Ed., CRC Press, Baton Rouge, Fl. 1984, p149.

2.   C. J. Kim and P. I. Lee, "Constant Rate Drug Release from Novel Anionic Gel Beads with Transient Composite Structure," *Proceed. Int. Symp. Control. Rel. Bioact. Mater.*, 19, 162 (1992).

3.   Y. Raghunathan, L. Amsel, O. Hinsvark, and W. Bryant, "Sustained-Release Drug Delivery System I: Coated Ion-Exchange Resin System for Phenylpropanolamine and Other Drugs", *J. Pharm. Sci.*, 70, 379 (1981).

4. J. E. Polli and G. L. Amidon, "In Vitro Characterization of Sodium Glycocholate Binding to Cholestyramine Resin," *J. Pharm. Sci.*, 84, 55 (1995).
5. G. M. Burke, R. W. Mendes, and S. S. Jambhekar, "Investigation of The Application of Ion Exchange Resin as a Sustained Release Drug Delivery System for Propranolol Hydrochloride," *Drug Dev. Ind. Pharm.*, 12, 713 (1986).
6. S. Motycke and J. G. Narin, "Influence of Wax Coating on Release Rate of Anions from Ion-Exchange Resin Beads," *J. Pharm. Sci.*, 67, 500 (1978).
7. W. J. Irwin, R. Michale, and P. J. Watts, "Drug Delivery by Ion-Exchange. Part VII: Release of Acidic Drugs from Anion Exchange Resinate Complexes," *Drug Dev. Ind. Pharm.*, 16, 883 (1990).
8. G. Garcia, D. Torres, B. Seijo, and J. L. Vila Jato, "In Vivo Evaluation of Nylon-Coated Diclofenac Resin Complex," *J. Control. Rel.*, 23, 201 (1993).
9. D. L. Spokel and J. C. Price, "Evaluation of Sustained Release Aqueous Suspensions Containing Micro-encapsulated Drug-Resin Complexes," *Drug Dev. Ind. Pharm.*, 15, 1275 (1989).
10. L. P. Amsel et al., "Recent Advances in Sustained-Release Technology using Ion Exchange Polymers," *Pharm. Technol.*, 8(4), 28 (1984).
11. C. J. Kim, "Swelling and Release Characteristics of Poly(Sulfopropyl Methacrylate Potassium-co-Hydroxyethyl methacrylate) Gels," *J. Macrom. Sci., Pure Appl. Chem.*, A31, 783 (1993).
12. W. J. Irwin, K. A. Belaid, and H. O. Olpar, "Drug Delivery by Ion Exchange. Part IV: Coated Resinate Complexes of Ester Prodrug of Propranolol,' *Drug Dev. Ind. Pharm.*, 14, 1307 (1988).
13. C. J. Kim, "Hydrogel Beads for Oral Drug Delivery Systems," *Chemtech*, 24(8), 36 (1994).
14. C. J. Kim and Y. N. Nujoma, "Drug Release from Erodible Polyelectrolyte gel Beads," *Eur. Polym. J.*, 31, 937 (1995).
15. C. J. Kim, "A Linear Drug Release from Erosion-Controlled Drug/resin Complex," *J. Appl. Polym. Sci.*, 54, 1179 (1994).
16. Y. N. Nujoma and C. J. Kim, "A Designer's Polymer as an Oral Drug Carrier (Tablet) with Pseudo-Zero-Order Release Kinetics," *J. Pharm. Sci.*, 85, 1091 (1996).
17. F. K. Wildman, <u>Goodale's Clinical Interpretation of Laboratory Tests</u>, 7th Edition, F. A. Davis Co., Philadelphia, PA, 1973, p276.
18. N. Konar and C. J. Kim, "Drug Release from Drug-Polyion Complex Tablets," *J. Control. Rel.* (in press).
19. N. Konar and C. J. Kim, "Watre Soluble Polycations for Oral Drug Carriers (Tablets)," *J. Pharm. Sci.*, 86, 1339 (1997).
20. N. Konar and C. J. Kim, "Water-Soluble Quaternary Amine Polymers as Controlled Release Carriers," *J. Appl. Polym. Sci.*, 69, 263 (1998).
21. G. E. Boyd, A. W. Adamson, and L. S. Myers, "The Exchange Adsorption of Ions from Aqueous Solution by Organic Zeolite. II. Kinetics," *J. Am. Chem. Soc.*, 69, 2836 (1947).
22. D. Reichenberg, "Properties of Ion Exchange Resins in Relation to their Structure. III. Kinetics of Exchange," *J. Am. Chem. Soc.*, 75, 589 (1953).

23. P. Gyselinck, H. Steyaert, R. Van Severn, and P. Braeckman, "Drug-Polymer Combinations. Part 2. Evaluation of some Mathematic Approaches to Drug Release from Resinate," *Pharmazie*, 37, 190 (1982).

24. R. Bhaskar, R. S. R. Murphy, B. D. Miglianli, and K. Viswanathay, "Novel Method to Evaluate Diffusion Controlled Release from Resinate," *Int. J. Pharm.*, 28, 59 (1986).

25. W. Holl and H. Sontheimer, "Ion Exchange Kinetics of Protonation of Weak Acid Ion Exchange Resins," *Chem. Eng. Sci.*, 32, 755 (1977).

26. M. S. Selim and R. C. Seagrave, "Solution of Moving-Boundary Transport Problems in Finite Media by Integral Transforms. III. The Elution Kinetics of the Copper Amine Complex from a Cation-Exchange Resins," *Ind. Eng. Chem. Fundl.*, 12, 14 (1973).

27. M. S. Selim and R. C. Seagrave, "Solution of Moving-Boundary Transport Problems in Finite Media by Integral Transforms. II. Problems with a Cylindrical or Spherical Moving Boundary," *Ind. Eng. Chem. Fundl.*, 12, 1 (1973).

28. C. J. Kim, "Application of Shrinking-Core Model for Ionization of Hydrophobic Ionic Beads," *Drug. Dev. Ind. Pharm.*, 22, 309 (1996).

29. L. T. Villa, O. D. Quiroga and G. V. Moraces, "The Shrinking Core Model for Non-Catalytic Gas-Solid Reactions with Arbitray Order with Respect to the Gaseous Reactant and General Boundary Conditions," *Trans. I. Chem. E.*, 70(A), 276 (1992).

30. G. Lapidus and M. D. Mosqueira, "The Effect of Product Solubility on the Leaching Kinetics of Non-Porous Minerals," *Hydrometal.*, 20, 49 (1988).

31. O. Levenspiel, Chemical Reaction Engineering, 2nd Ed., John Wiley & Son, New York, 1972.

32. Y. N. Nujoma, Ph.D. Dissertation, Temple University, Philadelphia, PA, 1998.

32. K. Tojo, J. A. Masi, and Y. W. Chien, "Hydrodynamic Characteriscs of an In-Vitro Permeation Cell," *Ind. Eng. Chem. Fundl.*, 24, 368 (1985).

34. P. I. Lee, "Interpretation of Drug-Release Kinetics from Hydrogel Matrices in terms of Time-Dependent Diffusion Coefficients," in Controlled Release Technology: Pharmaceutical Applications, W. R. Good and P. I. Lee (Eds.), ACS Symposium No. 348, American Chemical Society, Washington, DC, 1987, p71.

Chapter VII

Gradient Matrix Systems

Dosage forms based on polymeric matrix systems, described in chapters II-V, do not generally allow one to obtain zero-order release kinetics, which is inherent of matrix systems. In most cases, zero-order release kinetics provide constant blood plasma level for a prolonged period. It is beneficial to develop controlled-release dosage forms that demonstrate zero-order release kinetics based on monolithic matrix systems, which are less expensive to produce than other dosage forms. However, these matrix systems, as presented in preceding chapters, follow square root of time release kinetics. This phenomenon is a result of the deepening of the diffusion pathway and decreasing concentration distribution in the matrix as drug release proceeds. Furthermore, for cylindrical or spherical geometry, drug release decreases as the releasing surface area diminishes with the release time. For this case, the drug loading is uniform across the cross-section of the matrix.

VII.1. Theoretical Expressions

The method of non-uniform initial drug distribution has been developed for drug delivery systems to regulate release kinetics. Lee [1] presented a mathematical interpretation of concentration gradient matrix systems for controlled release delivery. Non-uniform drug distribution in which the drug concentration is lower at the surface and higher toward the core of the matrix compensates for diminishing surface area with time and increasing diffusion resistance with higher concentration. If the initial drug concentration distribution in a sphere is $f(r)$, the concentration distribution in the matrix with time can be expressed, following the derivations presented in previous sections, by [2]:

for a sphere:

$$C(r,t) = \frac{2a}{r} \sum_{n=1}^{\infty} e^{-Dn^2\pi^2 t/a^2} \sin\left(\frac{n\pi r}{a}\right) \times \left\{ \int_0^a r' f(r') \sin\left(\frac{n\pi r'}{a}\right) dr' \right\} \quad (7\text{-}1)$$

for a plane:

$$C(x,t) = \frac{2}{l} \sum_{n=0}^{\infty} e^{-D(2n+1)^2\pi^2 t/4l^2} \cos\left(\frac{(2n+1)\pi x}{l}\right) \times \left\{ \int_0^l f(x') \cos\left(\frac{(2n+1)\pi x'}{l}\right) dx' \right\} \quad (7\text{-}2)$$

The initial concentration distribution of drug in a matrix can be expressed by several theoretical forms, e.g. linear, parabolic, trigonometric, etc. [2]. Here, the linear distribution is presented as an example.

For a sphere, the initial concentration distribution is described by $C_o(a-r)/a$ and then the drug concentration distribution in the matrix is expressed by [2]:

$$C(r,t) = \frac{8aC_o}{r\pi^3} \sum_{n=0}^{\infty} \frac{1}{(2n+1)^3} e^{-D(2n+1)^2\pi^2 t/a^2} \sin\left(\frac{(2n+1)\pi r}{a}\right) \qquad (7\text{-}3)$$

For a slab, the initial concentration distribution is expressed by $C_o(l-|x|)/l$ and then the drug concentration distribution in the plane is [2]:

$$C(x,t) = \frac{8C_o}{\pi^2} \sum_{n=0}^{\infty} \frac{1}{(2n+1)^2} e^{-D(2n+1)^2\pi^2 t/4l^2} \cos\left(\frac{(2n+1)\pi x}{2l}\right) \qquad (7\text{-}4)$$

The amount of drug released at time t (flux) for the given geometry is represented by:

For a slab:

$$J(flux) = -D\frac{\partial C}{\partial x}\bigg|_{x=l} = \frac{4DC_o}{\pi} \sum_{n=0}^{\infty} \frac{(-1)^n}{(2n+1)} e^{-D(2n+1)^2\pi^2 t/4l^2} \qquad (7\text{-}5)$$

$$\frac{M_t}{M_\infty} = 1 - \frac{16}{\pi^2} \sum_{n=0}^{\infty} \frac{(-1)^n}{(2n+1)^3} e^{-D(2n+1)^2\pi^2 t/4l^2} \qquad (7\text{-}6)$$

Lee [1] introduced the sigmoidal, staircase and parabolic concentration distributions:

For sigmoidal profile:

$$f(\zeta) = \frac{1 - e^{-\frac{1}{2}\left(\frac{1-\zeta}{1-\zeta_c}\right)^2}}{1 - e^{-\frac{1}{2}\left(\frac{1}{1-\zeta_c}\right)^2}} \qquad (7\text{-}7)$$

where ζ_c is the initial location of the inflection point of the initial concentration distribution. Lee [1] has explored the special case of $\zeta_c = 0.4$.

For staircase functions:

$$f(\zeta) = \sum_{i=1}^{m} A_i\left[\Delta(\zeta - \zeta_{i-1}) - \Delta(\zeta - \zeta_i)\right] \qquad (7\text{-}8)$$

where Δ is the delta function defined as:

$$\Delta(\zeta - \zeta_i) = \begin{cases} 0 \\ 1 \end{cases} \qquad (7\text{-}9)$$

and where A_j is the drug concentration within each step, ζ_{i-1} is the beginning position of step j, and ζ_i, is the ending position j.

Generally the fractional release can be obtained by [1]:

For a slab:

$$\frac{M_t}{M_\infty} = 1 - \frac{\sum_{n=0}^{\infty} \frac{(-1)^{n+1}}{2n+1} I_1(n) e^{-\frac{(2n+1)^2 \pi^2 D t}{4l^2}}}{\sum_{n=0}^{\infty} \frac{(-1)^{n+1}}{2n+1} I_1(n)} \qquad (7\text{-}10)$$

where
$$I_1(n) = \int_0^1 f(\varsigma) \cos((n+1/2)\pi\varsigma) d\varsigma . \qquad (7\text{-}11)$$

For a sphere:

$$\frac{M_t}{M_\infty} = 1 - \frac{\sum_{n=1}^{\infty} \frac{(-1)^{n+1}}{n} I_2(n) e^{-\frac{n^2 \pi^2 D t}{r^2}}}{\sum_{n=1}^{\infty} \frac{(-1)^{n+1}}{n} I_2(n)} \qquad (7\text{-}12)$$

where
$$I_2(n) = \int_0^1 \varsigma f(\varsigma) \sin(n\pi\varsigma) d\varsigma \qquad (7\text{-}13)$$

The characteristic drug release patterns for the slab, cylinder, and sphere with the initial sigmoidal drug concentration distribution are illustrated in Fig. VII-1. The release rate follows close to zero-order kinetics up to 60% of release for the planar geometry while the release rate deviates from the zero-order kinetics for spherical geometry due to the decreasing surface area for drug release. A constant drug release rate can be obtained by use of a descending staircase distribution, resembling a sigmoidal profile, for the plane geometry, as presented in Fig. VII-2.

There are several approaches to implementing the concentration gradient matrix systems for controlled release dosage form design. The simplest way to demonstrate the validity of gradient matrix systems for constant release kinetics is to design a system by the lamination process. Each layer or film, containing different drug loading, is separately prepared and then laminated together. A laminated gradient system of 5 layers prepared with a mixture of Pluronic and cellulose acetate phthalate is

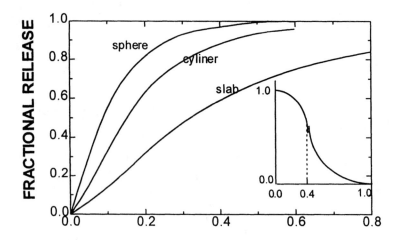

Figure VII-1. Release profiles from the matrices having the sigmoidal drug distribution. (Graph reconstructed from data by Lee [1].)

illustrated in Fig. VII-3. As Lee [3] noted, the system possessing a smooth inflection of the drug loading profile in the laminated matrix demonstrates zero-order release kinetics; whereas a gradient matrix system composed of steep inflections (Fig. VII-4) exhibits a drastic inflection in the release profile as well. Gradient matrix systems, in general, allow one to design temporal or pulsatile drug delivery systems [4].

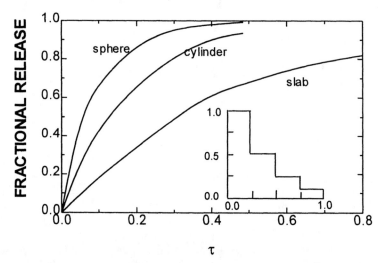

Figure VII-2.   Release profiles from the matrices having the descending drug distribution. (Graph reconstructed from data by Lee [1].)

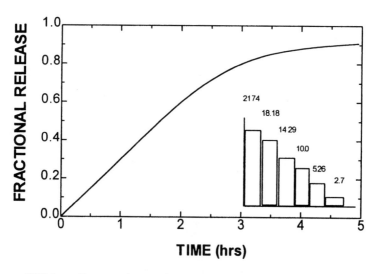

Figure VII-3. Drug release from a laminated film with a smooth inflection. (Graph reconstructed from data by Lee [3].)

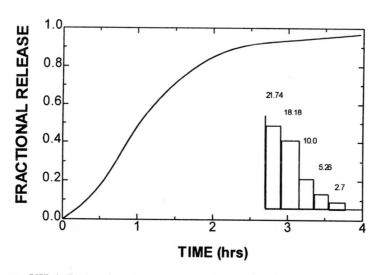

Figure VII-4. Drug release from a laminated film having a sharp inflection. (Graph reconstructed from data by Lee [3].)

VII.2. Hydrogel Beads

Lee [1] theoretically demonstrated the possibility of obtaining a zero-order release rate from spherical geometry by creating a concentration gradient across the radius. He confirmed the validity of the theory with drug release from PHEMA beads. Hydrogel beads prepared by suspension polymerization were purified and equilibrated with an aqueous alcoholic drug solution. During this loading process, the drug concentration profile generated inside the bead follows the pattern illustrated in Fig. VII-5. Eventually the drug concentration across the radius becomes homogeneous. The loaded swollen beads were filtered before being dried.

The release profile from homogeneous hydrogel beads follows Fickian kinetics as pointed out in Chapter II. Uniformly distributed drug loaded beads are subject to partial extraction with swelling solvents such as water, alcohol or acetone. During the partial extraction process, the drug diffuses out and generates the concentration gradient in a matrix, which furnishes the Fickian diffusion profile. During the extraction process, the initial uniform concentration distribution in the hydrogel beads becomes a sigmoidal distribution because drug release kinetics in a good swelling solvent is non-Fickian. Separating the hydrogel beads from the extraction medium and drying retains this sigmoidal distribution. During drug release from hydrogel beads prepared in this manner (non-uniform distribution), the limitations of increasing diffusion resistance and decreasing radial surface area at the penetration front counterbalance the increasing drug loading toward the core of the bead. Depending on the extraction medium and duration of extraction, a different gradient will be formed and a different release profile will be produced. Lee [5] showed by X-ray diffraction that the drug distribution in the extracted beads had a sigmoidal profile. Fig. VII-6 shows the effect of the extraction process on the release of oxprenolol HCl from poly(hydroxypropyl methacrylate) (PHPMA) beads. The release of oxprenolol HCl from an un-extracted PHPMA bead produces a square-root-of-time profile whereas that from an extracted PHMA bead demonstrates linear release kinetics up to 70% of drug release. A slight time lag or sigmoidal pattern is observed in the early stage of release. Drug release then slowly levels off as a result of the minimal osmotic force of dissolved drug in the matrix and further low swelling of the polymer.

The partial extraction process leads to an interesting evaluation of drug release from gradient matrix systems. Initially, one can consider a matrix in which the drug is in a dissolved state. However, if the matrix is swellable and the drug release is expressed by a time dependent diffusion coefficient as discussed in Chapter IV, then the concentration distribution within the matrix at the extraction time is given by:

$$C(r,t) = \frac{2a}{r} \sum_{m=1}^{\infty} e^{-m^2\pi^2\Psi} \sin\left(\frac{m\pi r}{a}\right) \qquad \text{for a sphere} \qquad (7\text{-}14)$$

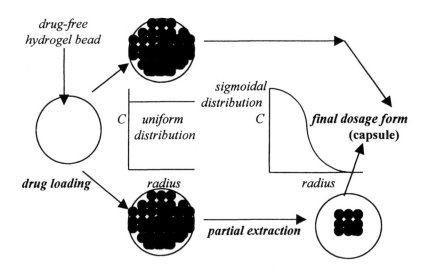

Figure VII-5. A process to produce a non-uniform drug distribution in a hydrogel bead [6].

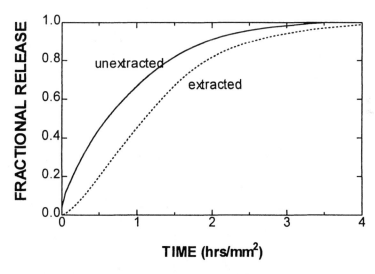

Figure VII-6. Effect of extraction on drug release from PHPMA hydrogel beads. (Graph reconstructed from data by Kim [6].)

where $\psi_e = \tau_e - \left(1 - \dfrac{D_{i,e}}{D_{\infty,e}}\right)\dfrac{D_{\infty,e}}{ka^2}\left[1 - e^{-\dfrac{ka^2}{D_{\infty,e}}\tau_e}\right]$ and $\tau_e = \dfrac{D_{\infty}t_e}{a^2}$ where t_e is

the extraction time, $D_{i,e}$ and $D_{\infty,e}$ are the initial and equilibrium drug diffusion coefficient in an extraction solvent, respectively, and k_e is the polymer relaxation rate constant in an extraction solvent. If $k_e \rightarrow 0$ or $k_e \rightarrow \infty$, equation (7-15) is reduced to equation (2-19) for a non-swellable sphere. The matrix possessing the concentration distribution given in equation (7-14) is immobilized and dried. The fractional release at time t for this gradient matrix placed in a dissolution medium is expressed as:

$$\frac{M_t}{M_\infty} = 1 - \left[\sum_{n=1}^{\infty}\frac{(-1)^{n+1}}{n}e^{-n^2\pi^2\psi}\sum_{m=1}^{\infty}e^{-m^2\pi^2\psi_e}\int_0^1 r'\sin\left(\frac{m\pi r'}{a}\right)\sin\left(\frac{n\pi r'}{a}\right)dr'\right]$$

$$\div \sum_{n=1}^{\infty}\frac{(-1)^{n+1}}{n}\sum_{m=1}^{\infty}e^{-m^2\pi^2\psi_e}\int_0^a r'\sin\left(\frac{m\pi r'}{a}\right)\sin\left(\frac{n\pi r'}{a}\right)dr' \qquad (7\text{-}15)$$

$$\frac{M_t}{M_\infty} = 1 - \left[\sum_{n=1}^{\infty}\frac{(-1)^{n+1}}{n}e^{-n^2\pi^2\psi}\sum_{m=1}^{\infty}e^{-m^2\pi^2\psi_e}\left(\frac{a\sin((m-n)\pi)}{2(m-n)\pi} - \frac{a\sin((m+n)\pi)}{2(m+n)\pi}\right)\right]$$

$$\div \sum_{n=1}^{\infty}\frac{(-1)^{n+1}}{n}\sum_{m=1}^{\infty}e^{-m^2\pi^2\psi_e}\left(\frac{a\sin((m-n)\pi)}{2(m-n)\pi} - \frac{a\sin((m+n)\pi)}{2(m+n)\pi}\right) \qquad (7\text{-}16)$$

$$\text{for} \qquad m \neq n$$

if $m=n$, then

$$\frac{M_t}{M_\infty} = 1 - \left[\sum_{n=1}^{\infty}\frac{(-1)^{n+1}}{n}e^{-n^2\pi^2\psi}\sum_{m=1}^{\infty}e^{-m^2\pi^2\psi_e}\left(\frac{a}{2r\pi} - \sin\left(\frac{2n\pi r}{a}\right)\right)\right]$$

$$\div \sum_{n=1}^{\infty}\frac{(-1)^{n+1}}{n}\sum_{m=1}^{\infty}e^{-m^2\pi^2\psi_e}\left(\frac{a}{2\pi r} - \sin\left(\frac{2m\pi r}{a}\right)\right) \qquad (7\text{-}17)$$

where

$$\psi = \tau - \left(1 - \frac{D_i}{D_\infty}\right)\frac{D_\infty}{ka^2}\left[1 - e^{-\frac{ka^2}{D_\infty}\tau}\right] \quad \text{and} \quad \tau = \frac{D_\infty t}{a^2}$$

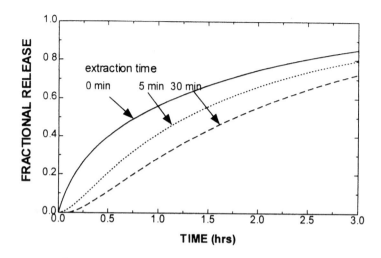

Figure VII-7. Effect of extraction time on the release of oxprenolol HCl from PHEMA beads. (Graph reconstructed from data by Lee [7].)

where D_i and D_∞ are the initial and equilibrium drug diffusion coefficient in a dissolution medium, respectively, and k is the polymer relaxation rate constant in a dissolution medium. As mentioned before, if $k \to 0$ or $k \to \infty$, the release of drug from the matrix is the same as for non-swellable systems. Some interesting situations arise for certain choices of the solvent used in the partial extraction of the drug from the matrix and the solvent used for the dissolution medium. Lee [7] showed linear drug release from spherical hydrogel beads in which the drug has been partially extracted with water, and the non-uniform gradient beads released the drug linearly in water. Water is a moderately good solvent for the PHEMA beads having a 40% degree of swelling. One may speculate as to whether a linear release can be achieved with a solvent, which is not good for swelling.

VII.3. Laminated Slabs and Films

Van Blommel et al. [8] developed a loading (concentration) gradient tablet, in which the inwardly increasing drug concentration may compensate for the increasing diffusion path resistance. As shown in Fig. VII-8, the gradient matrix tablet is fabricated by layering coatings of different drug concentrations so that the drug concentration increases from the surface to the core. To compensate for lower drug concentration layers, a non-active ingredient, xylitol, was added in the opposite order to that of the drug concentration gradient; i.e., the xylitol concentration is higher at the surface and lower in the center as shown in Fig. VII-9. From the composition shown

Table VII-1. Mean Drug Concentrations and Layer Thickness in Three-Layer Gradient Systems [8].

Inner-layer ACE/XYL/EC*	Middle-layer ACE/XYL/EC	Outer-layer ACE/XYL/EC	Mean layer thickness μm
1.91/1.83/3.33	1.91/1.83/3.33	1.91/1.83/3.33	270
3.33/0.50/3.33	2.08/1.75/3.33	0.33/3.25/3.33	270

*ACE/XYL/EC=acetaminophen/xylitol/ethylcellulose

in Table VII-1, experimental release data were obtained as presented in Fig. VII-8. Generally after an initial burst of drug from the immediate surface, the release follows zero-order kinetics.

Mitra [9] has developed a controlled release delivery system based on multi-layered polymeric composite film. The multi-layered films are prepared by sequential casting of solutions containing different drug concentrations or laminating thin films containing different drug loading. In this way, the concentration of the drug is increased from the surface layer to the core layer of the film. The multi-layered film design was capable of delivering quinidine gluconate at a zero-order rate over the entire release time. ***Transdermal Deponit TTS:*** This device [10] consists of three components as shown in Fig. VII-9. Component 2 (300 μm thickness) consists of a nitroglycerin-lactose-concentration gradient in a water-insoluble adhesive of polyisobutylene affixed to the impermeable backing foil in such a way that there are three different drug-dispersion, or reservoir, regions in the adhesive film (R_1 to R_3). Fig. VII-9 shows the *in-vitro* release of nitroglycerin from Deponit TTS over 24 hrs. After an initially higher release rate, the release rate leveled off to a reasonably constant release.

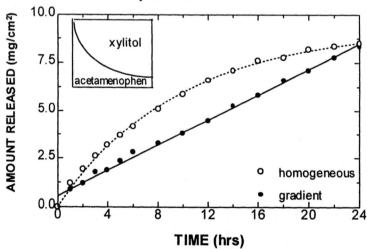

Figure VII-8. The release of acetaminophen from homogeneous and gradient matrices. (Graph reconstructed from data by van Blommel et al. [8].)

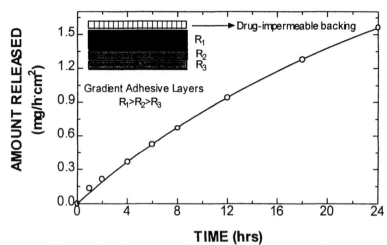

TIME (hrs)

Figure VII-9. The release of nitroglycerin from Deponit TTS. (Graph reconstructed from data by Wolff et al. [10].)

VII.4. Granules or Pellets

Although the nonuniform concentration gradient tablets and hydrogel beads described in the previous section demonstrate that the drug concentration gradient presents a linear drug release, it is not easy to apply the process to large-scale manufacturing. Small particles or granules are produced by a fluidization coating of nonpareil seed. Scott and Hollenbeck [11] have used gradient matrix system methods in order to control drug release from small particle dosage forms. It has been shown that the concentration gradient matrix system can generate zero-order release kinetics

Table VII-2. Formulas for the Matrix Suspension and Drug Solution [11].

Matrix suspension formula		Drug solution formula	
Eudragit RS 30D	80 g	Chlorpheniramine maleate	2.81 g
Talc	70 g	1/3 water, 2/3 ethanol	q.s. 25 ml
Triacetin	6 g		
Ethanol	75 g		
Water	19 g		
	Pump rate		
Time (min)	Matrix suspension (g/min)	Drug solution (ml/min)	
0 to 27	1.6	0.27	
27 to 61	1.6	0.151	
61 to 103	1.6	0.0733	
103 to 155	1.6	0.0201	

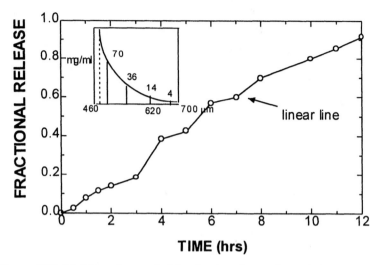

Figure VII-10. The release of chlorpheniramine maleate from granules with gradient drug concentration. (Graph reconstructed from data by Scott and Hollenbeck [11].)

with small granules. Non-pareil (sugar) beads were coated with pumping drug solution and matrix suspension, as shown in Table VII-2. Adjusting the drug solution concentration and the duration of coating for the specific coating solution created the concentration gradient. As shown in Fig. VII-10, the initial release profile is slow (or retarded), followed by a sharp increase of drug release because of higher drug loading in the next coating level. There is discontinuity of drug release due to the four discrete layers employed to approximate a continuous gradient [11]. These discontinuities take place when drug in each successive layer begins to diffuse out. Overall, the release profile is close to zero-order.

VII. 5. Megaloporous Matrix

Haan and Lerk [12] introduced the megaloporous system which has the property of releasing drug at a constant rate. The system is composed of two phases. One phase, the housing phase, controls liquid penetration into the system and the other phase, the restraining phase, delivers drug over an extended period of time. Upon contact with water, water-soluble ingredients of the housing phase leach out, producing large pores in the system, during water penetration into the inner parts of the system, the surface area of restraining phase increases. The drug in the restraining phase (drug containing phase) is exposed to the leaching solvent and the exposing rate

Table VII-3. Composition of the Restraining Phase and Housing Phase [12].

Restraining phase	5	6	Housing phase	
Eudragit RS	25.0		Carbomer	7.5
Theophylline anhydrous	44.0		PEG 6000	35.0
Cetyl alcohol	5.0		Mg stearate	1.8
Talc	25.0		Lactose	35.7
Particle size (mm)	0.6-0.71	1.4-1.6	CaH$_2$PO4	20.0

decreases with time but simultaneously the total pore surface area exposed to the solvent increases. The formulations are prepared as presented in Tables VII-3.

Theophylline release profiles from tablets composed of the housing phase (Table VII-3) in combination with the restraining phase (Table VII-3) arepresented in Fig. VII-11. An incorporation of 7.5% Carbomer 934P in the housing phase resulted in an increased and constant release rate up to 80% of release of the system. On the contrary, the release rate of theophylline from the system containing 1.8% of Mg stearate as the only insoluble excipient in the housing phase decreased with time [12]. Subsequent experiments have demonstrated that drug release profiles for a megaloporous system become non-linear as the portion of Carbomer in the housing phase is excessive (>25%). In this case, the housing phase governs the release kinetics having the decrease in a release rate with time. As the polymer content of the restraining phase is increased, the release rate of the drug from the megaloporous system decreased.

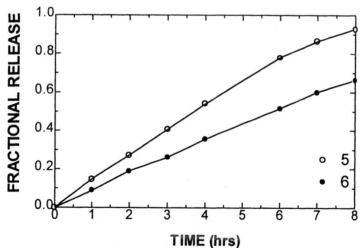

Figure VII-11. The release of theophylline from megaloporous matrices. (Graph reconstructed from data by Haan and Lerk [12].)

VII.6. Erodible Matrix

The same gradient matrix systems can be applied to the erodible systems. Here only a pure heterogeneous (surface erosion) mechanism having no diffusional process of drug is considered. For three types of geometry (slab, cylinder, and sphere) containing drug (dissolved or dispersed) and initial drug distribution in a matrix, $f(r)$, the fractional release of the drug may be expressed:

$$\frac{M_t}{M_\infty} = \frac{\int_S^a f(x)x^n dx}{\int_0^a f(r)x^n dx} \tag{7-18}$$

where $n=0$, 1, and 2 for a slab, cylinder, and sphere, respectively, and a is the radius or half-thickness of slab, and S is the erosion moving front. The concentration gradient function may be linear, parabolic, sigmoidal, and staircase. If the erosion rate is constant, the erosion front position rate is expressed by:

$$S = a - Bt \tag{7-19}$$

where B is the erosion rate constant. Then equation (7-18) can be rearranged as:

$$\frac{M_t}{M_\infty} = \frac{\int_{1-Bt/a}^1 f(\lambda)\lambda^n d\lambda}{\int_0^1 f(\lambda)\lambda^n d\lambda} \tag{7-20}$$

There are some differences in drug release profiles from erodible matrices containing non-uniform initial drug distribution compared to diffusion controlled matrix, as shown in Fig. VII-12. For a slab geometry, only uniform drug distribution furnishes constant release kinetics because of the constant releasing surface area whereas for a sphere, non-uniform drug distribution (staircase or sigmoidal) provides linear release profiles with and without delay because of decreasing releasing surface area with time. However, staircase or sigmoidal drug distribution for non-eroding matrix gives rise close to zero-order release kinetics for all geometry due to diffusion controlled process. From equation (7-20), constant release kinetics can be obtained from erosion controlled matrices with an initial drug concentration distribution expressed by [1]:

$$f(r) = \frac{1}{[r(or,l)]^n} \tag{7-21}$$

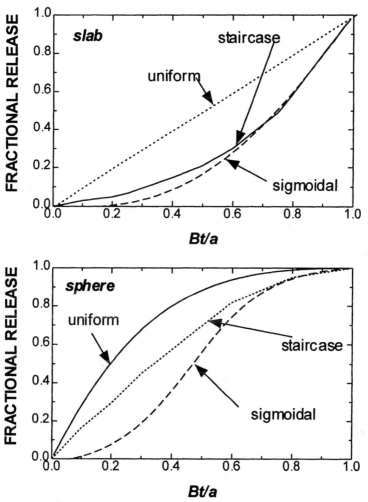

Figure VII-12. Effect of initial drug distribution in erosion controlled matrices on release kinetics. (Graph reconstructed from data by Lee [1].)

where $n = 0$, 1, and 2 are for slab, cylinder, and sphere, respectively.

Unlike diffusion controlled gradient matrices, pulsatile drug delivery systems can be fabricated by inserting drug-free layers in a laminated film and varying drug concentration in each layer. The drug concentration in each layer of composite sphere and cylinder should be designed in an increasing manner toward the core to achieve the same pulse rate [4].

References

1. P. I. Lee, "Initial Concentration Distribution as a Mechanism for Regulating Drug Release From Diffusion Controlled and Surface Erosion Controlled Matrix Systems," *J. Control. Rel.*, 4, 1 (1986).
2. H. S. Carslaw and J. C. Jaegar, <u>Conduction of Heat in Solids</u>, Clarendon Press, Oxford, 1959.
3. P. I. Lee, US Patent 4,729,190 (March 1988).
4. P. I. Lee, "Diffusion-Controlled Matrix Systems," In Treatise on Controlled Drug Delivery, A. Kydonieus (Eds.), Marcel Dekker, New York, 1992, p155.
5. P. I. Lee, "Novel Approach to Zero-Order Drug Delivery via Immobilized Nonuniform Drug Distribution in Glassy Hydrogels," *J. Pharm. Sci.*, 73, 1344 (1984).
6. C. J. Kim, "Hydrogel Beads for Oral Drug Delivery Systems," *Chemtech*, 24(8), 36 (1994).
7. P. I. Lee, "Effect of Non-Uniform Initial Drug Concentration Distribution on the Kinetics of Drug Release from Glassy Hydrogel Matrices," *Polymer*, 25, 973 (1984).
8. E. M. G. van Bommel, J. G. Fokkens, and D. J. A. Crommelen, "A Gradient Matrix System as a Controlled Release Device: Release from a Slab Model System," *J. Control. Rel.*, 10, 283 (1989).
9. S. B. Mitra, "Oral Sustained Release Drug Delivery System Using Polymer Film Composites," *Polymer Preprint*, 24, 51 (1983).
10. M. Wolff, G. Cordes, and V. Luckow, "In Vitro and In Vivo-Release of Nitroglycerin from a New Transdermal Therapeutic System," *Pharm. Res.*, 2, 23 (1985).
11. D. C. Scott and R. G. Hollenbeck, "Design and Manufacture of a Zero-Order Sustained-Release Pellet Dosage Form Through Nonuniform Drug Distribution in a Diffusional Matrix," *Pharm. Res.*, 8, 156 (1991).
12. P. D. Haan and C. F. Lerk, "The Effects of Polymer Content and Distribution on Drug Release Characteristics of the Megaloporous System," *Acta Pharm. Technol.*, 33, 149 (1987).

Chapter VIII

Osmotically Controlled Systems

VIII.1. Osmosis

Solvent from a solution of lower concentration will move spontaneously to a higher concentration solution across an ideal semi-permeable membrane, which is permeable to solvent but impermeable to solute. This phenomenon is called osmosis. The flow of solvent can be reduced by applying pressure to the higher concentration solution side of the membrane as shown in Fig. VIII-1. At a certain pressure, equilibrium is reached so that the movement of water ceases. This pressure is called the osmotic pressure, which is solely a property of the solution. If a pressure greater than the osmotic pressure is applied to the higher concentration side, the flow of solvent will be reversed, i.e., the solvent now moves from the higher concentration solution to the lower concentration solution. This phenomenon is called reverse osmosis. Osmotic pressure may be considered a measure of the difference between the nature of the solution and the pure solvent. It often poses a problem in diffusion-controlled devices. Of particular concern is the osmotic pressure of a water-soluble drug in a hydrogel matrix. The matrix is distorted by expanding the hydrogel beyond its swelling capacity, thus causing rupture. Drug release is also affected because the osmotic pressure acts as a driving force. Initially there is a large amount of drug present in the hydrogel matrix. When this drug comes in contact with the dissolution medium, it dissolves and produces a significant osmotic pressure. As a result, drug release is accelerated during early time release. However, a later time drug release slows down because there is a lower amount of dissolved drug and, therefore, a reduced osmotic pressure. A drop in osmotic pressure causes the dimensions of the matrix to shrink. Osmotic pressure can be successfully used in drug delivery systems by confining it in a mechanical device and concentrating the pressure at a single site.

When equilibrium is reached, the chemical potentials of the pure solvent (or dilute solution), μ_A^*, and the concentrated solution, μ_A, are equal,

$$\mu_A^*(p) = \mu_A(x_A, \pi + p) \tag{8-1}$$

where x_A is the concentration of solute, π is the osmotic pressure, and p is the experimental pressure. The right-hand side of equation (8-1) can be rewritten in terms of the pure solvent by:

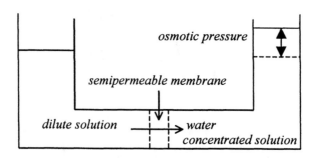

Figure VIII-1. Osmosis process [1].

$$\mu_A(x_A, \pi + p) = \mu_A^*(\pi + p) + RT \ln x_A \tag{8-2}$$

where R and T are the gas constant and temperature, respectively. However, we may express the chemical potential of the concentrated solution only due to solvent:

$$\mu_A^*(\pi + p) = \mu_A^*(p) + \int_p^{\pi+p} V_m dp \tag{8-3}$$

where V_m is the volume of solvent. Substitution of equations (8-2) and (8-3) into (8-1) yields:

$$-RT \ln(1 - x_A) = \int_p^{\pi+p} V_m dp \tag{8-4}$$

For the dilute solutions, $\ln(1 - x_A) = -x_A$. If constant molar volume of the solvent is assumed, then from equation (8-4) the van't Hoff equation is obtained:

$$\pi V = nRT \tag{8-5}$$

Table VIII-1. Typical osmotic pressure [1].

Compound	Concentration mg/l	moles/l	Osmotic Pressure psi at 25°C
NaCl	35000	0.6	398
NaCl	1000	0.0171	11.4
Na_2SO_4	1000	0.0071	6.0
$MgCl_2$	1000	0.0105	9.7
Sucrose	1000	0.0029	1.4
Dextrose	1000	0.0055	2.0

As shown in Table VIII-1, the osmotic pressure caused by solutes is very high and that from an ionic salt is much higher than that from a nonionic solute. Theoretically the osmotic pressure of an ionic salt is given by:

$$\pi V = inRT \qquad (8\text{-}6)$$

where i is the number of ions that compose the salt.

Problem VIII-1: Calculate the osmotic pressure of sucrose and phenobarbital sodium (i=2.0) [2]. C_s=100 g/l, M = 254.2 g/l, Temp.=37°C [2].
Solution:

$$\pi = 2.0 \; \frac{nRT}{V} = 2.0 \; \frac{(100)(0.08205)(310)}{254.2} = 20.0 \text{ atm}$$

VIII.2. Elementary Osmotic Pump Systems (OROS®)

After experimenting with several osmotic pressure driven drug delivery systems [3,4], Alza Corporation developed the OROS® elementary pump shown in Fig. VIII-2. This system is prepared by compressing drug powder into a hard tablet, coating the tablet with cellulose derivatives to form a semi-permeable membrane, and then drilling an orifice in the coating with a laser.

The volumetric flow of solvent (water) across the semi-permeable membrane is given by the non-equilibrium thermodynamics of the reverse osmosis process as [5]:

$$\frac{dV}{dt} = \frac{A}{h} L_p (\sigma \Delta \pi - \Delta p) \qquad (8\text{-}7)$$

where $\Delta \pi$ and Δp are the osmotic and hydrostatic pressure difference, respectively, between the high and low concentration sides of the membrane, L_p is the permeability coefficient of the semi-permeable membrane, σ is the reflection coefficient, A is the membrane surface area, and h is the membrane thickness.

The solute delivery rate, dm/dt, is equal to the product of the volume flow rate and drug concentration written as:

$$\frac{dm}{dt} = \frac{dV}{dt} C \qquad (8\text{-}8)$$

where C is the solute concentration in the outgoing fluid. When the osmotic pressure inside the membrane is very large compared to the pressure outside the membrane and $\Delta \pi \gg \Delta p$, equation (8-7) simplifies to:

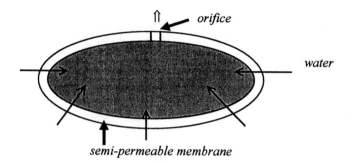

Figure VIII-2. The elementary osmotic pump [5].

$$\frac{dV}{dt} = \frac{A}{h} L_p \sigma \pi = \frac{A}{h} k \pi \tag{8-9}$$

where $k = \sigma L_p$.

**Zero-order rate and mass delivered at zero-order**: As long as the un-dissolved drug remains in the osmotic tablet, the release rate is zero-order. If the concentration of the drug is equal to the drug's solubility in water, C_s, and the osmotic pressure generated by this saturated solution is π_s, then

$$\left(\frac{dm}{dt}\right)_z = \frac{A}{h} k \pi_s C_s \tag{8-10}$$

The time for which drug is delivered under zero-order conditions is given by:

$$t_z = m_t (1 - \frac{C_s}{\rho}) \frac{1}{(dm/dt)_z} \tag{8-11}$$

where t_z is the time at which all of the solid in the core has been dissolved.

The total mass in the core, m_t, is the sum of the mass delivered at zero-order, m_z, and the mass delivered at non-zero-order rate, m_{nz}, after which the entire solid drug has dissolved, given by:

$$m_{nz} = C_s V \tag{8-12}$$

$$m_t = \rho V \tag{8-13}$$

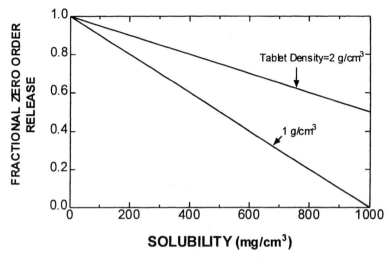

Figure VIII-3. Percentage of drug content delivered at a constant rate.

where V and ρ are the volume and density of the osmotic tablet, respectively. Combining equations (8-12) and (8-13) gives:

$$\frac{m_z}{m_t} = 1 - \frac{C_s}{\rho} \tag{8-14}$$

Fig. VIII-3 shows the effect of the drug's solubility and bulk density of drug on the percentage of drug delivered at a constant rate.

Non-zero release rate: As soon as all of the solid has dissolved, the solute concentration drops below saturation, and the osmotic pressure and the drug delivery rate decline as a function of time.

From t_z and afterwards, the delivery rate (non-zero order) is described by [5]:

$$\left(\frac{dm}{dt}\right)_{nz} = \frac{(dm/dt)_z}{\left[1 + \dfrac{1}{C_s V}\left(\dfrac{dm}{dt}\right)_z (t - t_z)\right]^2} \tag{8-15}$$

which indicates that the release rate declines parabolically with respect to time as shown in Fig. VIII-4. The concentration at time t after t_z is calculated by [5]:

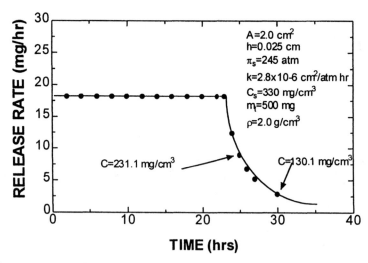

Figure VIII-4. Theoretical delivery rate of KCl from an elementary osmotic pump [5].

$$C = \frac{C_s V}{V + (t - t_z)F_s} \qquad (8\text{-}16)$$

where $F_s = AL_p\pi_s/h$.

An advantage of the osmotic pump delivery device is that the delivery rate is not influenced by physiological and experimental conditions as shown in Figs. VIII-5 and VIII-6. Due to the semi-permeable membrane, ions do not readily cross over but water does. The permeation of water through the membrane is not dependent upon stirring rate because water permeation is a property of the membrane and the osmotic pressure gradient across it.

With this consideration, even a drug with a pH-dependent solubility can be delivered at a constant rate regardless of the pH of the delivery medium. As an example, Theeuwes [5] demonstrated that the release rate of phenobarbitol sodium was independent of the pH.

However, with this type of device there is a problem in delivering drug with low water solubility because the osmotic pressure generated by the drug solution is not sufficient to drive the drug release. As a result, the percentage of the total mass delivered at zero-order is less with a drug of low solubility. In this case, osmagents, such as glucose and NaCl, are added to the device to increase the osmotic pressure. In order to maintain a zero-order rate for a given release period, the ratio of drug to osmagent must be equal to the

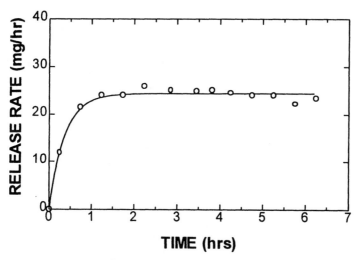

Figure VIII-5. Effect of the hydrodynamic conditions on the delivery rate of KCl from an OROS pump. (Graph reconstructed from data by Theeuwes [5].)

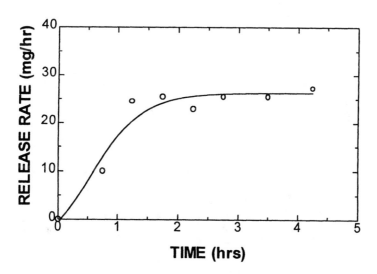

Figure VIII-6. Effect of pH conditions on the delivery rate of sodium phenobarbital from an OROS pump. (Graph reconstructed from data by Theeuwes [5].)

Table VIII-2. Solubilities of Salbutamol Sulfate and NaCl [6].

Solute in Solvent	Solubility (mg/ml)
Salbutamol in water	275
Salbutamol in saturated NaCl	16
Sodium chloride in water	321
NaCl in saturated salbutamol	320

ratio of the solubility of drug to osmagent. However, if the drug solubility is too low (i.e. < 1%) and the amount of drug to be administered is large, the usefulness of the elementary osmotic pump device is limited due to the tablet size needed to accommodate the amount of drug. Other modifications of the osmotic pump have been developed to address this situation and are discussed in the next section.

Alternatively, a highly water-soluble drug may allow a higher percentage of drugs to be delivered at zero-order, but the length of delivery is short because the drug concentration quickly falls below saturation. For this situation, a solubility modulated osmotic pump device has been developed to increase the duration of delivery time while maintaining a reasonable zero-order rate [6]. As shown in Table VIII-2, the solubility of salbutamol sulfate in water is 275 mg/ml while it is 16 mg/ml in saturated NaCl. The solubility of NaCl is not significantly different in water and saturated salbutamol sulfate. When salbutamol sulfate and NaCl are formulated into an osmotic pump tablet, the release of salbutamol sulfate can be extended to 12-24 hrs

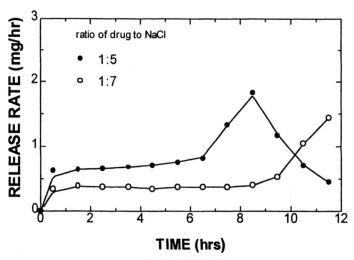

Figure VIII-7. Release rate of salbutamol sulfate from the OROS system containing various proportions of salbutamol sulfate and NaCl. (Graph reconstructed from data by Magruder et al. [6].)

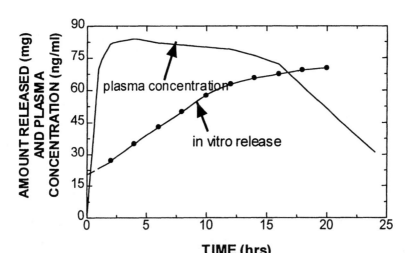

TIME (hrs)
Figure VIII-8. Delivery of phenylpropanolamine HCl from an OROS pump. (a) *In vitro* release, (b) *in vivo* mean plasma concentration. (Graph reconstructed from data by Good and Lee [7].)

depending upon the ratio of salbutamol sulfate to NaCl as presented in Fig. VIII-7. Delayed pulse doses of drug are observed due to the higher solubility of salbutamol sulfate in a dilute NaCl solution.

Accutrim® [7]: This osmotic pump tablet is a pill used to control appetite. It is employed in weight loss programs. Phenylpropranolamine HCl and NaCl are compressed to form a hard tablet and coated with cellulose acetate to form a semi-permeable membrane. The release of drug from this tablet follows zero-order kinetics, as shown in Fig. VIII-8. There is constant drug release of up to 60-70% of the dose with a plateau when a sub-saturation concentration level of drug is reached. However, this zero-order release rate may not affect the serum blood drug concentration near the therapeutic level. This shortcoming is attributed to the pharmacokinetics of phenylpropranol amine HCl since the elimination of the drug from the body is much slower than the absorption rate. In order to address this drawback, an immediate dose is coated on the outside of the semi-permeable membrane. The immediate dose provides a rapid achievement of therapeutic levels after which the zero-order release rate maintains this level for a expected time periods up to 12 hrs.

As expected from equation (8-7), drug release is strongly dependent upon the osmotic pressure difference between the inside and the outside of the tablet. As shown in Fig. VIII-9, when an osmotic pressure equilibrium is established between the external and internal environments of the tablet, the rate release goes to zero.

This type of osmotic pump has been applied to other drugs (i.e.

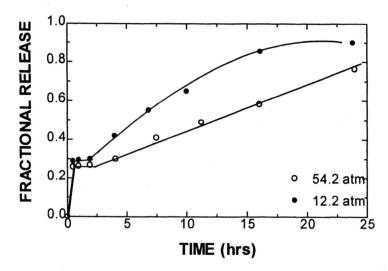

Figure VIII-9. The effect of the differential osmotic pressure on the release profile of phenylpropanolamine HCl. (Graph reconstructed from data by Liu et al. [8].)

indomethacin) [9]. Due to the low solubility of indomethacin in acidic conditions, potassium bicarbonate is incorporated into the tablet. This maintains a neutral or weakly basic pH of the drug solution in the core and prevents precipitation of indomethacin upon contact with gastric fluid. The system delivers 80% of the drug at a constant rate. Delivery rates are independent of stirring rate and pH of the dissolution medium as observed in the release of KCl from the OROS pump (Fig. VIII-10).

VIII.3. Micro-Porous Osmotic Pumps (MPOP)

Fabricating an osmotic pump with a single orifice is a costly process because the hole must be produced consistently with a laser drill. Zetner et al. [10-13] developed an osmotic pump device based upon a micro-porous membrane rather than a non-porous semi-permeable membrane as shown in Fig. VIII-11. In this device, drugs, as well as water, freely diffuse through the membrane. A fraction of the drug and the osmogent diffuses through the micro-porous membrane. Incorporating water-soluble substances in the coating solution (i.e. polyethylene glycol and lactose) forms the micro-porous structure of the membrane. Upon contact with water, the water-soluble substances from the membrane leach out, leaving behind a micro-porous morphology. This device delivers drug by both osmotic pressure and diffusion mechanisms. The delivery rate of drug is expressed by [5]:

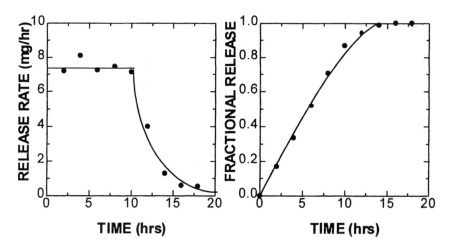

Figure VIII-10. Experimental and theoretical release rate (a) and cumulative release (b) of indomethacin from OROS pump. (Graph reconstructed from data by Theeuwes et al. [9].)

$$\left(\frac{dm}{dt} \right)_z = \frac{A}{h} k\pi_s C_s + \frac{A}{h} PC_s \qquad (8\text{-}17)$$

where P is the permeability of the membrane. A rigorous mathematical interpretation of the non-zero-order release rate for both the osmotic pump and membrane diffusion has been presented by Theeuwes [5] and is expressed by:

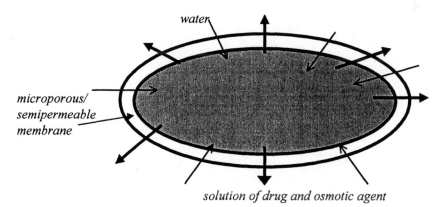

Figure VIII-11. Schematic diagram of the porosity controlled osmotic pump [11].

$$t - t_z = \frac{Vh}{AP} \ln\left[\frac{F_s \dfrac{C}{C_s} + \dfrac{AP}{h}}{\left(F_s + \dfrac{AP}{h}\right)\dfrac{C}{C_s}}\right] \qquad (8\text{-}18)$$

The non-zero order delivery rate is given by:

$$\frac{dm}{dt} = \frac{F_s}{C_s} C^2 + \frac{A}{h} PC \qquad (8\text{-}19)$$

As indicated in equation (8-17), the release rate is controlled by [10]: (1) the level of leachable additives incorporated into the membrane which affect membrane permeability, (2) the nature of the polymer membrane, (3) the thickness and surface area of the membrane, (4) the solubility and osmotic pressure of the core, and (5) the drug load in the core. The most common polymers used for the micro-porous membrane are cellulose acetate, ethyl cellulose and Eudragit® LS and RS. A scanning electron microscope showed that the micro-porous membrane is a sponge-like structure consisting of numerous open and closed pores that form an interconnected network structure [10]. The release profile of KCl from the micro-porous osmotic pump in water is shown in Fig. VIII-12. As we observed for the OROS® device, the drug release is linear over almost 100% of the 6 hrs dose interval. Like the OROS® system, the release rate of KCl is inversely proportional to the thickness of the membrane due to the increase of inter-membrane diffusion length.

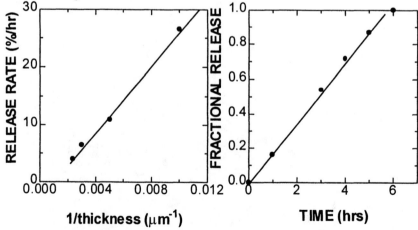

Figure VIII-12. Release profile of KCl and effect of membrane thickness on the release rate. (Graph reconstructed from data by Appel and Zentner [14].)

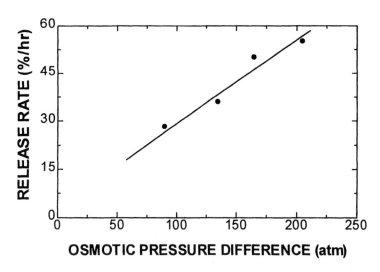

Figure VIII-13. Effect of osmotic pressure on the release rate of KCl from the porosity controlled osmotic pump. (Graph reconstructed from data by Appel and Zentner [14].)

In addition, the release rate of KCl from MPOP device is driven by the osmotic pressure difference across the membrane, as shown in Fig. VIII-13. Figures (VIII-12) and (VIII-13) show that the MPOP is controlled by the osmotic pumping and diffusion through the membrane.

As discussed previously for salbutamol sulfate, solubility modulated delivery may be achieved for the porosity controlled osmotic pump. The solubility of diltiazem HCl varies in NaCl solution as presented in Table VIII-3. The release kinetics of diltiazem HCl follow a zero-order rate for 70% of the release time and are not affected by the pH of the dissolution medium.

Table VIII-3. Effect of NaC Solution on the Solubility of Diltiazem HCl [12].

Solubility of Diltiazem HCl (mg/ml)	Sodium Chloride Concentration (M)	Theoretical Release Profile (% zero-order)[a]
>590	0	<51
545± 12	0.25	55
395± 29	0.50	67
278± 10	0.75	77
155± 20	1.00	87
40± 5	1.20	99

[a] Based on diltiazem HCl density = 1.2 g/cm^3

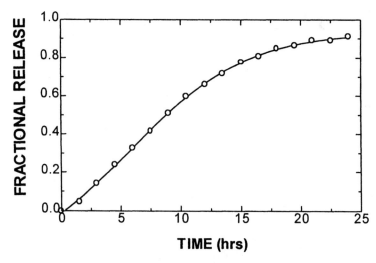

Figure VIII-14. Release of diltiazem HCl from the porosity controlled osmotic pump. (Graph reconstructed from data by Zentner et al. [12].)

VIII.4. Push-Pull

As mentioned in the previous section, the simple OROS® system is well suited for a moderately water-soluble drug. For a poorly water-soluble drug (<1%), the delivery rate is very slow because of the small osmotic pressure gradient. Even if an osmogent is incorporated into the core, the osmotic pressure gradient is not increased enough to effect a sufficient delivery rate because the ratio of drug to osmogent concentration is not equal to the ratio of drug solubility to osmogent concentration. To deal with this problem, Alza developed another osmotic pump system shown in Fig. VIII-15. This device consists of two compartments: a water-swellable polymer layer and a drug layer. The core is coated with a non-porous semi-permeable membrane as described in the OROS® system. When the "push-pull" device is in contact with water, both layers pull water from the dissolution medium. Due to the low solubility of the drug, a drug suspension is produced in the top layer while a hydrophilic polymer in the bottom layer expands toward the top layer to push the suspended drug through the orifice.

Fig. VIII-16 shows a comparative *in-vivo* study of nifedipine release from: Adalat Retard tablets and the push-pull osmotic pump (Procardia® XL). After 6 hours of oral administration of nifedipine by Procaria® XL, the mean plasma concentration of nifedipine reaches 20 ng/ml and remains at this concentration for up to 24 hrs; Adalat Retard tablets produce plasma concentrations which climb very quickly to 95 ng/ml followed by a rapid

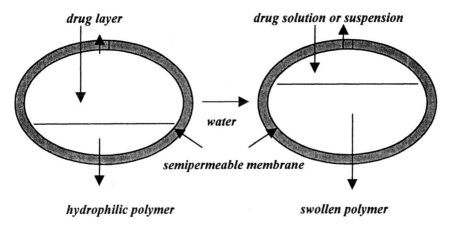

Figure VIII-15. Schematic diagram of the push-pull osmotic pump [15].

decline. Within 12 hrs of oral administration of Adalat Retard, the drug concentration level falls below 20 ng/ml.

A similar push-pull osmotic pump device has been applied to delivery of anti-parasite drugs for cattle. As shown in Fig. VIII-18, the basic concept is the same as the original push-pull system but on a larger scale. This dosage form differs: there is a placebo partition layer between the swellable polymer and drug compartments. The partition promotes uniform movement of drug solution to the exit port by the expansion of the swelling

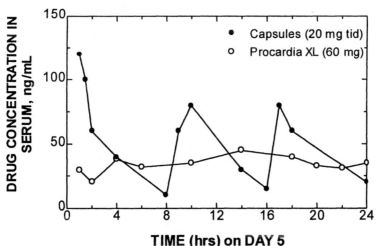

TIME (hrs) on DAY 5

Figure VIII-16. Comparative mean blood drug concentration profile of nifedipine. (Graph reconstructed from data by Alza Corporation [15].)

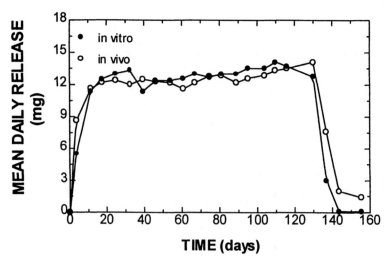

Figure VIII-17. *In-vivo* and *in-vitro* mean ivermectin profile. (Graph reconstructed from data by Zingerman et al. [16].)

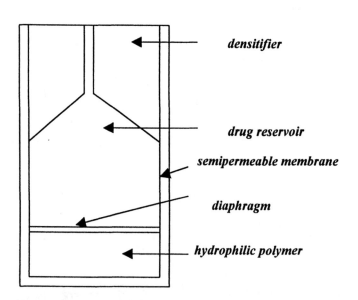

Figure VIII-18. Schematic diagram of Ivomec SR Bolus [16].

polymer. Another important difference is the density element, which provides the mass necessary to retain the dosage form in the cattle's stomach [16].

Release rates of ivermectin (IVOMEC SR Bolus) *in vivo* and *in vitro* are presented in Fig. VIII-17. On average, this device maintains a constant release rate of approximately 12 mg/day for 130 days. The *in vivo* rate of drug release is slower than *in vitro* probably due to the different chemical activity of water in the rumen contents (i.e. osmotic pressure difference) [16].

Similarly, Pope et al. [17] showed that a specially weighted mini-osmotic pump (ALZET 2ML4) delivered ivermectin at a controlled rate and predictable levels of drug in plasma could be maintained.

Problem VIII-2: Design an osmotic pump system for a drug which has a solubility of 330 mg/cm^3. The drug is ionic (i=1.9) and its molecular weight is 95.3. The semi-permeable membrane surface area is 2.2 cm^2, its thickness is 0.025 cm, and its permeability (L_p) is 2.8x10-6 cm^2/atm/hr. The total mass of the drug to be delivered is 500 mg and the density of the drug core is 2g/cm^3. Calculate the zero-order release rate and the time t_z. Also calculate the time at which the drug's release rate is 3.5 mg/hr.

Solution:

$$\pi = \frac{n}{V} RT = \frac{297}{74.6} \text{(mole/l)} \times 0.082 \text{(l atm/mole K)} \times 310.16 \text{(mole)}$$

$$= 101.3 \text{ atm}$$

$$\left(\frac{dm}{dt}\right)_z = \frac{A}{h} k\pi_s C_s$$

$$= (1.97 \text{ cm}^2/0.025 \text{ cm})(2.7\times10^{-6} \text{ cm}^2/\text{atm hr})(297 \text{ mg/cm}^3)(101.3 \text{ atm})$$
$$= 6.4 \text{ mg/hr}$$

$$t_z = m_t(1 - C_s / \rho)/(dm/dt)_z$$
$$= 475 \text{ mg } (1 - 297 \text{ mg/cm}^3/1900 \text{ mg/cm}^3)/ 6.4 \text{ mg/hr} = 62.6 \text{ hrs}$$

$$\left(\frac{dm}{dt}\right)_{nz} = \frac{(dm/dt)_z}{\left[1 + \frac{1}{C_s V}\left(\frac{dm}{dt}\right)_z (t - t_z)\right]^2} = \frac{6.4}{[1 + 0.0862(t - 62.5)]^2} = 3.1 \text{ (mg/hr)}$$

$t = 67.67$ hr $=$ time at which the release rate is 3.1 mg/hr

$$F_s = \frac{A}{h} L_p \pi_s = (1.97 \text{ cm}^2/0.025 \text{ cm})(2.7\times10^{-6} \text{ cm}^2/\text{atm hr})(101.3 \text{ atm}) = 0.0216 \text{ cm}^3/\text{hr}$$

$$C = \frac{C_s V}{V + (t - t_z) F_s}$$

=(297 mg/ml/0.25 ml)/[0.25 ml + (67.67 – 62.6)(hr)(0.021 cm^3/hr]
= 206.3 mg/ml

206.3 mg/cm^3 = drug concentration at release rate of 3.1 mg/hr.

References

1.   J. E. Curver, "Membrane Processes," in Physicochemical Processes for Water Quality Control W. J. Weber, Jr. (Ed.), Wiley-Interscience, New York, 1972. p235.
2.   A. Martin, J. Swarbrich, and A. Cammarata, (Eds.), Physical Pharmacy, 3rd Edition, Lea & Febiger, Philadelphia, PA, 1983. p591.
3.   T. Higuchi and H. M. Leeper, "Improved Osmotic Dispenser Employing Magnesium Sulfate and Magnesium Chloride," U.S. Patent 3,760,804 (Sept. 1973).
4.   T. Higuchi, "Osmotic Dispenser with Collapsible Supply Container," U.S. Patent 3,760,805 (Sept. 1973).
5.   F. Theeuwes, "Elementary Osmotic Pump," J. Pharm. Sci., 64, 1987 (1975).
6.   P. R. Magruder, B. Barclay, P. S. L. Wong, and F. Theeuwes, U.S. Patent 4,751,071 (June 1988).
7.   W. R. Good and P. I. Lee, "Membrane-Controlled Reservoir Drug Delivery Systems," in Medical Applications of Controlled Release, Vol. I, R. S. Langer and D. L. Wise (Eds.), CRC Press, Baton Rouge, Fl. 1984. p1.
8.   F. Liu, M. Farber and Y. Chien, "Comparative Release of Phenypropranolamine HCl from Long-Acting Appetite Suppressant Products: Accutrim vs. Dexatrim," Drug Dev. Ind. Pharm., 10, 1639 (1984).
9.   F. Theeuwes, D. Dawanson, P. Wong, P. Bonsen, V. Place, K. Heimlich, and K. C. Kwan, "Elementary Osmotic Pump for Indomethacin," J. Pharm. Sci., 72, 253 (1983).
10. G. M. Zentner, G. S. Rork, and K. J. Himmelstein, "The Controlled Porosity Osmotic Pump," J. Control. Rel., 1, 269 (1985).
11. G. M. Zentner, G. S. Rork, and K. J. Himmelstein, "Osmotic Flow Through Controlled Porosity Film: An Approach to Delivery of Water Soluble Compounds," J. Control. Rel., 2, 217 (1985).
12. G. M. Zentner, G. A. McClelland, and S. C. Sutton, "Controlled Porosity Solubility- and Resin-Modulated Osmotic Drug Delivery Systems for Release of Diltiazem Hydrogen Chloride," J. Control. Rel., 16, 237 (1991).
13. A. G. Thrombe, G. M. Zentner, and K. J. Himmelstein, "Mechanism of Water Transport in Controlled Porosity Osmotic Devices," J. Membr. Sci., 40, 279 (1989).

14. L. E. Appel and G. M. Zentner, "Use of Modified Ethylcellulose Lattices for Microporous Coating of Osmotic Tablets," *Pharm. Res.*, 8, 600 (1991).
15. Alza Technology, Alza Corporation, Palo Alto, CA., 1992. p6.
16. J. R. Zingerman, J. R. Cardinal, J. Holste, B. Eckenhoff, and J. Wright, "The In Vitro and In Vivo Performance of an Osmotically Controlled Delivery System - IVOMEC SR Bolus," *Proceed. Intern. Symp. Control. Rel. Bioact. Mater.*, 19, 82 (1992).
17. D.G. Pope, P. K. Wilkinson, J. R. Egerton, and J. Conroy, "Oral Controlled-Release Delivery of Ivermectin in Cattle via an Osmotic Pump," *J. Pharm. Sci.*, 74, 1108 (1985).

Chapter IX

Geometrically Modified Systems

The diffusion-controlled monolithic matrix systems discussed in the previous sections have some advantages over other systems especially when compared to the fabrication of reservoir systems. A major drawback is that they do not inherently possess zero-order release kinetics. However, these systems can overcome the diminishing release rate as the drug diffuses from longer diffusion length or lower drug concentration distribution. This problem is especially severe for spherical and cylindrical shaped devices. A possible solution to obtaining zero-order release of drugs is to modify the matrix geometry. Examples of alternative geometries, e.g. pie, hemisphere or cone are illustrated here. Most of these devices find application in agriculture or large animals rather than in humans.

IX.1. Pie Shaped, Perforated Tablets (Coated and Uncoated), and Multi-Hole Systems

Brooke and Washkuhn [1] presented the pie (or prism) shaped device to deliver a drug at a zero-order rate. Dissolution from a solid drug or diffusion from a polymer matrix may be used to control the release of its drug contents. As illustrated in Fig. IX-1, this device has a slot width a, an effective slot length L, and an angle 2θ. The release of stearic acid from a pie shaped device in methanol is constant for 400 hrs as shown in Fig. IX-2.

Lipper and Higuchi [2] presented a theoretical expression for release of a drug from pie-shaped devices. The flux J, for diffusion path length s, is given by:

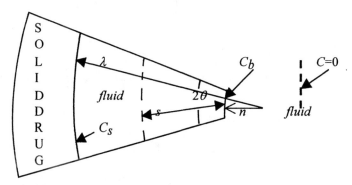

Figure IX-1. Cross-sectional view of a pie-shaped device [1].

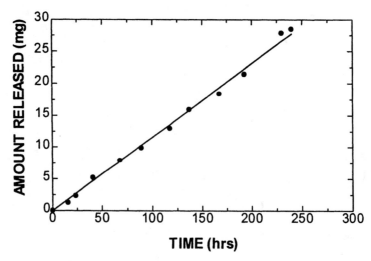

Figure IX-2. The release of stearic acid from the pie-shaped device [1]. (Graph reconstructed from data by Brooke and Washkuhn [1].)

$$J = 2\theta LD(s + n)\frac{dC}{ds} \tag{9-1}$$

where D is the diffusion coefficient of the drug in the dissolution medium, s is the diffusion path length, n is the opening radius, and C is the drug concentration. At a pseudo-steady state (constant flux), integration of equation (9-1) with respect to both distance and concentration yields:

$$J = \frac{2\theta LD(C_s - C_b)}{\ln\dfrac{\lambda}{n}} \tag{9-2}$$

where C_s and C_b are the drug concentration at the drug dissolution moving front and at the opening, respectively, and λ is the distance between the center of the pie device and the moving front.

However, diffusion from the opening of the device into the dissolution medium is expressed for sink conditions by:

$$J = \frac{2\theta LDnC_b}{h} \tag{9-3}$$

where h is the stagnant film thickness.

By solving equations (9-2) and (9-3) for C_b, and taking into account the mass dissolved at time t, $M = (\lambda^2 - n^2)L\theta\rho$, the following relationship between the mass dissolved and time can be obtained:

$$t = \frac{\left(\dfrac{h}{n} - \dfrac{1}{2}\right)M + \left(\dfrac{M + L\theta\rho n^2}{2}\right)\ln\left(\dfrac{M}{L\theta\rho n^2} + 1\right)}{2\theta LDC_s} \tag{9-4}$$

or

$$t = \frac{\left(\dfrac{h}{n} - \dfrac{1}{2}\right)(\lambda^2 - n^2)\rho + \lambda^2\rho\ln\dfrac{\lambda}{n}}{2DC_s} \tag{9-5}$$

However, if one considers the mass dissolved in the diffusion layer between λ and 0, the following equation may be derived for relating λ and M_r:

$$M_r = (\lambda^2 - n^2)\left[L\theta\rho - L\theta C_s + \frac{L\theta C_s}{2\left(\dfrac{h}{n} + \ln\dfrac{\lambda}{n}\right)}\right] - \frac{L\theta C_s n^2}{\dfrac{h}{n} + \ln\dfrac{\lambda}{n}} \tag{9-6}$$

Thus, M_r versus t can be generated by equations (9-5) and (9-6).

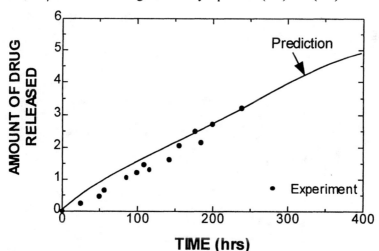

Figure IX-3. Cumulative release of stearic acid from a pie-shaped device. (Graph reconstructed from data by Lipper and Higuchi [2].)

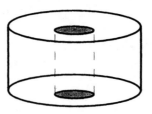

Figure IX-4. Cross-sectional view of a coated/perforated device [3].

Fig. IX-3 shows that the release data is in good agreement with the predicted profile although the experimental data is more linear.

Various authors have extended the method of geometrical modification to the design of specific delivery systems. Hanssen et al [3] and Conte et al. [4] developed the *perforated, coated tablet* (PCT) and Boettner et al. [5] presented the multi-perforated trilaminate. A single perforated tablet, as shown in Fig. IX-4, is made by direct compression of drug and other excipients (magnesium stearate and lactose). Dipping or spraying a polymer solution [poly(ethylene-co-vinyl acetate)] coats the tablet in which a single hole is drilled through the center from top to bottom. The core matrix may be non-porous.

Fig. IX-5 shows the effect of the size of the drilled hole on the release of sodium benzoate. As observed for other configurations, the release of the drug is linear because the inner releasing surface area increases as the dissolution front moves. However, Hansson et al. [3] observed a significant decrease in the dissolution rate and deviation from zero-order when a water-insoluble polymer is incorporated into the core matrix. Conte et al. [4] fabricated perforated coated tablets with a central hole by spraying a coating solution. In the perforated-coated tablets consisting of hydrophobic polymer, the drug is released only from the central hole, and the increase of surface area counterbalanced the increase of the diffusion length resistance with time, giving a constant release rate. During the coating operation, however, the inner surface of the central hole may be coated to form a film [4]. Equation (9-6) can be modified to calculate the amount of drug released from perforated-coated tablets by replacing θ with π as:

$$M_r = (\lambda^2 - n^2) \left[L\pi\rho - L\pi C_s + \frac{L\pi C_s}{2\left(\dfrac{h}{n} + \ln\dfrac{\lambda}{n}\right)} \right] - \frac{L\pi C_s n^2}{\dfrac{h}{n} + \ln\dfrac{\lambda}{n}} \qquad (9\text{-}7)$$

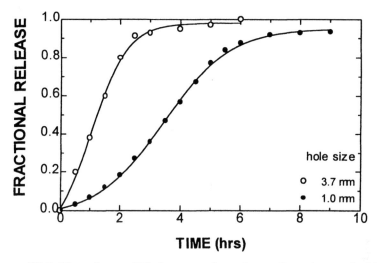

Figure IX-5. The release of Na benzoate from the perforated-coated tablets. (Graph reconstructed from data by Hanssen et al. [3].)

The *multi-perforated device* is similar to the single perforated tablet but consists of a core matrix with drug/polymer and top/bottom coated layers, which are impermeable to the drug. Circular perforations are punched from the top to the bottom as shown in Fig. IX-6. The drug is released through the perforated holes and uncoated sides. The number of perforations and the device's size control the amount of drug released over time. A device, which can be rolled and taped with water-soluble adhesive, has been used for delivery of morantel tartrate in cattle. Boettner et al. [5] adopted the concept used for the pie-shaped device. The device consists of the core sheet containing poly(ethylene-co-vinyl acetate) (PEVA) and a drug laminated with the top and bottom films of PEVA. Numerous holes are punched through the trilaminated sheet. Model equations have been developed to predict the release of drug from the multi-perforations as follows for a coated edge:

$$M_r = N(\lambda^2 - n^2)L\pi\varepsilon\left[\rho - C_s + \frac{C_s}{2\left(\frac{h\varepsilon}{n\tau} + \ln\frac{\lambda}{n}\right)}\right] - \frac{NL\pi\varepsilon C_s n^2}{\frac{h\varepsilon}{n\tau} + \ln\frac{\lambda}{n}} \qquad (9\text{-}8)$$

$$t = \frac{\left(\frac{h\varepsilon}{n\tau} - \frac{1}{2}\right)(\lambda^2 - n^2)\rho\tau + \lambda^2\tau\rho\ln\frac{\lambda}{n}}{2DC_s} \qquad (9\text{-}9)$$

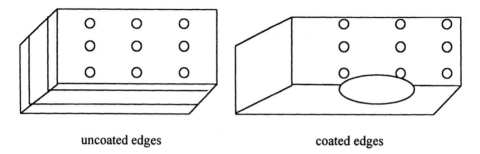

uncoated edges   coated edges

Figure X-6. Schematic diagram of morantel sustained release trilaminate [5].

and for an un-coated edge,

$$M_r = N(\lambda^2 - n^2)L\pi\varepsilon\left[\rho - C_s + \frac{C_s}{2\left(\dfrac{h\varepsilon}{n\tau} + \ln\dfrac{\lambda}{n}\right)}\right] - \left[\frac{NL\pi\varepsilon C_s}{\dfrac{h\varepsilon}{n\tau} + \ln\dfrac{\lambda}{n}}\right]$$

$$+ \quad S\left[\frac{D\varepsilon(2A - \varepsilon C_s)C_s t}{\tau}\right]^{\frac{1}{2}} \quad (9\text{-}10)$$

where ε and τ are the porosity and tortuosity of the matrix, respectively, N is the number of holes, and S is the surface perimeter of the edges. Fig. IX-7 shows *in-vitro* and *in-vivo* performance and the model predictions of the release of morantel from the controlled release trilaminate.

Kim [6] proposed simple un-coated-compressed (swellable/erodible) tablets with a central hole (*donut-shaped*). The release of theophylline from donut-shaped tablets is zero order (80-90% release) before rapidly decreasing, as shown in Fig. IX-8. As the hole size is increased from $\frac{7}{16}$" to $\frac{5}{32}$", the release rate increases and the release time is shortened. The observed behavior of erosion boundaries and diffusion fronts during drug release from the donut-shaped tablets is shown in Fig. IX-9. It is evident that the decrease of releasing surface area from the outer surface is compensated for by the increase of releasing surface area from the central hole. This results in a constant lateral releasing surface area as:

initial surface area = $\pi(a^2+b^2)L$ = surface area at time t = $\pi\{(a+x)^2+(b-x)^2\}L$
$$= \pi(a^2+b^2)L$$

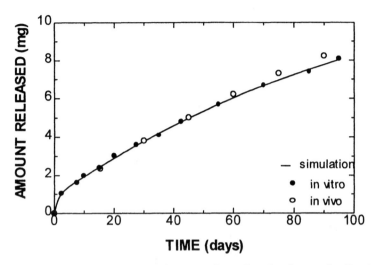

Figure IX-7. *In-vitro, in-vivo* release, and predicted release of trilaminated morantel controlled release sheets. (Graph reconstructed from data by Boettner et al. [5].)

At the later stage of drug release, the swollen gel thickness of the donut-shaped tablet is thin enough to be broken by fast stirring. However, if the hole size is smaller than 7/16", the hole collapses during drug release due to the inward swelling of the polymer from the central hole. As a result, the

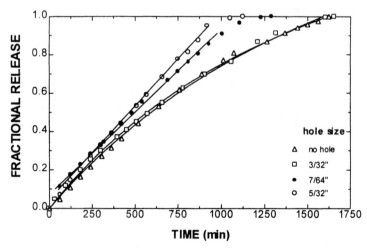

Figure IX-8. The release of theophylline from donut-shaped tablets. (Graph reconstructed from data by Kim [6].)

erosion front　　　　　　　　　　　　　*diffusion front*

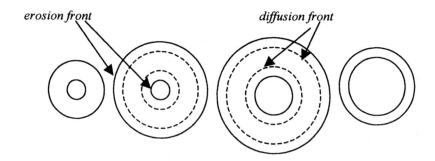

Figure IX-9. Schematic diagram of releasing surface area boundaries [6].

drug release from a small hole donut-shaped tablet tends to follow the drug release from the tablet without a hole.

　　　Kim [7] has developed *coated, donut-shaped tablets*, an improvement of perforated-coated and donut-shaped tablet. Water-soluble polymers and swellable/erodible polymers have been employed in perforated-coated tablets. In this design, drug diffusion and/or polymer erosion govern drug release kinetics, providing parabolic or linear release profiles. If the drug carrier is highly erodible, the parabolic release kinetics is expected by:

$$\frac{M_t}{M_\infty} = \frac{\left(a + \frac{k_e}{C_o}t\right)^2 - a^2}{r_o^2 - a^2} \tag{9-11}$$

where k_e is the erosion rate constant, r_o is the outer radius, a is the central hole radius, and L is the tablet thickness.

　　　Fig. IX-10 shows the drug loading on the release of diltiazem HCl from coated, donut-shaped tablets with a 3/16" hole. Release profiles become parabolic at high loading (59% and 49% w/w). At high loading, the dissolution of drug or a combination of drug dissolution and polymer erosion controls drug release expressed by equation (9-11). However, for a drug loading level less than 45%, drug release is linear and is governed primarily by the erosion of the polymer (HPMC E5). The diffusion of a freely water-soluble drug (diltiazem HCl) from the coated, donut-shaped tablet significantly contributed to the overall release kinetics.

IX.2. Cone-Shaped and Hemisphere Systems

The cone-shaped device, as shown in Fig. IX-11, was introduced by Nelson et al. [8]. It is based on the same concept that releasing surface area increases as the drug dissolution front moves inward. The device consists of a non-permeable lateral side and backing, and the drug is either suspended or dispersed in the matrix. The drug is then released through a small hole at the bottom of the cone. As water (or dissolution medium) penetrates the device through the hole, a drug-depleted layer forms between the opening of the hole (a) and the solid suspension interface (r). As for the pie-shaped device, the releasing interfacial surface area [$\pi r^2(1-\cos \phi)$] increases with increasing diffusion path length ($r-a$).

Nelson et al. [8] treated the release of drug from the device as a pseudo-steady state diffusion in a hollow sphere with a declination angle ϕ. The release rate from a hollow sphere is given by:

$$\frac{d}{dr}\left(r^2\frac{dc}{dr}\right) = 0 \tag{9-12}$$

Applying the moving dissolution interface r instead of b for the cone-shaped device gives the release rate (R) of:

$$R = 4\pi D\frac{ab}{a-b}C_s \tag{9-13}$$

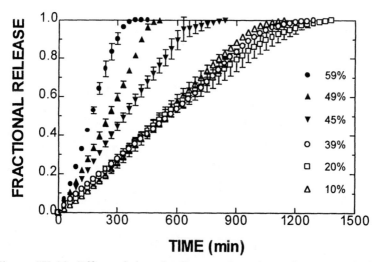

Figure IX-10. Effect of drug loading on the release from coated, donut-shaped tablets. (Graph reconstructed from data by Kim [7].)

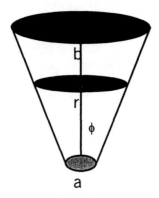

Figure IX-11. Cross-sectional view of a cone-shaped device [8].

and for $b \gg a$, $R = 4\pi DaC_s$ (9-14)

Equation (9-14) indicates that the release rate into a perfect sink from a hollow sphere loaded with a dispersed drug would be constant in contrast to the $\sqrt{t}$ dependence of release from a dispersed matrix system. The amount of drug release over time, M_t can be expressed as:

$$M_t = \frac{2}{3}\pi S(1 - \cos\phi)(r^3 - a^3)$$ (9-15)

where S is the concentration of suspended drug. Differentiating equation (9-15) with respect to time yields:

$$\frac{dM_t}{dt} = 2\pi S(1 - \cos\phi)r^2 \frac{dr}{dt}$$ (9-16)

The flux from Fick's first law becomes:

$$\frac{dM_t}{dt} = 2\pi D(1 - \cos\phi)r^2 \frac{dc}{dr}$$ (9-17)

Combining equations (9-16) and (9-17) yields:

$$\frac{dr}{dt} = \frac{D}{S}\frac{dc}{dr}$$ (9-18)

The radial concentration gradient, dc/dr, is then given by:

$$\frac{dc}{dr} = \frac{aC_s}{r(r-a)} \tag{9-19}$$

Substituting equation (9-19) into (9-18) and integrating for the radius from a to r and time from 0 to t gives:

$$\frac{r^3}{3a^3} - \frac{r^2}{2a^2} + \frac{1}{6} = \frac{DC_s}{Sa^2}t \tag{9-20}$$

Equations (9-15) and (9-20) are used to calculate M_t versus time t for the entire release period. Fig. IX-12 illustrates the experimental release profile of ethyl p- aminobenzoate suspended in a silicone elastomer base for device declination angles of 13.5°, 17.5°, and 20°. It shows that after a burst period of 8-12 hrs, zero-order release profiles are observed. A comparison of the experimental data with the simulated profile (Fig. IX-12) shows good agreement. Also a reasonable agreement between the experiment and predicted results is observed for different loading levels.

An interesting aspect of this cone-shaped device is that when the declination angle is 90°, the device becomes a *hemisphere*. Hsieh et al. [9] studied the release kinetics from a hemispheric matrix as presented in Fig. IX-13. Except for the brief burst period as mentioned with the cone-shaped device, the release rate is nearly zero-order. It can be seen from equation (9-17) that dM_t/dt is constant if $r \gg a$.

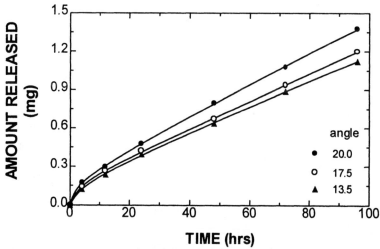

Figure IX-12. The release of ethyl p-aminobenzoate from a cone-shaped device. (Graph reconstructed from data by Nelson et al. [8].)

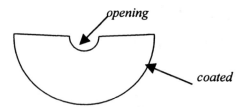

Figure IX-13. A hemisphere design [9].

The amount of drug released from a hemispheric device is given by setting $\phi=45°$:

$$M_t = \frac{2}{3}\pi S(r^3 - a^3)$$ (9-21)

The release of bovine serum albumin from an inwardly releasing hemisphere device is shown in Fig. IX-14.

Siegal [10] applied the hemispheric device for a system where the drug concentration in the hemisphere matrix is below the drug's solubility. Fick's second law is given by:

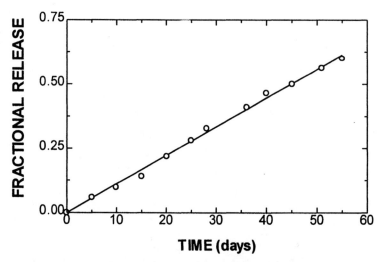

Figure IX-14. The release of serum albumin from a hemisphere device. (Graph reconstructed from data by Hsieh et al. [9].)

$$\frac{\partial C}{\partial t} = \frac{D}{r^2}\frac{\partial}{\partial r}\left(r^2\frac{\partial C}{\partial r}\right) \qquad a < r < R \tag{9-22}$$

Initial and boundary conditions are:

$$C(r,0) = 0 \tag{9-23}$$

$$C(a,t) = 0 \tag{9-24}$$

$$\frac{\partial C(R,t)}{\partial r} = 0 \tag{9-25}$$

The above equations are solved using giving [10]:

$$C(r,t) = 2C_o\left(\frac{\alpha}{1-\alpha}\right)\left(\frac{R}{r}\right)\sum_{n=1}^{\infty}\frac{c_n}{\lambda_n}\sin\lambda_n\frac{r-a}{R}\exp\left(-\lambda_n^2 Dt/R^2\right) \tag{9-26}$$

where

$$c_n = \left[1 - \frac{\sin 2\lambda_n(1-\alpha)}{2\lambda_n(1-\alpha)}\right]^{-1} \tag{9-27}$$

with

$$\alpha = a/R$$

and λ_n is the nth positive root of:

$$\lambda_n = \tan\lambda_n(1-\alpha) \tag{9-28}$$

The fractional release at time t is then given by [10]:

$$\frac{M_t}{M_\infty} = \frac{6\alpha^2}{(1-\alpha)(1-\alpha^3)}\sum_{n=1}^{\infty}\frac{c_n}{\lambda_n^2}\left(1 - \exp(-\lambda_n^2 Dt/R^2)\right) \tag{9-29}$$

As $\alpha \to 0$,

$$\lambda_1 \approx \sqrt{\frac{3\alpha}{(1-\alpha)^3}} \tag{9-30}$$

$$\lambda_n \approx \frac{(2n-1)\pi}{2(1-\alpha)} \qquad n > 1 \tag{9-31}$$

An approximate solution then can be obtained as [10]:

$$\left(\frac{M_t}{M_\infty}\right)_{approx} = 1 - \exp\left(-\frac{\lambda_1^2 Dt}{R^2}\right) \tag{9-32}$$

      Fig. IX-15 shows the fractional release for M_t / M_∞ and $M_t / M_\infty|_{approx}$ with the dimensionless time (Dt / R^2). $M_t / M_\infty|_{approx}$ is in excellent agreement with M_t / M_∞ at all values of α.

      The devices discussed in this section use the principle of increasing the surface area at the dissolution front with time or diffusion distances. Other configurational geometries have been proposed such as clover, flying saucer, multi-hole systems etc. [11-13].

IX.3. Multi-Layer Tablet and Cylinder Systems

      Hydrophilic polymers have been used to extend drug release. A swelling/erosion or erosion process may be used to control drug release kinetics. If the drug diffusion process is a major contribution to the overall release kinetics, even well designed dosage forms cannot provide the zero-order release through control by the degree and the rate of swelling of the hydrophilic polymers. In addition, one may have difficulty in obtaining zero-order kinetics from tablet geometry, due to decreasing release area. Conte et

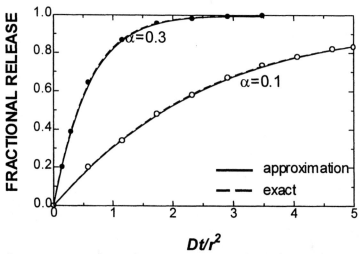

Figure IX-15. Fractional release function and approximate function vs. a dimensionless time (Dt / r^2). (Graph reconstructed from data by Siegal [10].)

al. [14] developed a multi-layer tablet system (Geomatrix®) as shown in Fig.IX-16. A core tablet is sandwiched between two barrier layers. When a hydrophilic swellable/erodible polymer is used, zero-order release kinetics are obtained. However, zero-order release kinetics also depends on the solubility of drugs. If a hydrophilic swellable polymer is used for the two barrier layers, the drug release rate is controlled by several mechanisms. Upon contact with water, the polymer is hydrated and the drug diffuses laterally through the swollen gel. When water penetrates through the barrier layer, the drug also diffuses through it. At this point the swollen barrier layer acts as a membrane. Initially, the entire drug release is controlled by the diffusion of drug through the swollen barriers because the total lateral surface area is greater than the radial surface area. Core tablet hydration is delayed due to the drug-free barrier layers. In addition, the thickness of the swollen barrier layers diminishes with time, causing the diffusion resistance of the membrane to decrease. This counterbalances the effect of the reduced concentration of the drug in the core tablet on the drug release kinetics, leading to the prolonged zero-order release. However, the kinetics of drug release from the multi-layered tablet systems is dependent on the drug solubility. As drug solubility decreases, more linear release kinetics is observed [15]. Fig. IX-17 shows the release of diltiazem HCl from triple-layer tablets made of polyethylene oxide. Others modified the structure of the outer layer [16]. This multi-layered tablet system was evaluated much earlier with a water-impermeable barrier layer and core tablet (PVC or Eudragit® RS or RL) [17]. Chidanbaram et al. [18] developed a triple-layer tablet system consisting of water-insoluble core matrix and two water-soluble barrier layers. As the barrier layer swells and erodes, the core tablet exposes more surface area with time, producing a linear release profile.

One of problems encountered when developing controlled release dosage forms based on tablet geometry is that of formulating tablets containing different dose levels with identical release kinetics. The tablet design requires changing the formulation and tablet size. Therefore, each

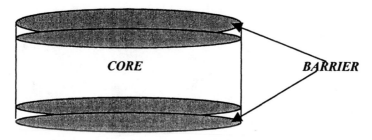

Figure IX-16. Schematic diagram of triple-layer tablets (Geomatrix®) [14].

tablet requires a unique formulation for each dose level. Conte et al. [19] developed small tablets with multi-layer system design which can be placed in a hard gelatin capsule. In this system, the drug release characteristics of different dose levels display the same release profile.

This multi-layered tablet system has been further extended to press-coat tablets. The press-coated tablet system consists of an outer low drug (or drug-free) content layer and a high drug content core [20]. The mixture of excipients for the bottom layer is compressed with a flat-faced punch followed by placing the core tablet in the middle of the bottom layer. The rest of the mixture is then poured into the die forming the side and top layer. The schematic structure of the press-coated tablet is shown in Fig. IX-18. The outer barrier delays drug release from the press-coated systems for a considerable period of time depending on the thickness of the dry coat and the type of materials. The barrier is able to slow down the hydration/swelling process of the core tablet for a long period of time. In addition, the outer barrier layer serves as a controlling membrane producing a linear release profile. When the drug concentration in the core falls below its solubility level, the drug release rate decreases. Because the barrier layer thickness decreases with time, the diffusion resistance in the barrier membrane also decreases.

Gopferich and Langer [21] proposed implants consisting of multiple layers of a heterogeneous eroding polymer to release drugs one after another. Such an implant is composed of a core containing one drug encased within a polymer containing a second drug. Obviously, the drug is first released from the outer layer followed by release of the second drug from the core after a delay. It can be clearly seen that a composite cylindrical implant can deliver

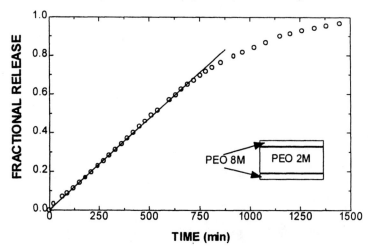

Figure IX-17. Release of diltiazem HCl from triple-layer tablet systems made of different molecular weight of PEO [16].

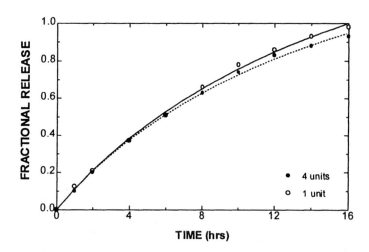

Figure IX-18. Release of diltiazem HCl from small triple-layer tablets representing different dose levels. (Graph reconstructed from data by Conte et al [19].)

two drugs consecutively, as shown in Fig. IX-20. Gopferich and Langer [22] also developed a theoretical model to predict the drug release and erosion of the composite polyanhydride implants (cylinders). To extend the time lag between the start of drug release from the outer layer and the onset of release

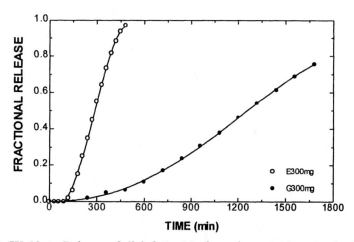

Figure IX-19. Release of diclofenac Na from dry-coated encased tablets. (Graph reconstructed from data by Conte et al. [20].)

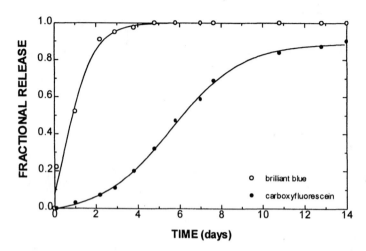

Figure IX-20. Release of drugs from composite cylindrical implant. (Graph reconstructed from data by Gopferich and Langer [21].)

for the second drug, a drug-free layer can be incorporated into the composite implant. Such systems may be useful for vaccination, to reduce resistance problems that occur in tumor therapy (e.g. cytostatics), and local antibiotic therapy [21].

References

1. D. Brooke and R. J. Washkuhn, "Zero-Order Drug Delivery System: Theory and Preliminary Testing," *J. Pharm. Sci.*, 66, 159 (1977).
2. R. A. Lipper and W. I. Higuchi, "Analysis of Theoretical Behavior of a Proposed Zero-Order Drug Delivery System," *J. Pharm. Sci.*, 66, 163 (1977).
3. A. G. Hansson, A. Giardino, J. R. Cardinal, and W. Curatolo, "Perforated Coated Tablets for Controlled Release of Drugs at a Constant Rate," *J. Pharm. Sci.*, 77, 322 (1988).
4. M. E. Sangalli, U. Conte, A. Gazzaniga, and A. La Manna, "Inert Monolithic Device with Central Hole for Constant Drug Release," *Proceed. Int. Symp. Control. Rel. Bioact. Mater.*, 20, 316 (1993).
5. W. A. Boettner, A. J. Aguiar, J. R. Cardinal, A. C. Curtiss, G. R. Ranade, J. A. Richards, and W. F. Sokol, "The Morantel Sustained Release Trilaminate: A Device for the Controlled Ruminal Delivery of Morantel to Cattle," *J. Control. Rel.*, 8, 23 (1988).
6. C. J. Kim, "Compressed Donut-Shaped Tablets with Zero-Order Release Kinetics," *Pharm. Res.*, 12, 1045 (1995).

7. C. J. Kim, "Release Kinetics of Coated, Donut-Shaped Tablets for Water Soluble Drugs," *Eur. J. Pharm. Sci.* (in press).

8. K. G. Nelson, S. J. Smith, and R. M. Bennet, "Constant-Release Diffusion Systems: Rate Control by Means of Geometric Configuration," in Controlled-Release Technology: Pharmaceutical Applications, P. I. Lee and W. R. Good (Eds.), ACS Symposium Series No. 348, 1987, pp324.

9. D. S. Hsieh, W. D. Rhine, and R. S. Langer, "Zero-Order Controlled Release Polymer Matrices for Macro- and Micromolecules," *J. Pharm. Sci.*, 72, 17 (1983).

10. R. A. Siegal, "Equations for Inward Hemispheric Release below Drug Solubility," *Proceed. Int. Symp. Control. Rel. Bioact. Mater.*, 23, 117 (1996).

11. D. O. Cooney, "Effect of Geometry on the Dissolution of Pharmaceutical Tablets and Other Solids: Surface Detachment Kinetics Controlling," *AIChEJ*, 18, 446 (1972).

12. A. Nangia, T. Molloy, B. J. Fahie, and S. K. Chopra, "Novel Regulated Release System Based on Geometric Configuration," *Proceed. Int. Symp. Control. Rel. Bioact. Mater.*, 22, 294 (1995).

13. W.-Y. Kuu and S. H. Yalkowsky, "Multiple-Hole Approach to Zero-Order Release," *J. Pharm. Sci.*, 74, 926 (1985).

14. U. Conte, L. Maggi, P. Colombo, and A. La Manna, "Multi-Layered Hydrophilic Matrices as Constant Release Devices (Geomatrix® Systems)," J. Control. Rel., 26, 39 (1993).

15. U. Conte, L. Maggi, and A. La Manna, "A Multi-Layer Matrix Tablet Design for Constant Drug Release," *Proceed. Int. Symp. Control. Rel. Bioact. Mater.*, 19, 369 (1992).

16. C. J. Kim, Unpublished data.

17. R. A. Fassihi and W. A. Ritschel, "Multiple-Layer Direct-Compression, Controlled Release System: In Vitro and In-Vivo Evaluation," *J. Pharm. Sci.*, 82, 750 (1993).

18. N. Chidambaram, W. Porter, K. Flood, and Y. Qin, "Formulation and Characterization of New Layered Diffusional Matrices for Zero-Order Sustained Release," *J. Control. Rel.*, 52, 149 (1998).

19. U. Conte, L. Maggi, and A. La Manna, "Geomatrix® Technology for the Extended Release of Drugs at a Constant Rate," *Proceed. Int. Symp. Control. Rel. Bioact. Mater.*, 20, 350 (1993).

20. L. Maggi, M. L. Torre, P. Giunchedi, U. Conte, and A. La Manna, "New Oral Systems for Timing-Release of Drugs," *Proceed. Int. Symp. Control. Rel. Bioact. Mater.*, 20, 366 (1993).

21. A. Gopferich and R. Langer, "Programmable Drug Delivery Implants," *Proceed. Int. Symp. Control. Rel. Bioact. Mater.*, 22, 63 (1995).

22. A. Gopferich and R. Langer, "Modeling of Polymer Erosion," *Macromolecules*, 26, 4105 (1993).

Chapter X

Other Systems

X.1. Hydrodynamically Balanced Systems

Hydrodynamically balanced systems (HBS) are designed to prolong the residence time of CRDF in the GI tract and maximize absorption. For many drugs, the solubility of the drug and its release rate from CRDF depend on the pH of the dissolution medium. For instance, the solubility of chlodiazeperoxide HCl is approximately 150 mg/ml in an acidic environment while, in a weak acid or neutral pH, it is below 0.1 mg/ml as shown in Fig. X-1. As the CRDF passes through the GI tract, the rate of release changes. One way to alter these variations in the release rate is to keep the drug carrier in a constant environment (especially a constant pH). For these systems, the CRDF remains in the stomach for a long period of time and the drug in the solution is absorbed in the stomach or upper small intestine. In order to accomplish this objective, the bulk density of the CRDF should be lighter than that of the stomach content and should remain buoyant on the surface of the stomach fluid. One may call this as a floating (tablet or capsule) system. The CRDF should have the following characteristics [1]:

1. It must maintain its structural integrity.
2. Its bulk density must be lower than that of the gastric contents.
3. The drug carrier should release the drug for a long period of time.

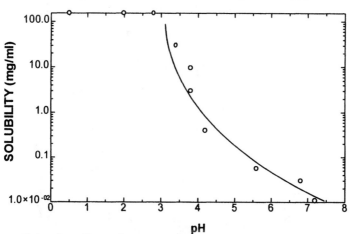

Figure X-1. The effect of pH on the solubility of chlodiazeperoxide HCl. (Graph reconstructed from data by Seth and Tossounian [2].)

269

The HBS CRDF is prepared by incorporating gel-forming hydro-colloids such as HPMC, excipients, hydrogenated fatty materials, etc. When the tablet or capsule comes into contact with gastric fluid, the gel layer forms on the surface. Like the swelling/erosion systems discussed in Chapter V, the gel layer grows until the pseudo-steady state is reached. The tablet floats due to the lower density of CRDF than that of gastric fluid and the drug diffuses out through the gel layer by diffusion.

The HBS is most suitable for drugs that are (a) insoluble in intestinal fluid and (b) exhibit site-specific absorption in the intestinal tract such as Valium, chlordiaperoxide HCl and Levadopa. Erni and Held [3] showed the radioactivity of a radio-labeled CRDF in the stomach, indicating that the HBS remains in the stomach for up to 6 hrs compared to the less than 2 hrs for conventional tablets. Seth and Tossounian [2], and Erni and Held [3] presented evidence by a gamma scintiographic method that the HBS dosage form remains even though the stomach is half-filled. The release of chlordiaperoxide HCl from the HBS is fitted via the square-root-of-time relationship as shown in Fig. X-2.

Hydrodynamically balanced systems (floating dosage forms), described above, may be single-unit tablets or multi-unit capsules. A single-unit floating dosage form may move into the small intestine in a short time. Ichikawa et al. [4] prepared a multiple-unit capsule of oral floating dosage forms by using carbon dioxide generated by an effervescent chemical (sodium bicarbonate). Fig. X-3 shows the structural diagram of a floating beadlet. First, the sustained release granule is prepared by coating nonpareil seeds with a drug and excipients. Secondly, effervescent layers containing sodium carbonate, talc, silicic acid and hydroxypropylcellulose are coated on the

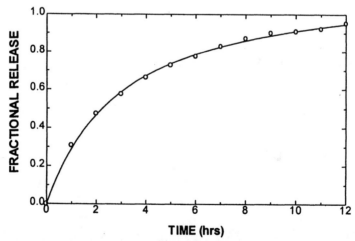

Figure X-2. The release of chlordiaperoxide HCl from the HBS. (Graph reconstructed from data by Seth and Tossounian [2].)

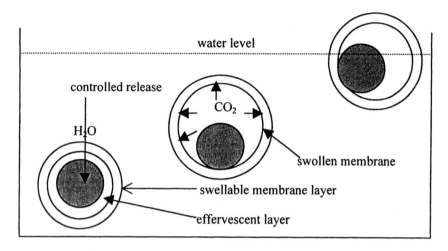

Figure X-3. Schematic diagram of floating micro-particles [4].

sustained release granules, followed successively by coating with other chemicals such as tartaric acid, silicic acid, talc, and calcium stearate. Finally, the swellable membrane layers consisting of poly(vinyl acetate) and shellac along with other excipients are coated on effervescent coated sustained release granules.

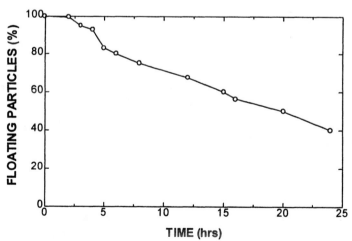

Figure X-4. Floating and sedimentation pattern of the micro-particles. (Graph reconstructed from data by Ichikawa et al. [4].)

Upon contact with water, micro-particles sink to the bottom and water then diffuses into the matrix's effervescent layers. Carbon dioxide gas is generated at the inner layers by the neutralization between sodium bicarbonate and tartaric acid, as illustrated in Fig. X-3. After that, the micro-particles are floating and the drug is released from the particles. The density of the particles changes from 1.42 g/ml to 0.54 g/ml. The number of swellable membrane layers and the composition of the swellable membrane layer affect the floating of the particles. Floating patterns of the floating micro-particle system, based on photographic observation of the particle, are shown in Fig. X-4. After 5 hrs, the number of floating micro-particles decreases to 85% due to the penetration of water into the swollen particles and the escape of carbon dioxide, resulting in the increase in the density of the particle. About 50% of the particles remain floating after 24 hours release. The drug release rate is zero order as shown in Fig. X-5 and is not influenced by the portion of the swellable layer (compared to total weight of the micro-particles) up to 13 w% [4]. Increasing the percentage of the swellable membrane layer from 13 to 25 w% results in decreasing the release rate and increasing the lag time of release [4].

X.2. Time-Controlled Releasing Systems

Many types of oral CRDFs described in the previous sections have continuous release patterns. However, it is often necessary to release a drug at a specific site in the GI tract or immediately after a certain period of time. The development of the CRDFs whose release profile has a time lag, followed

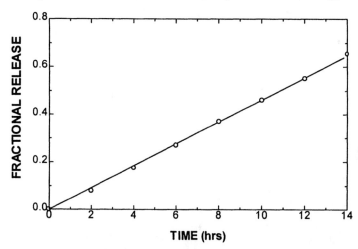

Figure X-5. The release of p-aminobenzoic acid from the floating micro-particles. (Graph was recconstructed from data by Ichikawa et al. [4].)

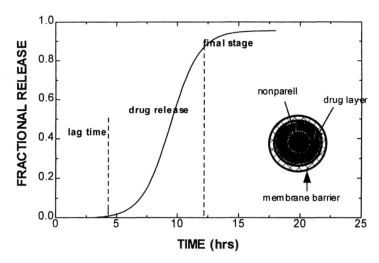

Figure X-6. Typical release profile of TCRS.

by an appropriate release stage and a final stage, as illustrated in Fig. X-6, should effectively achieve the following [5]:

1) Drugs are released at a specific part of the GI tract or to be delivered to the colon.

2) Drugs are administrated to heal diseases, which undergo pulsed or circadian rhythms.

3) Plasma level of drugs can be prolonged for a day by blending different kinds of time-controlled releasing systems (TCRS) having different time lag.

Osawa et al. [5] designed TCRS granules as presented in Fig. X-6 (insert). Nonpareils are coated with drugs by spraying aqueous drug/polyvinylpyrrolidone followed by spraying Eudragit® RS to form controlled release membranes before being dried. The membrane thickness or the concentration of polymer in the second coating solution determines the time lag.

The release of diltiazem HCl from TCRS is illustrated in Fig. X-7. The drug was released after a time lag, which increases with the increase of membrane thickness or coating percent. The release rate after the lag time was not influenced by the coating thickness or coating percent. As shown in Fig. X-7, one may blend two different particles having different time lags to obtain the desirable release profiles. Ueda et al. [6] incorporated an additional hydrophilic/swellable layer between the drug layer and the polymer membrane. In this case, water infiltrates through the polymer membrane followed by the hydration of the hydrophilic polymer. Swelling pressure

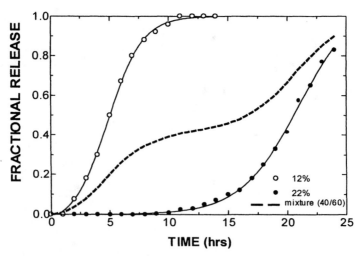

Figure X-7. The release of diltiazem HCl from TCRS and theoretical profile of the blend of 12% and 22% coated particles. (Graph reconstructed from data by Osawa et al. [5].)

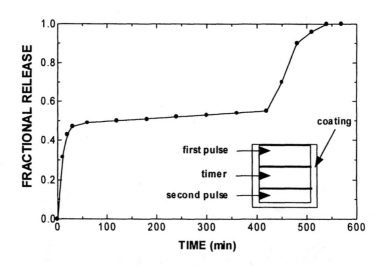

Figure X-8. The release of diclofenac Na from the pulsatile delivery system and its schematic design. (Graph was reconstructed from data by Conte et al. [7].)

exerts against the membrane, which is exploded, and subsequently fast drug release is encountered.

Conte et al. [7] developed TCRS with a tablet form. Erodible barriers are layered onto an inner core matrix by a dry coat press. The barrier layer contains active drugs. The drug is then delivered after a definite time lag. This time lag is determined by varying the barrier layer polymer type (e.g. HPMC E and K series) and thickness. Conte et al. [7] proposed a pulsatile delivery tablet. It consisted of a three-layer tablet. The first layer releases a drug immediately (first pulse) followed by exposing the second layer to the aqueous medium. The second layer hydrates and erodes slowly. This allows a pre-programmed time delay before the second release pulse. As shown in Fig. X-8, the first pulse is released in a short time (15-30 min) followed by no drug release before the second pulse is quickly delivered. The polymer materials and the amount of the materials incorporated determine the pre-programmed time delay. Crison et al. [8] designed the PORT® capsule system enabling the release of its content at pre-programmed times, allowing site-specific release of drugs and reduction of dose frequency. The system, as shown in Fig. X-9, is composed of a hard gelatin capsule coated with a semi-permeable membrane, a water-insoluble plug, and an osmotic charge mixed with a drug. The permeability of the membrane, the size of the plug, and the composition of the osmotic charge govern the release of the drug. Similarly, Pusicap® has been developed to release its content at a pre-determined time or place within the gastro-intestinal tract. The device consists of a water impermeable capsule with a hydrogel plug under which drug is located. Upon contact with water, the hydrogel plug swells and is ejected from the device at a specific time, dependent upon the plug size. The contents of the capsule are released after the plug ejection.

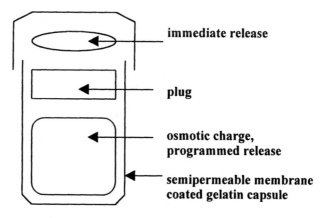

Figure X-9. Design of PORT® system [8].

References

1. Y. W. Chien, Novel Drug Delivery Systems, 2nd Edition, Marcel Dekker, New York, 1992, p164.
2. P. R. Seth and J. L. Tossounian, "The Hydrodynamically-Balanced System: A Novel Drug Delivery System for Oral Use," *Drug Dev. Ind. Pharm.*, 10, 313 (1984).
3. W. Erni and K. Held, "The Hydrodynamically Balanced System: A Novel Principle of Controlled Drug Release," *Eur. Neurol.*, 27 (suppl.), 21 (1987).
4. M. Ichikawa, S. Watanabe, and Y. Miyake, "A New Multiple-Unit Oral Floating Dosage Form. I. Preparation and In-Vitro Evaluation of Floating and Sustained-Release Characteristics," *J. Pharm. Sci.*, 80, 1062 (1991).
5. T. Osawa, H. Takahata, T. Maejima, M. Kobayashi, and K. Noda, "Sigmoidal-Releasing system (SRS) as a Novel Oral Controlled Release Formulation," *Procced. Int. Symp. Control. Rel. Bioact. Mater.*, 18, 405 (1991).
6. S. Ueda, R. Ibuki, T. Hata, and Y. Ueda, "Design and Development of Time-Controlled Explosion System (TES) as a Controlled Drug Release System," *Procced. Int. Symp. Control. Rel. Bioact. Mater.*, 15, 450 (1988).
7. U. Conte, L. Maggi, and P. Giunchedi, "A New Production Technology for a Pulsatile Delivery Device," *Procced. Int. Symp. Control. Rel. Bioact. Mater.*, 19, 103 (1992).
8. J. R. Crison, P. R. Siersma, M. D. Taylor, and G. L. Amidon, "Programmable Oral Release Technology PORT System®: A Novel Dosage Form for Time and Site Specific Oral Drug Delivery," *Procced. Int. Symp. Control. Rel. Bioact. Mater.*, 22, 278 (1995).
9. J. S. Binnis, H. N. Stevens, M. Bakhsha, and C. G. Wilson, "Colon Targeted Release Using Pulsicap™ Delivery System," *Proceed. Int. Symp. Control. Rel. Bioact. Mater.*, 21, 260 (1994).

Chapter XI

Pharmacokinetic Considerations in the Design of Controlled Release Dosage Forms

Delivery of a drug from dosage forms into the human body can be described by the sequences of the absorption, distribution and elimination of drugs. Release kinetics from a CRDF must conform to physiological constraints and the route of administration. In this chapter, the selection criteria for dosage forms are discussed and the mechanistic prediction of *in-vivo* performance of the CRDF is carried out with examples of commercial products.

For oral administration of a CRDF, a one-compartment model or a two-compartment model is usually applied. Of note the CRDF releases its contents (drug) much slower than by drug absorption through the GI bio-membrane (the release process is a rate-determining step). It is assumed that the absorption, distribution, and elimination (metabolism and excretion) of drugs in the body are described by first-order processes. This leads to a linear set of ordinary differential equations (pharmacokinetic models).

XI. 1. One-Compartment Model

The transport of a drug into the body for a one-compartment model is shown in Fig. XI-1. Mathematical expressions for the drug content of each compartment can be written as:

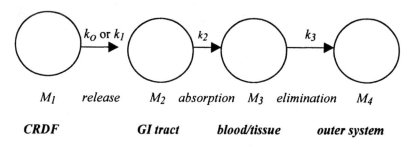

k_O or k_1 k_2 k_3

M_1 *release* M_2 *absorption* M_3 *elimination* M_4

CRDF   **GI tract**   **blood/tissue**   **outer system**

Figure XI-1. A one-compartment model.

$$\frac{dM_1}{dt} = -R(t) \tag{11-1}$$

$$\frac{dM_2}{dt} = R(t) - k_2 M_2 \tag{11-2}$$

$$\frac{dM_3}{dt} = k_2 M_2 - k_3 M_3 \tag{11-3}$$

$$\frac{dM_d}{dt} = k_3 M_3 \tag{11-4}$$

where M_1, M_2, M_3, and M_4 denote the amount of drug present in the CRDF, GI tract, blood/tissue, and outer body, respectively; $R(t)$ is the release rate of the drug from the CRDF, and k_2 and k_3 are the rate constants for the absorption and elimination of drug, respectively. $R(t)$ (zero-order rate constant, k_o, or first-order rate constant, k_1) dictates the profile of the drug in blood plasma with respect to time within any dose duration. The amount of the drug or drug concentration in the body can be predicted by solving equations (11-1)-(11-3).

XI.1.1. Zero-order release kinetics

The amount of drug absorbed in the body after a single dose of the CRDF exhibiting zero-order release kinetics ($R(t) = k_o$) is obtained by solving equations (11-1)-(11-3) with the initial condition ($M_3 = 0$ at $t=0$) as:

$$M_3 = k_o \left(\frac{1}{k_3} + \frac{1}{k_2 - k_3} e^{-k_2 t} - \frac{k_2}{(k_2 - k_3)k_3} e^{-k_3 t} \right) \tag{11-5}$$

When $k_2 \gg k_3$ and $k_o \ll k_2$, in which k_o is the rate determining constant, equation (11-5) reduces:

$$M_3 = \frac{k_o}{k_3}(1 - e^{-k_3 t}) \quad \text{or} \quad C_3 = \frac{k_o}{V k_3}(1 - e^{-k_3 t}) \tag{11-6}$$

where C_3 and V are the drug concentration in the body and the volume distribution, respectively.

Equation (11-6) shows that the drug concentration profiles in the body from the CRDF with zero-order release kinetics are governed by the drug release rate (or rate constant) and the elimination rate constant. Fig. XI-

2 illustrates the influence of both the rate constants (release and elimination) on the drug concentration profiles. For a given elimination rate constant ($k_3 =$ 0.28/hr, which is equal to the drug's half-life of 2.5 hr), the drug profile is directly proportional to the release rate from the CRDF. This is an inherent property of zero-order release CRDFs and can be predicted from equation (11-6) in which the steady state drug level is solely dependent upon the elimination rate constant (k_3).

It takes approximately 20 hrs to obtain the steady state drug concentration level for drugs with a half-life of 2.5 hrs. For drugs with a much longer half-life, the steady state level is not likely to be achieved within the 24 hr time frame by a single dose. Fig. XI-3 clearly demonstrates the effect of the elimination rate constant (or half-life) on the drug concentration profile in the body. The shorter the half-life of the drug, the earlier the drug concentration level approaches toward the steady state level. However, the true steady state of the drug concentration in the body takes place when the release rate of the drug from the CRDF equals the elimination rate of the drug [1,2]. It is important to remember that the drug concentration level in the body declines at a first-order rate (solely elimination) after release from the CRDF is completed or the CRDF is out of the body. As seen in Fig. XI-4, if the declining concentration profile is mirror-imaged with the early portion of the drug concentration profile of the subsequent dose, the steady state level is maintained with repetitive doses. For drugs with a longer half-life, the drug will accumulate in the body with repetitive doses until a steady state level is obtained. In general, 4 to 5 half-lives of the drug are required to reach a steady state drug concentration in the body [1,3].

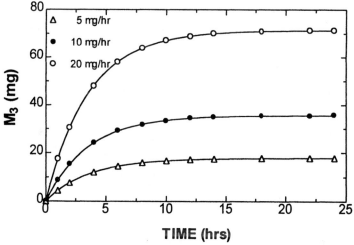

Figure XI-2. Amount of drug in the blood plasma from a single dose of a zero-order release CRDF with k_3 = 0.28/hr.

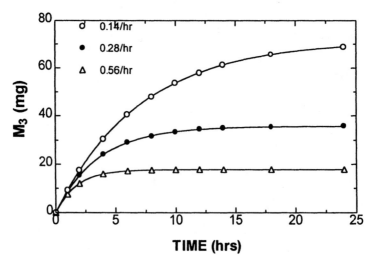

Figure XI-3. Amount of drug in the blood plasma from a single dose of a zero-order release CRDF with k_O=10 mg/hr.

Some CRDFs have a dual zero order release (faster zero order release followed by slower zero order release or vice versa), as expressed by:

$$R(t) = k_o' t \qquad\qquad 0 < t \le t_o \qquad\qquad (11\text{-}7a)$$

$$= k_o' \left[t - \frac{T}{T - t_o}(t - t_o) \right] \qquad t_o < t \le T \qquad (11\text{-}7b)$$

where T is the total release time and $k_o' = 2M_T / Tt_o$ in which M_T is the total amount of drug in the CRDF. The drug concentration in the body is given by [4]:

$$C(t) = G(t) \qquad\qquad 0 < t \le t_o \qquad\qquad (11\text{-}8a)$$

$$= G(t) - H(t) \qquad\qquad t_o < t \le T \qquad\qquad (11\text{-}8b)$$

where

$$G(t) = \frac{2M_T}{Vk_3(k_2 - k_3)Tt_o} \left[(k_2 - k_3)t + \frac{k_3}{k_2}(1 - e^{-k_2 t}) - \frac{k_2}{k_3}(1 - e^{-k_3 t}) \right] \qquad (11\text{-}8c)$$

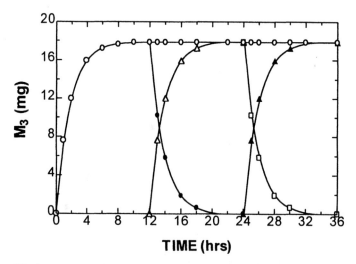

Figure XI-4. Amount of drug in the blood plasma from repeated doses of a zero-order CRDF with the mirror images of one dose and the subsequent dose.

$$H(t) = \frac{2M_T}{Vk_3(k_2 - k_3)(T - t_o)t_o}$$

$$\times \left[(k_2 - k_3)(t - t_o) + \frac{k_3}{k_2}(1 - e^{-k_2(t - t_o)}) - \frac{k_2}{k_3}(1 - e^{-k_3(t - t_o)}) \right] \tag{11-8d}$$

When a CRDF has released its entire drug, or when the CRDF is eliminated from the body before its complete release, the drug concentration in the body declines as:

$$C_3 = C_{3,T}e^{-k_3(t - t^*)} + \frac{k_2 X(t^*)}{V(k_2 - k_3)}\left(e^{-k_3(t - t^*)} - e^{-k_2(t - t^*)} \right) \tag{11-9}$$

where t^* is the residence time of the CRDF in the body and

$$X(t^*) = \frac{M_T}{k_2 t^*}\left(1 - e^{-k_2 t^*} \right) \tag{11-10}$$

XI.1.2. *Zero-order release kinetics with an immediate release dose*

For a drug with a long half-life (longer than 4 hrs), the drug concentration does not reach a plateau level with a single dose. To achieve a rapid onset of the plateau level (less than 2 hrs) with a single dose requires administering the CRDF with an immediate release dose. The drug concentration in the body after administration of the CRDF with an immediate release dose, can be predicted from equations (11-1)-(11-3) with initial conditions ($M_3 = M_o$ at $t = 0$) as follows:

$$C_3 = \frac{k_o}{Vk_3}\left(1 - e^{-k_3 t}\right) - \frac{k_o - k_2 M_o}{(k_3 - k_2)V}\left(e^{-k_2 t} - e^{-k_3 t}\right) \tag{11-11}$$

The second term of equation (11-11) represents the contribution of the immediate release dose. In general, $k_o - k_2 M_o \cong -k_2 M_o$ leads to a simple form of equation (11-11) [5,6]. As demonstrated in the previous section, the plateau drug level is not achievable by a single dose for drugs with long half-lives. With aid of an immediate release dose, the steady state level is reached within a little more than 1 hr as illustrated in Fig. XI-5.

There have been several methods proposed to calculate the amount of drug for the immediate release dose and constant release dose. They can be calculated by using the mass balance equations for the unchanged active drug in the whole system at steady state conditions of the drug concentration as follows [6]:

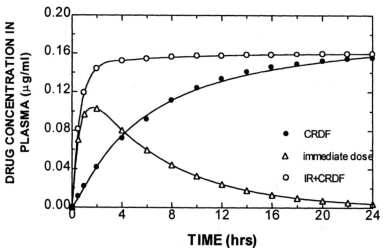

Figure XI-5.   The drug concentration in the blood plasma from a zero-order release CRDF and a zero-order release with an immediate release (k_o=3 mg/hr, k_2=1.6/hr, k_3=0.15/hr, V=125 L, and M_o=18.5 mg).

$$\int R(t)dt = M_2 + M_3 + M_4 \qquad (11\text{-}12)$$

Equation (11-12) states that the total amount of drug released from the CRDF should equal the summation of the amount of drug remaining in the GI tract, absorbed drug, and eliminated drug. The amount of eliminated drug can be obtained by integrating equation (11-4) ($M_4 = k_3 M_3 t$). In addition, at the steady state condition ($dM_3 / dt = 0$) equation (11-3) yields:

$$k_2 M_2 = k_3 M_3 \qquad (11\text{-}13)$$

Thus equation (11-12) gives:

$$\int R(t)dt = M_2 + M_3 + k_3 M_3 t$$
$$= \frac{(k_2 + k_3)VC_{3,s}}{k_2} + k_3 VC_{3,s}t \qquad (11\text{-}14)$$

where $C_{3,s}$ is the steady state drug concentration in the body (or target plasma level).

Equation (11-14) clearly indicates that the release from the CRDF should be zero order with $k_3 VC_{3,s}$ and the first term of the right-hand side of equation (11-14) provides the optimum immediate dose:

$$M_o = \frac{k_2 + k_3}{k_2} VC_{3,s} \qquad (11\text{-}15)$$

As an example of the application of equation (11-14), Lee [6] used phenylpropranolamine HCl. Pharmacokinetic parameters for the drug are $k_2 = 1.58 / hr$, $k_3 = 0.159 / hr$ and $V = 245.6 L$. For the steady state drug concentration of 80 μg/ml, the zero-order release rate should be $k_o = 3.12$ mg/hr while the optimum immediate release dose is $M_o = 21.6$ mg from equation (11-15). Fig. XI-5 clearly illustrates the importance of the immediate release dose to the early onset of the steady state drug concentration.

For drugs with long half-lives, however, equation (11-11) fails to provide the plateau drug concentration level following repeated dose of CRDF with an immediate release dose. The plateau concentration level can be achieved after 4 to 5 doses of zero-order release CRDF without an immediate release dose [2]. Fig. XI-6 demonstrates that by successive dosing of the CRDF with an immediate release dose, the plateau level of drug concentration in the body cannot be achieved and the drug concentration increases shortly after consecutive doses as well. Several approaches have been suggested to prevent the fluctuation in drug concentration due to zero-order release with an immediate release dose [2]. However, these are not practical due to patient compliance issues.

XI.1.3. First-order release kinetics

The amount of drug absorbed in the body following the administration of a single dose of CRDF exhibiting first-order release kinetics [$R(t) = k_1 M_1$, where k_1 is the first-order release rate constant] is given by equation (11-16):

$$M_3 = k_1 M_{1,T} \left(\frac{e^{-k_1 t}}{(k_2 - k_1)(k_3 - k_1)} + \frac{e^{-k_2 t}}{(k_1 - k_2)(k_3 - k_2)} + \frac{e^{-k_3 t}}{(k_2 - k_3)(k_1 - k_3)} \right) \quad (11\text{-}16)$$

where $M_{1,T}$ is the total amount of drug in the CRDF. When $k_2 \gg k_1$ and $k_2 \gg k_3$, equation (11-16) yields

$$M_3 = \frac{k_1 M_{1,T}}{k_1 - k_3} \left(e^{-k_3 t} - e^{-k_1 t} \right) \quad \text{or} \quad C_3 = \frac{k_1 M_{1,T}}{V(k_1 - k_3)} \left(e^{-k_3 t} - e^{-k_1 t} \right) \quad (11\text{-}17)$$

Equation (11-17) is the same form as for first-order absorption kinetics except that k_1 instead of k_2 is used.

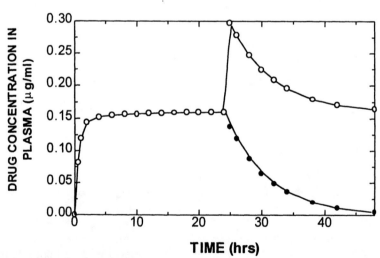

Figure XI-6. Simulated drug concentration of zero-order release CRDF with a bolus after consecutive dose.

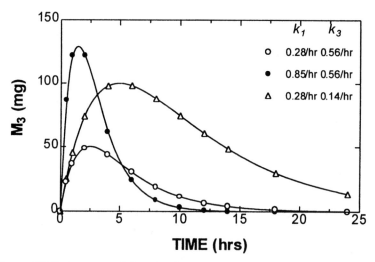

Figure XI-7. Amount of drug in the blood plasma from a first-order release CRDF.

As previously demonstrated for zero-order release CRDF, the plasma drug concentration is influenced by both the drug release and elimination rate constants as presented in Fig. XI-7. For a given release rate constant ($k_1 = 0.28$/hr), the drug concentration profiles in the body are significantly affected by the half-life of the drug. However, if k_3 is greater than k_1, apparent elimination slopes among the curves generated by $k_3 > k_1$ cases are identical, which means that the apparent elimination slope is governed by the drug release rate constant (flip-flop model) [2,3].

For a given elimination rate constant, the drug concentration extends for a longer time with a lower maximum level as k_1 decreases. As shown in Fig. XI-7, the CRDF exhibiting first-order release provides the maximum drug concentration (C_{max}) at T_{max}. Because of this phenomenon, a ten-fold decrease in the release rate results in only a 2.2 fold increase in T_{max} [2,3]. However, it takes a much longer time for the drug concentration to fall below the minimum therapeutic level than with conventional release dosage forms. If the C_{max} is critical for drugs exhibiting a well-defined minimum therapeutic level ($C_{t,min}$), immediate release doses can be added to the CRDF. The drug concentration profile for this formulation is expressed by [1]:

$$C_3 = \frac{k_1 M_{1,T}}{V(k_1 - k_3)}\left(e^{-k_3 t} - e^{-k_1 t}\right) + \frac{k_2 M_o}{V(k_3 - k_2)}\left(e^{-k_2 t} - e^{-k_3 t}\right) \qquad (11\text{-}18)$$

The immediate release dose is then calculated by [1]:

$$\frac{M_{1,T}}{M_o} = \left(\frac{k_2}{k_3}\right)^{\frac{k_3}{(k_3-k_2)}} \left(\frac{k_1}{k_3}\right)^{\frac{k_3}{(k_1-k_3)}}$$

(11-19)

As shown in previous chapters, first-order release CRDFs displaying square-root-of-time or non-zero-order kinetics have been common products. The products should be designed so that the drug accumulation in the body from repetitive doses is minimized by choosing dosing interval equal to 4 times the first-order release rate half-life [3]. For this dosing interval, approximately 6% of the previous dose remains in the GI system when the next dose is administered [2]. The time course of drug concentration in the body can be calculated from [1,3]:

$$C_n = \frac{k_1 M_{1,T}}{V(k_1 - k_3)} \left[\left(\frac{1-e^{-nk_3\tau}}{1-e^{-k_3\tau}}\right) e^{-k_3 t} - \left(\frac{1-e^{-nk_1\tau}}{1-e^{-k_1\tau}}\right) e^{-k_1 t} \right]$$

(11-20)

where n and τ are the number of repeated doses and the dosing time interval, respectively. As shown in Fig. XI-8, a first-order release CRDF provides a reasonable drug concentration in the plasma with less fluctuation within the therapeutic window, when compared to conventional dosage forms.

XI.1.4. *Zero-order release followed by first-order release*

The approaches described in the preceding sections with regard to zero order release CRDF are idealistic for real dosage form designs. Even though a CRDF is well designed with osmotically controlled, membrane controlled, or other governing principles to provide zero-order release kinetics for a prolonged time, the major controlling mechanisms fall short of maintaining a linear release beyond a certain time (t_z). Up to $t = t_z$, the drug concentration profile is given by equation (11-6), and for $t \geq t_z$, is expressed by [1]:

$$C_3 = AM_z[(k_3 - k_2)e^{-k_1\omega} - (k_3 - k_1)e^{-k\omega} + (k_2 - k_1)e^{-k_3\omega}]$$
$$+ \frac{k_2 M_{2,z}}{(k_3 - k_2)V}\left(e^{-k_2\omega} - e^{-k_3\omega}\right) + \frac{M_{3,z}}{V}e^{-k_3\omega}$$

(11-21)

in which $\omega = t - t_z$

(11-22a)

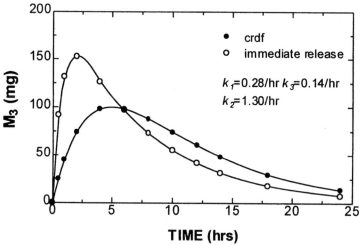

Figure XI-8. Simulated comparative drug concentration profile between first-order CRDF and immediate release dose form.

$$A = \frac{k_1 k_2}{V(k_2 - k_1)(k_3 - k_1)(k_3 - k_2)} \qquad (11\text{-}22b)$$

$$M_z = M_{1,T} - M_o - k_o t \qquad (11\text{-}22c)$$

$$M_{2,z} = \frac{k_o}{k_3}(1 - e^{-k_2 t_z}) + M_o e^{-k_2 t_z} \qquad (11\text{-}22d)$$

$$M_{3,z} = \frac{k_o}{k_3}\left(1 - e^{-k_3 t_z}\right) - \frac{(k_o - k_2 M_o)}{k_3 - k_2}\left(e^{-k_2 t_z} - e^{-k_3 t_z}\right) \qquad (11\text{-}22e)$$

Good and Lee [6] demonstrated the utility of equations (11-6) and (11-22e) with an immediate release dose for designing CRDF of phenylpropanolamine HCl. The overall constraints on the CRDF design of phenylpropanolamine HCl are as follows:

1. The immediate release dose is 21.6 mg.
2. 42.7 mg is delivered at a 3.12 mg/hr for 13.7 hrs.
3. 10.7 mg is delivered by a first-order rate according to eq. (11-23).

Using these constraints and pharmacokinetic parameters for phenylpropanolamine HCl (k_2, k_3 and V), the simulated drug concentration

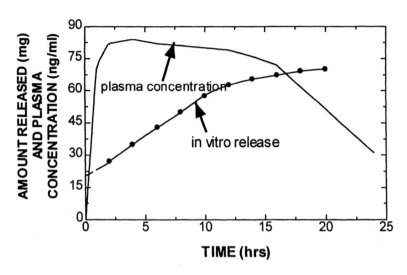

Figure XI-9. *In-vitro* release and theoretical plasma concentration of phenylpropranolamine HCl from an OROS® system for a bolus followed by a constant release. (Graph reconstructed from data by Good and Lee [6].)

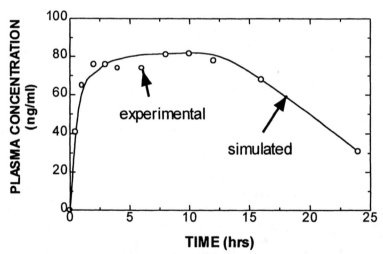

Figure XI-10. Simulated and experimental plasma concentration of phenylpropanolamine HCl. (Graph reconstructed from data by Good and Lee [6].)

profile and simulated *in-vitro* release kinetics are illustrated in Fig. XI-9. Based upon the above concept, an elementary osmotic pump system for phenylpropranolamine HCl has been developed with the pharmacokinetics in mind and with modified constants (M_o = 20 mg, 3.5 mg/hr zero order rate for 12.5 hrs, and 11.5 mg for non-zero order rate). Because of using the osmotic pump system, after zero-order rate is completed, the drug release is not simply first-order as described by equation (11-11). Rather the following equation applies (see Chapter VIII):

$$R(t) = \frac{k_o}{(1 + k_o(t - t_z)/C_s V_r)^2} \tag{11-23}$$

where V_r is the volume of the osmotic pump tablet and C_s is the drug solubility in water. Equation (11-23) describes the quadratic decline of the drug release rate due to decreasing osmotic pressure and drug concentration. Equations (11-2), (11-3) and (11-10) are solved numerically (i.e. Runge-Kutta 4th order) after substituting equation (11-22) into equation (11-2). Fig. XI-10 shows the *in-vivo* plasma concentration in good agreement with the model.

XI.2. Two-Compartment Model with Zero-Order Release Kinetics

The transport of a drug in the body is illustrated in Fig. XII-10 for a two-compartment model. Assuming first-order absorption and elimination, the distribution of the drug in the body for a two-compartment model can be described by:

$$\frac{dM_1}{dt} = -R(t) \tag{11-1}$$

$$\frac{dM_2}{dt} = R(t) - k_2 M_2 \tag{11-2}$$

$$\frac{dM_3}{dt} = k_2 M_2 + k_{21} M_5 - k_3 M_3 - k_{12} M_3 \tag{11-24}$$

$$\frac{dM_4}{dt} = k_3 M_3 \tag{11-25}$$

$$\frac{dM_5}{dt} = k_{12} M_3 - k_{21} M_5 \tag{11-26}$$

where M_5 represents the amount of drug in the peripheral compartment, and k_{12} and k_{21} are the forward rate constant from the central compartment to the peripheral compartment and the backward rate constant from the peripheral compartment to the central compartment, respectively.

If a CRDF exhibits zero-order release kinetics, the drug concentration profile in the central compartment can be expressed by [1,5]:

$$C_3 = \frac{1}{V_c}\left[\frac{k_o}{k_3} - \frac{k_o(k_{21}-k_2)}{(\alpha-k_2)(\beta-k_2)}e^{-k_2 t}\right.$$
$$\left. + \frac{k_o k_2(k_{21}-\alpha)}{\alpha(k_2-\alpha)(\alpha-\beta)}e^{-\alpha t} + \frac{k_o k_2(k_{21}-\beta)}{\beta(\beta-k_2)(\alpha-\beta)}e^{-\beta t}\right] \tag{11-27}$$

where
$$\alpha + \beta = k_3 + k_{12} + k_{21} \tag{11-28a}$$

$$\alpha\beta = k_3 k_{21} \tag{11-28b}$$

and V_c is the volume distribution of the central compartment. As observed for the one-compartment model, the plasma concentration in the central compartment is influenced by the elimination rate constant k_3. In order to obtain plateau concentration level rapidly for a short half-life drug, a bolus dose may be added to the CRDF. In this design, the drug concentration in the central compartment is given by [1,5]:

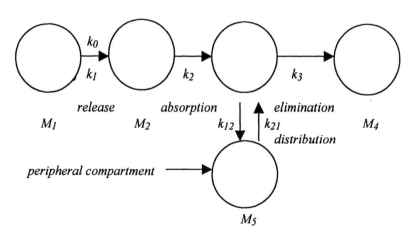

Figure XI-11. A two-compartment model.

$$C_3 = \frac{k_2 M_o}{V_c}\left(\frac{(k_{21}-k_2)}{(\beta-k_2)(\alpha-k_2)}e^{-k_2 t} + \frac{(k_{21}-\alpha)}{(k_2-\alpha)(\beta-\alpha)}e^{-\alpha t} + \frac{(k_{21}-\beta)}{(k_2-\beta)(\alpha-\beta)}e^{-\beta t}\right) +$$

$$\frac{1}{V_c}\left[\frac{k_o}{k_3} - \frac{k_o(k_{21}-k_2)}{(\alpha-k_2)(\beta-k_2)}e^{-k_2 t} + \frac{k_o k_2(k_{21}-\alpha)}{\alpha(k_2-\alpha)(\alpha-\beta)}e^{-\alpha t} + \frac{k_o k_2(k_{21}-\beta)}{\beta(\beta-k_2)(\alpha-\beta)}e^{-\beta t}\right]$$

$$(11\text{-}29)$$

The amount of the bolus dose can be determined from mass balance of the drug in the body. At steady state,

$$\frac{dM_3}{dt} = 0 = k_2 M_2 + k_{21}M_4 - (k_{12}+k_3)M_3 \qquad (11\text{-}30a)$$

$$M_2 = \frac{(k_{12}+k_3)M_3 - k_{21}M_4}{k_2} \qquad (11\text{-}30b)$$

$$\frac{dM_4}{dt} = 0 = k_{12}M_3 - k_{21}M_4 \qquad (11\text{-}30c)$$

$$k_{12}M_3 = k_{21}M_4 \qquad (11\text{-}30d)$$

the amount of drug released is the sum of all drugs distributed in the body and the eliminated from the body as follows:

$$\int R(t)dt = M_2 + M_3 + M_4 + M_5$$

$$= V_c C_3\left[\frac{k_3}{k_2} + 1 + \left(\frac{k_{12}}{k_{21}}\right)^2\right] + k_3 V_c C_3 t \qquad (11\text{-}31)$$

Therefore the optimum amount of the bolus dose can be found as:

$$M_o = V_c C_3\left[\frac{k_3}{k_2} + 1 + \left(\frac{k_{12}}{k_{21}}\right)^2\right] \qquad (11\text{-}32)$$

Fig. XI-12 shows the effect of bolus on the drug concentration in the central compartment.

If a CRDF exhibits dual zero-order release kinetics, described by equation (11-1), the drug concentration in the central compartment is given by:

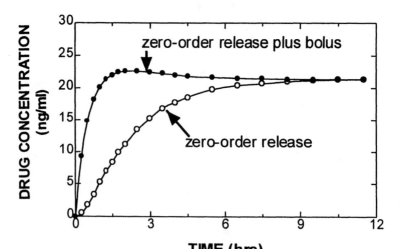

Figure XI-12.   Simulated drug concentration in body of zero-order release CRDF with and without bolus.

$$C_3 = G(t) \qquad\qquad 0 < t \le t_o \qquad\qquad (11\text{-}33a)$$

$$= G(t) - H(t) \qquad\qquad t_o < t \le T \qquad\qquad (11\text{-}33b)$$

where

$$G(t) = \frac{2k_2 M_T}{V_c T t_o}\left[\frac{k_{21}}{k_2 \alpha \beta}\left(t + \frac{1}{k_{21}} - \frac{1}{k_2} - \frac{1}{\alpha} - \frac{1}{\beta}\right) + \frac{k_{21} - k_2}{k_2^2(\alpha - k_2)(\beta - k_2)}e^{-k_2 t}\right.$$
$$\left. + \frac{k_{21} - \alpha}{\alpha^2(k_2 - \alpha)(\beta - \alpha)}e^{-\alpha t} + \frac{k_{21} - \beta}{\beta^2(k_2 - \beta)(\alpha - \beta)}e^{-\beta t}\right] \qquad (11\text{-}33c)$$

$$H(t) = \frac{2k_2 M_T}{V_c(T - t_o)t_o}\left[\frac{k_{21}}{k_2 \alpha \beta}\left(t - t_o + \frac{1}{k_{21}} - \frac{1}{k_2} - \frac{1}{\alpha} - \frac{1}{\beta}\right)\right.$$
$$\left. + \frac{k_{21} - k_2}{k_2^2(\alpha - k_2)(\beta - k_2)}e^{-k_2(t - t_o)} + \frac{\dfrac{k_{21} - \alpha}{\alpha^2(k_2 - \alpha)(\beta - \alpha)}e^{-\alpha(t - t_o)}}{} \right. \qquad (11\text{-}33d)$$
$$\left. + \frac{k_{21} - \beta}{\beta^2(k_2 - \beta)(\alpha - \beta)}e^{-\beta(t - t_o)}\right]$$

Young et al. [7] designed a CRDF for a drug which exhibits two-compartment model kinetics based on the above theory [i.e., equations (11-

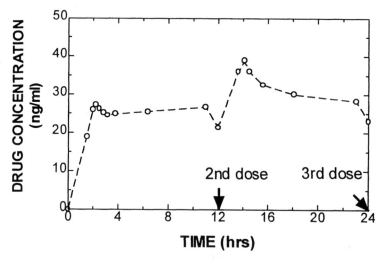

Figure XI-13. Simulated drug concentration after three consecutive doses. (Graph reconstructed from data by Lu et al. [1].)

33a), (11-33b), (11-33c), and (11-33d)]. The drug has the following pharmacokinetic parameters: $V_c = 891\,\text{L}$, $k_{21} = 0.223\,/\text{hr}$, $k_2 = 3.31\,/\text{hr}$, $\alpha = 0.407/\text{hr}$, and $\beta = 0.158\,/\text{hr}$. A dual zero-order rate dosage form provides fast release of a 36 mg dose for 2 hrs followed by a slow release of a 60 mg dose at 2.5 hrs for the next 8.5 hrs. Fig. XI-13 shows the simulated plasma concentration in the central compartment.

XI.3. Application of Pharmacokinetics to Transdermal Delivery Systems

The transport of a drug delivered by a transdermal delivery system through the skin is depicted in Fig. XI-14. Assuming that the viable epidermis, epidermis and body tissue is a single compartment, the change of the amount of drug in the body is given by:

$$\frac{dM_3}{dt} = -k_3 M_3 + SJ\big|_{x=0} \tag{11-34}$$

where S is the surface area of transdermal patch and $J\big|_{x=0}$ is the flux of drug across the stratum cornea.

$$J\big|_{x=0} = D\frac{\partial c}{\partial x}\bigg|_{x=0} \tag{11-35}$$

The diffusion of drug through the stratum cornea is described by:

$$\frac{\partial c}{\partial t} = D\frac{\partial^2 c}{\partial x^2} \tag{11-36}$$

$$c(t = 0) = 0 \tag{11-37a}$$

$$c(x = 0) = 0 \tag{11-37b}$$

$$c(x = L) = c_{sc} \tag{11-37c}$$

where c is the drug concentration in the stratum cornea, x the distance, and c_{sc} is the drug concentration at the surface of stratum cornea.

The drug concentration profile in the stratum cornea can be obtained by solving equations (11-36) and (11-37a,b and c) as follows [7]:

$$\frac{c}{c_{sc}} = \frac{x}{L} + \frac{2}{\pi}\sum_{n=1}^{\infty}\frac{(-1)^n}{n}e^{-k_3 t}\sin\left(\frac{n\pi x}{L}\right) \tag{11-38}$$

The drug concentration in the body is then given by solving equations (11-34), (11-35) and (11-38) [7]:

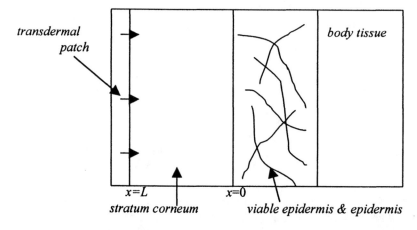

Figure XI-14. Schematic pathway of transdermal therapeutic system.

$$C_3 = \frac{SDc_{sc}}{LV}\left[\frac{1-e^{-k_3 t}}{k_3} + 2\sum_{n=1}^{\infty}\frac{(-1)^n}{k_3-X}\left(e^{-Xt}-e^{-k_3 t}\right)\right] + \frac{C_o}{V}e^{-k_3 t} \quad (11\text{-}39)$$

where $X = n^2\pi^2 D/L^2$, and C_o is the initial total amount of drug in the body.

After the patch is removed from skin, the initial and boundary conditions become:

$$c(t=0) = c_{sc}\left[\frac{x}{L} + \frac{2}{\pi}\sum_{n=1}^{\infty}\frac{(-1)^n}{n}e^{-k_3 t}\sin\left(\frac{n\pi x}{L}\right)\right] \quad (11\text{-}40a)$$

$$c(x=0) = 0 \quad (11\text{-}40b)$$

$$c(x=L) = 0 \quad (11\text{-}40c)$$

The drug concentration in the body is then given by [7]:

$$C_3 = \frac{SD}{LV_c}\sum_{n=1}^{\infty}\frac{1}{k_3-X}e^{-Xt} + \left(C_{3t} - \frac{SDc_{sc}}{V_c L}\sum_{n=1}^{\infty}\frac{(-1)^n}{k_3-X}e^{-k_3 t}\right) \quad (11\text{-}41)$$

where C_{3t} is the drug concentration in the body at the time of patch removal.

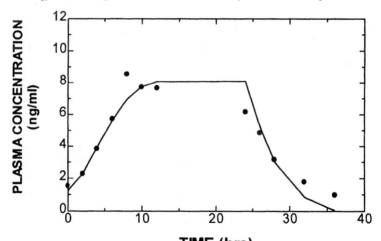

Figure XI-15. Plasma concentration of nicotine between model prediction (-) and experiments (surface area: 20 cm^2). (Graph reconstructed from data by Young et al. [7].)

The plasma drug concentration simulated for the model described by equations (11-39) and (11-41) is illustrated in Fig. XI-15 along with the *in-vivo* clinical data for transdermal delivery of nicotine [7].

Guy [8] developed the mathematical equation describing transdermal delivery systems based on the two-compartment model. Drug releases at the first-order rate (k_1') from the adhesive layer containing a dose (M_∞) followed by the zero-order release rate (k_o) from the transdermal system. The plasma concentration in the central compartment is [8]:

$$
C_s = \frac{S k_o k_1 k_2}{V_c}\left[\frac{1}{\alpha\beta\varepsilon} - \frac{e^{-\alpha t}}{(\alpha-\varepsilon)\alpha(\alpha-\beta)} - \frac{e^{-\beta t}}{(\beta-\varepsilon)\beta(\beta-\alpha)} - \frac{e^{-\varepsilon t}}{(\varepsilon-\beta)\varepsilon(\varepsilon-\alpha)}\right]
$$

$$
+ \frac{M_\infty k_1' k_1 k_2}{V_c}\left[\begin{array}{c} \dfrac{e^{-\alpha t}}{(\beta-\alpha)(\alpha-\varpi)(\alpha-\mu)} + \dfrac{e^{-\beta t}}{(\alpha-\beta)(\beta-\varpi)(\beta-\mu)} \\[3mm] - \dfrac{e^{-\varpi t}}{(\alpha-\varpi)(\varpi-\beta)(\varpi-\mu)} + \dfrac{e^{-\mu t}}{(\alpha-\mu)(\mu-\beta)(\mu-\varpi)} \end{array}\right]
$$

$$(11\text{-}42)$$

where $\varepsilon = k_1 + k_r$, $\varpi + \mu = k_1' + k_r + k_1$, $\varpi\mu = k_1' k_1$, and k_r is the partition coefficient of the drug for the transdermal device and the skin. The first term of the right-hand side in equation (11-42) describes the release kinetics of zero-order portion whereas the second term accounts for the first-order dose from the adhesive layer.

The mathematical equations described above are valuable tools to understand the role of basic physicochemical processes of percutaneous absorption [8]. One should consult Ref. [9,10] for further comprehensive models.

References

1. F.-Y. Lu, N. C. Sambol, R. P. Giannini, and C. Y. Liu, "Pharmacokinetics of Oral Extended-Release Dosage Forms. I. Release Kinetics, Concentration, and Absorbed Fraction," *Pharm. Res.*, 12, 720 (1995).
2. P. G. Welling, "Oral Controlled Drug Administration: Pharmacokinetic Considerations," *Drug Dev. Ind. Pharm.*, 9, 1185 (1983).
3. M. Gibaldi and D. Perrier, Pharmacokinetics, Marcel Dekker, New York, 1975.
4. W. A. Ritschel, "Biopharmaceutic and Pharmacokinetic Aspects in the Design of Controlled Release Peroral Drug Delivery Systems," *Drug Dev. Ind. Pharm.*, 15, 1073 (1989).
5. J. G. Wagner, Mathematical Modeling of Pharmacokinetics, Technomic Publ., Lancaster. PA. 1996.

6. W. R. Good and P. I. Lee, "Membrane-Controlled Reservoir Drug Delivery Systems," in Medical Applications of Controlled Release, Vol. I, R. S. Langer and D. L. Wise (Eds.), CRC Press, Baton Rouge, Fl., 1984, p1.

7. M.-J. Young, Y. Chang, and D. C.-H. Cheng, "Mathematical Modeling of Matrix Type Transdermal Therapeutic System," *Proceed. Int. Symp. Control. Rel. Bioact. Mater.*, 21, 443 (1994).

8. R. Guy, "The Modeling of Skin Absorption and Controlled Drug Delivery to the Skin,"

9. K. D. McCarley and A. L. Bunge, "Physiologically Relevant One-Compartment Pharmacokinetic Models for Skin. 1. Development of Models," *J. Pharm. Sci.*, 87, 470 (1998).

10. M. B. Reddy, K. D. McCarley, and A. L. Bunge, "Physiologically Relevant One-Compartment Pharmacokinetic Models for Skin. 2. Comparison of Models When Combined with a Systemic Pharmacokinetic Model," *J. Pharm. Sci.*, 87, 482 (1998).

Index